61
ARISTOTLE:
HISTORIA ANIMALIUM
BOOK X

ARISTOTLE

HISTORIA ANIMALIUM BOOK X

ENDOXON, TOPOS, AND *DIALECTIC*
ON ὑπὲρ τοῦ μὴ γεννᾶν

EDITED WITH INTRODUCTION,
TRANSLATION, AND COMMENTARY

BY
LESLEY DEAN-JONES
University of Texas, Austin

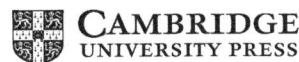

CAMBRIDGE
UNIVERSITY PRESS

CAMBRIDGE
UNIVERSITY PRESS

University Printing House, Cambridge CB2 8BS, United Kingdom

One Liberty Plaza, 20th Floor, New York, NY 10006, USA

477 Williamstown Road, Port Melbourne, VIC 3207, Australia

314–321, 3rd Floor, Plot 3, Splendor Forum, Jasola District Centre,
New Delhi – 110025, India

79 Anson Road, #06–04/06, Singapore 079906

Cambridge University Press is part of the University of Cambridge.

It furthers the University's mission by disseminating knowledge in the pursuit of
education, learning, and research at the highest international levels of excellence.

www.cambridge.org
Information on this title: www.cambridge.org/9781107015159
DOI: 10.1017/9781139057721

First published 2023

Printed in the United Kingdom by T J Books Ltd, Padstow Cornwall

A catalogue record for this publication is available from the British Library.

Library of Congress Cataloging-in-Publication Data
NAMES: Aristotle. | Dean-Jones, Lesley, editor.
TITLE: Historia animalium book X / Aristotle ; edited with introduction,
translation, and commentary by Lesley Dean-Jones, University of Texas,
Austin.
OTHER TITLES: Historia animalium. Book 10. English
DESCRIPTION: Cambridge, United Kingdom ; New York, NY : Cambridge
University Press, 2020. | Series: Cambridge classical texts and
commentaries ; 61 | Includes bibliographical references and index.
IDENTIFIERS: LCCN 2019059919 | ISBN 9781107015159 (hardback) | ISBN
9781139057721 (epub)
SUBJECTS: LCSH: Zoology–Pre-Linnean works.
CLASSIFICATION: LCC QL41 .A7416 2020 | DDC 590–dc23
LC record available at https://lccn.loc.gov/2019059919

ISBN 978-1-107-01515-9 Hardback

For Geoffrey Lloyd
with thanks

CONTENTS

CONTENTS

PREFACE

On p. 15 of my 1994 book *Women's Bodies in Classical Greek Science*, I described *HA* X as "the work of a later Hippocratic doctor writing under the influence of Aristotle," but like many scholars I did not make much use of *HA* X at all. Although I agreed that there was some Aristotelian influence on the work, I interpreted it as an explicit attempt to argue against his contention that a woman did not contribute "seed" to conception as a man did, so when David Balme's argument that *HA* X enshrined an early form of Aristotle's reproductive theory began to gain traction, I decided to do a full translation and commentary on the basis of Balme's 2002 text. The more I worked on the text the more confused I became. After a while I was forced to change my idea about the relative chronology of *HA* X and *GA* because it became clear that in *GA* Aristotle was explicitly arguing against arguments found in *HA* X. This led me to rethinking the relationship of the last two chapters (Chapters 6 and 7) to the rest of *HA* X because they contained material found in *GA*. I classified them first as addenda written at the end of the papyrus by a later follower of Aristotle. But then I realized that although they contained material found in the *GA*, the presentation of the material had to have preceded Aristotle's theories of generation as expressed in *GA*, so I took them to be notes by Aristotle himself which he reused in the *GA*. It was at this stage I published the article "Clinical Gynecology and Aristotle's Biology" in *Apeiron*. As I continued to work on the text I began to feel there was something Aristotelian about the first five chapters after all, and searches in the *TLG* confirmed my suspicion that the text was laced with distinctive Aristotelian phrases, though I still could not—and cannot—believe the content was genuinely Aristotelian. I concluded that the first five chapters were a summary by Aristotle of a text originally written by a practicing physician who assumed that women did contribute "seed" to conception in an analogous way to a man. I thought Aristotle had made a few random notes on the summary, some of which were possible objections to this theory, in what are now Chapters 6 and 7. The paragraph at the end of what is Chapter 5 in Balme's text still had me scratching my head. It was not until I started to read more widely about Aristotle's expressed methodological principles on the use of the earlier theories of others, *endoxa*, that I realized that the dense paragraph was a *topos* directing the shape of the objections to the theory of female seed as expressed in the first five chapters, so the notes of Chapters 6 and 7 are not so random after all. They deal, in an inconclusive *dialectic*, with the possibility that uterine mole, a condition Aristotle attributes to an overly cool mixture of male and female "seed" in *GA*, is analogous to avian wind-eggs. I have here outlined the process by which my ms. reached the form it has because I realize how unprecedented a summary with written notes would be for ancient Greece in the fourth century BCE. I did not begin with this view of *HA* X myself, and it largely revealed itself to me before I knew that Aristotle had outlined this very procedure in his own works. Unprecedented it may be, but perhaps it should not have been entirely unexpected.

The book has had a long gestation and several people have contributed to its nativity. Jim Hankinson and I collaborated on a draft of the translation and a prospectus of the work in 2004/5. Much in the book has changed since then, and it should not be assumed that Jim agrees with all the arguments I put forward, but his voice can still be heard in phrases throughout the translation and in many parts of the Introduction, and I am grateful to him for his continued interest in and support of the project. Philip van der Eijk gave some valuable feedback and comments on an early stage of the ms., and again I am grateful to him for his support. George Conklin met with me weekly for several months for a painstaking read through of the whole ms. at a relatively late stage and made many valuable suggestions and frequently challenged me to rethink or clarify a position. He has since read a revised version of the whole work and made further valuable comments and suggestions. In the Spring semester of 2015 I taught a graduate seminar on Aristotle's Biology at The University of Texas at Austin to students from Classics, Philosophy, Comparative Literature and English. Two weeks were spent discussing the ms. of the book as it stood at that time, and the many different points of view and the lively questions they engendered contributed to my later shaping of the work. Sam Ross proofread the ms for me before I submitted it to CUP and his curiosity about the content led to some further revisions. I gave only two presentations on the material in the book before I submitted it to Cambridge University Press: the Blechler Lecture at the University of South Carolina and at a conference at Notre Dame University. I benefitted enormously from the comments of the two anonymous referees to whom Cambridge University Press sent the ms. I am also deeply indebted to Michael Reeve for his painstaking editorial oversight in the preparation of the ms. for publication, including two very insightful suggestions for textual emendations, both of which I have adopted. Sarah Starkey was an invaluable, and patient, guide and editor in the final stages of preparing the printed text. I wish also to thank Pam Scholefield for preparing the General Index and Zafeirios Adramerinas for preparing the Index Locorum.

Until the Spring of 1982 I was completely unaware of the riches of ancient Greek medical and biological texts. I became enthralled by them thanks to a brilliant seminar offered by a visiting professor from Cambridge, now Professor Sir Geoffrey Lloyd. He continued to shape my scholarly development in supervising my Ph.D. thesis and beyond. Although I have become more of a "splitter" than a "lumper" in my view of the Aristotelian Corpus, I dedicate this work to him in gratitude for the joy I have found in my scholarly life.

NOTE ON THE TEXT

My text is based on that of David Balme's 2002 volume in the *Cambridge Classical Texts and Commentaries* series.[1] Balme collated all twenty-six of the mss. containing *HA*, though he did not include all the readings of clearly inferior mss. in the app. crit. (p. 6).[2] He deliberately produced a very conservative text in which "no editorial conjectures from Aldus onwards have been admitted to the text, but those that seem worth considering are given in the apparatus or in the commentary," (p. 4). Balme's adherence to the manuscript tradition produced a very helpful base text, but there are clearly many cruces where the received text is not just "more difficult sometimes and more roughly expressed" but confused, contradictory or unintelligible and easily corrected by a small emendation. Having experienced myself the errors that can creep in when copying a text even at just one remove, I find myself in sympathy with Haupt as quoted by Housman 1922, p. 77, "If the sense requires it, I am prepared to write *Constantinopolitanus* where the MSS. have the monosyllabic interjection *o*." This is especially true if, as I think is the case with *HA* X, the nature of the text was misunderstood by the very first copyists.

Because he treats the mss. tradition of *HA* X in the context of the transmission of the entire *HA*, Balme's explanation of the relative importance of the mss. for *HA* X can be a little misleading. He recognizes that D^a is the source of all the other

---

[1] I am in full agreement with Balme's decision to return to the original mss. order of the books. What was originally Book IX has been referred to as Book VII by all editors since Theodore Gaza placed it to follow Book VI in his 1476 translation. Following Balme I refer to this book as *HA* IX(VII), though I hope very soon a modern consensus can be reached and we can drop the bracketed reference to Gaza's ordering.

[2] I will not here replicate Balme's very full discussion in his Introduction of the mss. tradition and editorial history of *HA*. I am limiting my remarks to what is necessary to understand the sigla and their significance.

extant Greek mss. of *HA* X and is superior to them (p. 22). When he discusses the mss. of the *HA* as a whole, on the other hand, he states "there is no 'best' MS or family, whose readings should automatically carry more weight. D^a has the best claim, but there are reasons against trusting it" (p. 35). The reasons are that mss. of the α and γ families tend to agree with each other against the β family (of which D^a is the archetype) and that D^a exhibits more "diorthosis," i.e., hypercorrection, than other mss. In the context of *HA* I–IX, where the α and γ families have different histories of transmission, these are good reasons for not automatically acceding to D^a's readings, but in the context of *HA* X any alternate readings in the other eight mss. which contain the work are either errors or conjectures on the part of the copyists. Their readings have no independent authority.

D^a (Vat. gr. 262) was copied some time in the fourteenth century; S^c (Taur. C I 9 (56)) was copied, probably directly, from D^a by George Chrysokokkes at Constantinople early in the fifteenth century; Francesco Filelfo brought S^c to Italy in the 1420s, where Bessarion had Book 10 copied from it into G^a (Marc. gr. 212, from the α family of mss.),[3] and Andronicus Callistus into L^c (Ambros. I.56 sup., from the γ family). Bessarion then had Q (Marc. gr. 200) copied from G^a followed by F^a (Marc. gr. 207) from Q; X^c (Laur. 87.27) is a copy of F^a. Some time in the second half of the fifteenth century (after Theodore of Gaza's Latin translation) D^a arrived in Italy and R^c (Utin. VI,1, which followed the ordering of Gaza's books but retained Book X)

---

[3] At the end of *HA* X in G^a a copyist made two marginal notes, the first noting that he had found a tenth book of the *HA* in Latin—though he quotes the opening words in Greek—commenting that he did not know if a Greek version existed, the second that he had found a Greek copy and was about to transcribe it into the ms. However, the Greek that follows is in a new hand and the opening words are slightly different from those quoted in the first marginal note. The Greek may be a translation of the Latin of Guil.; see Balme 2002, p. 18.

was copied from it. John Rhosus copied V^c (Neap. III D 5) from it in 1493, with the original ordering of book numbers.⁴ So, the stemma for *HA* X looks like this:

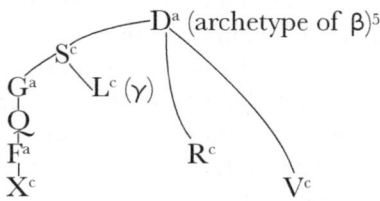

We do, though, have two independent witnesses of a different ms. tradition prior to D^a. An Arabic translation/paraphrase (possibly of a Syriac intermediary) of a Greek ms. of the α family was made in the ninth century,⁶ and in the thirteenth century. Michael Scot made a Latin translation of a different Arabic translation, though this was again more of a paraphrase in many places, especially in Book X.⁷ A Latin translation of

---

⁴ See Balme 2002, pp. 1–48, and Berger 2005, pp. 107–20.

⁵ O^c, T^c, U^c, and I^c are also members of the β family, but do not contain Book X. O^c is a simple copy of D^a which contains *HA* I–IX and the annotation ἔτι λείπει added in a later hand after Book IX. T^c is copied from O^c and so also omits Book X. U^c is the first of a pair of mss. of which V^c is the second. U^c contains *HA* I–V and V^c *HA* VI–X. I^c contains only *HA* I and a short excerpt from *HA* III. O^c is the only member of the β family to deliberately omit *HA* X, probably under the influence of Gaza, since O^c also reorders the books of the *HA* to that of Gaza's translation. The translation was printed in 1476 and Harlfinger dates O^c to 1470, so O^c would seem to have had access to the draft of Gaza's translation which was finished in 1458. It is ironic that within half a century of the marginal note in G^a celebrating the discovery of the tenth book of the *HA*, a direct descendant of the ms. that provided that book should be the first to deliberately omit it.

⁶ Filius 2018 was published too late to be used in the preparation of my text.

⁷ Filius 2007, p. 33. For *HA* X Balme consulted three mss. of Scot's text plus Rudberg's collated transcript. Aafke van Oppenraay is currently preparing an edition of Scot's translation and checked several readings for Gotthelf in his preparation of Balme's text. At the beginning of *HA* X in one of

the *HA* was made from the Greek later in the thirteenth century by William of Moerbeke (Guil.).⁸ He may have had access to two mss. for his translation of Books I–IX: the ninth-century Wᶜ (only a small portion of which is extant, not including *HA* X), which is independent of the α, β, and γ families of mss., and the twelfth-century Cᵃ, from the α family.⁹ Wᶜ seems to have been his sole source for Book X.¹⁰

the earliest mss. of Scot's translation a later annotator has written "totus iste liber est necessarius"; see van Oppenraay 2003, p. 393. Where I make independent references to Scot, I have used Rudberg's transcription.

⁸ Rudberg, pp. 79–87, argued that Book X was translated by someone other than Guil. He based this on his belief that Guil.'s exemplar was Cᵃ, which did not contain Book X, the fact that in two mss. of Guil. *HA* X is separated from the first nine books of the *HA* for no good reason, and what he considered to be a greater number of errors in the translation of Book X from that of the other nine books. However, since every other ms. of Guil. does have the tenth book immediately following the ninth and the two mss. that do not are later, it seems quite possible, as Balme 1991, p. 47 suggests, that the separation was made under Gaza's influence. Given that we cannot compare Guil.'s translation directly with his exemplar, the difficult nature of the Greek of *HA* X in some parts, and the fact that some of what Rudberg considers errors provide some useful readings, there seems no reason to attribute it to anybody other than Guil. Berger does not discuss this possibility. Anyway, Rudberg himself believes that Book X was added to Guil.'s translation "ziemlich bald nach" (p. 87). As with Scot, where I make independent reference to Guil. I have used Rudberg's transcription.

⁹ It is interesting that Cᵃ does show ten books in the *HA* by dividing Book II into two books at 504b12, at the transition from birds to fishes in the discussion of the external parts of ovipara. *HA* II is not a long book and other aspects of birds and fishes are covered in the same books in the *HA*, so it suggests that the copyist had some reason for thinking that there should be ten books in the *HA*, though the decision to make a division at 504b12 seems completely arbitrary.

¹⁰ Berger 2005, pp. 184–5; see Balme 2002, p. 44, n. 46. There are many mss. of Guil. The best is Toletanus 47.10, Guil. (Tz); the other important mss. are cited as Guil. cett. Citations to these mss. were provided to Gotthelf in his preparation of Balme's ms. for publication by Beullens and Bossier; see Balme 2002, p. 43, n. 45.

In the fourth century CE, Oribasius compiled a medical compendium of excerpts from famous physicians. In a fourteenth-century ms. of this work, Paris 2237, are included several excerpts from Aristotle's *HA*, including long sections from *HA* X.5 and 7, 636b39–637a10, 638a10–26, and 638b7–37.[11] Even if these sections were copied into Oribasius in the fourteenth century, they constitute an independent witness to parts of *HA* X, and obviously if they originated with Oribasius himself they are even more important. No editor, including Balme, has previously used these readings in compiling a text.

Consequently, in my app. crit. I will cite *descripti* readings that differ from those of D^a only if I adopt them in my text, treating them as conjectures. Apart from that, with the exception of my own conjectures, the bulk of my app. crit. is taken from Balme, with the addition of readings found in Oribasius. The readings of Scot and Guil. are those found in Balme's app. crit., as are most of the conjectures of earlier scholars, though I have added a very few which Balme missed. While I have included many of these conjectures into my text, the text remains basically that of D^a.

---

[11] Berger 2005, pp. 29–31. Like all the extant Greek mss., Guil. and Scot, Oribasius includes 636b39–637a10 after 638b37, though it is clearly misplaced there; see Balme 1991, p. 511. Berger believes the scribe omitted 638a26–b7 because of a similarity in the clauses πολὺν δὲ χρόνον ἐμμένει at 638a26 and τὸν χρόνον ποιοῦσι πολύν at 638b7. This is a coincidence, certainly, and may be the case, but it is a long way for the eye to skip. For reasons in the content of the passage that could explain Oribasius' omission see notes ad. loc.

ABBREVIATIONS

The titles of Aristotelian and Hippocratic works are abbreviated according to the system in LSJ. For Hippocratic references, the numbers in brackets refer to volume, page, and line number in É. Littré, *Oeuvres complètes d'Hippocrate* (Paris 1839–61). While this is no longer the most up-to-date text for the Hippocratic treatises, it functions as a reference point in the same way as Stephanus and Bekker pages. The best editions are usually in the *Corpus Medicorum Graecorum* series, but to date this does not include many of the gynecological works. Modern texts for other Hippocratic gynecological works are listed below:

Mul. I & II	Loeb 11 (2018), Potter
Nat. Mul.	Budé 12.1 (2008), Bourbon
	Loeb 10 (2012), Potter
Steril.	Loeb 10 (2012), Potter
Genit. & Nat. Puer.	Budé 11 (1972/2003), Joly
	Loeb 10 (2012), Potter
Sept./Oct.	CMG 1.2.1 (1968), Grensemann
	Budé 11 (1972/2003), Joly
	Loeb 9 (2010), Potter
Superf.	CMG 1.2.2 (1973), Lienau
	Loeb 9 (2010), Potter
Virg.	Loeb 9 (2010), Potter
Foet.	Loeb 9 (2010), Potter
Exsect.	Loeb 9 (2010), Potter

INTRODUCTION

1 DEBATE OVER THE AUTHENTICITY OF *HA* X

Among the extant Aristotelian writings are ten books that have survived under the title *Historia Animalium* or *Researches into Animals* (henceforth *HA*). Some of the ancient catalogues of Aristotle's works list ten books in the *HA*, some only nine. Among the latter, but not the former, there is also mention of a treatise ὑπὲρ τοῦ μὴ γεννᾶν (*On Failure to Reproduce*). It seems almost certain that this title refers to Book X, which deals exclusively with human sterility and fertility, and therefore that it was originally meant to stand as an independent work, a fact which explains its evident failure to fit in with the overall schema of the *HA*. Theodore Gaza's 1476 translation was made from several mss. which included Book X, including those of the β family and possibly Guil., but he deliberately omitted it.[1] The consensus of scholarly opinion since then has been that the text we possess as *HA* X was originally composed as a separate freestanding treatise, *On Failure to Reproduce*.

---

[1] In the initial preparation of the third volume of the Aldine *editio princeps* (1497), the editor printed only *HA* I–IX, following Gaza's reordering. However, *HA* X is included on unnumbered pages at the end of the volume with the note *En tibi lector carissime fragmenta ea, quae Gaza in prooemio de animalibus in nonnullis codicibus tum graecis tum latinis inueniri ait. quae suo fortasse loco impressa legeres, si suo tempore in manus nostras uenisset. nunc uero hoc loco adiecta maluimus quam te iisdem qualibuscumque fraudari*, "Here, dear reader, are those fragments which Gaza, in the introduction to *On Animals*, said were found in some manuscripts, first Greek then Latin. Perhaps you might have read these printed at that place <i.e., alongside *On Animals*> if it had come into our hands at that time. But now, we prefer to include them at this juncture rather than to defraud you of them, whatever their merits might be"; see Balme 2002, p. 36. Balme remarks that the Aldine's inclusion of Book X "may even suggest a reaction against Gaza" (p. 38), but the rebuke seems aimed rather at the deliberate exclusion of any work transmitted in a ms. as Aristotle's rather than an argument that it is part of the *HA*.

I

The addition of *Non Gen.* as the tenth book of the *HA* seems to have been made by Andronicus in the first century BCE; at least Andronicus' catalogue is the earliest to make no mention of ὑπὲρ τοῦ μὴ γεννᾶν and list ten books for the *HA*.[2] Balme states that our extant mss. "all presumably deriv[e] from post-Andronican archetype[s]," and assumes that Book X "was deliberately omitted by some later" mss. Rudberg finds it hard to believe that once a book had become part of the *HA* it would be deliberately omitted and argues that ὑπὲρ τοῦ μὴ γεννᾶν was first added to the *HA* by an Arabic translator and found its way back into the Greek tradition as a back translation from the Latin translations of the Arabic.[3] The last four words of Book IX(VII) as they have come down to us in most mss. (προϊούσης δὴ τῆς ἡλικίας) argue for Balme's interpretation.

HA X in Dᵃ (and therefore in all extant Greek mss. of the book) begins προϊούσης δὲ τῆς ἡλικίας, "But as this time of life proceeds." Contrary to most modern editors, Balme believes that προϊούσης δὴ τῆς ἡλικίας was originally the conclusion of Book IX(VII) and that a copyist repeated the words at the beginning of Book X to show that it should follow on from IX.[4] A similar precaution to indicate the order of books was taken between Books II and III (γ family exc. Mᶜ and Zᶜ), III and IV (Kᶜ of the γ family), IV and V (γ family exc. Mᶜ), V and VI (γ family exc. Mᶜ), and VI and VII(VIII) (α family and Eᵃ of the γ family), but in all five cases the opening words of the succeeding book are appended to the end of the preceding, which would argue for the original position of προϊούσης δὲ τῆς ἡλικίας being the beginning of *Non Gen.*[5] If the device of

[2] Balme 1985, pp. 191–2. For the role, or non-role, of Andronicus in shaping the Aristotelian Corpus, see Barnes 1997.
[3] Rudberg 1911, pp. 47–61. There is no merit at all in this suggestion. The Greek is not nearly as strange as Rudberg asserts, and the inclusion of sections of the treatise in Oribasius also argues against an Arabic origin.
[4] Balme 1985, p. 192. He believes that the phrase fits better in Book IX(VII). This will be discussed below, pp. 109–10.
[5] Rudberg 1911, pp. 59–60, recognizes this but does not account for it.

repetition is meant to ensure that the books are read or copied in order, this is a little more logical than repeating the final words of one book at the beginning of the next; it directs the copyist or reader to which book they should move on to rather than which book they ought to have copied/read before the one in their hand. A further argument against Book IX(VII) having been the original locus for the phrase is that in D^a it appears only at the beginning of *Non Gen.*, not at the end of IX(VII), and the tradition from which D^a descended diverged from the α and γ families before the practice of anticipating at the end of one book the opening words of the following book was instituted; there are no connective repetitions between any books of *HA* in D^a. Guil.'s thirteenth-century translation was based on W^c, a ninth-century ms. independent of the α, β, and γ families, of which only a portion is extant, not including Book X. Like D^a, Guil. shows no connective transitions between the books of *HA* and translates the phrase προϊούσης δὲ τῆς ἡλικίας only at the beginning of X.

The ninth-century Arabic version of Ibn al-Batriq, which Scot translated into Latin, derives ultimately from a Greek exemplar much earlier than any of our extant mss., and may itself be a translation of a Syriac version. The original Greek exemplar seems to have been related most closely to the α family.[6] The Latin indicates the presence of a version of προϊούσης δὲ τῆς ἡλικίας both at the end of IX and the beginning of Book X.[7] Scot translates the phrase at the end of Book IX(VII)— where the topic is the occasions when convulsions are particularly dangerous for infants—simply as "and when they are prolonged," *et quando prolongatur*, taking convulsions rather than ἡλικία to be the subject of the participle, while in the opening of Book X he translates it more literally as "and when their age increases," *etiam quando inierint etatem*. This implies that the

---

[6] Balme 2002, pp. 40–1.
[7] But unlike the mss. of the α and γ families it shows no other example of connective repetition between other books in the *HA*.

phrase appeared in both positions in the Arabic tradition and that the Arabic translator did not interpret the phrase as a connective repetition, probably because there were no other examples of this in the Greek ms. before him. There are no other connective repetitions in Scot's translation, which argues for this being the first one to be added in the *HA*. A second one was added in the archetype of the α family (and Eᵃ of the γ family) between Book VI and VII(VIII), another juncture where there is an abrupt change of subject (from modes of generation to the differences between animals in accord with their environment and nutrition). That this repetition is missing in Scot's Arabic exemplar implies that the Greek ms. the Arabic translated, predated the archetype of our extant mss. in the α family.

It could be argued that because προϊούσης δὴ τῆς ἡλικίας are the last words of Book *HA* IX(VII) in all of the mss. of the α and γ families, not just those into which Book X was copied from Dᵃ, the end of Book IX(VII) was their original position. However, the use of the particles argues against this. The phrase appears with the variation δή for the δέ which shows at the beginning of *HA* X, except in Gᵃ and Q, where the particle is missing altogether. The δέ at the beginning of *HA* X functions to connect the whole book to what preceded it. δέ could not stand in the phrase at the end of Book IX(VII) because a genitive absolute is subordinate, not paratactic, to the main clause and so does not need a conjunction. δή can be connective, but here would have more of an emphatic force, except that the emphatic use of δή does not seem to be common with the participle.[8] The use of the particles makes it more likely that the phrase was copied from the beginning of Book X and adapted to the end of Book IX(VII) than vice versa. Gᵃ and Q's solution of simply omitting δέ was the better adaptation.

In Dᵃ and Wᶜ, Guil.'s lost Greek exemplar, the connection of Book X to the *HA* was maintained without the inclusion of its

---

[8] Denniston cites only three examples (pp. 215–16), none of them a genitive absolute. The most common use of δή with the participle is in conjunction with ὡς (p. 230).

4

opening words at the end of Book IX(VII), so the repetition of the phrase was not coincident with the combining of ὑπὲρ τοῦ μὴ γεννᾶν and *HA*. If the connection was initially made in the Arabic tradition, as Rudberg argues, we would have to explain why ὑπὲρ τοῦ μὴ γεννᾶν's opening words are not found at the end of *HA* IX(VII) in D^a and W^c (translated in a different way in each place as they are in Scot), but are found in all the Greek mss. which did not see the treatise as part of the *HA*. The addition of the phrase to the end of Book IX(VII) would seem to have come about after the initial connection of ὑπὲρ τοῦ μὴ γεννᾶν when, in the tradition followed elsewhere in *HA* by the α and γ families, repetition of the opening phrase of the next book was used to ensure the correct ordering of books, and the Arabic translation was made from a ms. in this tradition. Given the anomalous nature of the content of *HA* X and the fact that the early catalogues list only nine books in the *HA*, it is ironic but not inexplicable that despite this precaution Book X was deliberately dropped in the α and γ families but retained in D^a and W^c which did not have the repetition. When Bessarion had Book X copied from S^c into G^a and Andronicus Callistus copied it into L^c, they did not excise these last four words from Book IX(VII), understanding them to be an example of connective repetition.

Gaza, who used mss. from all three families in his translation, explicitly rejected Book X, but he also omitted the phrase from Book IX(VII) when he rearranged the order of the *HA*, showing that he considered the phrase προϊούσης δὴ τῆς ἡλικίας to have originated in Book X and to have no essential meaning for the topic discussed at the end of Book IX(VII). In fact, the words are somewhat contradictory at the end of Book IX(VII). Aristotle is there explaining why babies are not named until the seventh day after birth, because as they get older their chance of surviving convulsions increases. He says that in those babies for whom convulsions begin from the back the condition is particularly dangerous, ἐπικίνδυνον δὲ καὶ ὅσοις τῶν παιδίων οἱ

5

σπασμοὶ ἐκ τοῦ νώτου ἄρχονται.[9] If, unlike other convulsions, these get worse as the child gets older, we might expect the contrast to be more marked. The words, then, are not well suited to end Book IX(VII).

However, the phrase does not work very well either as the introit to an independent treatise. Quite apart from the δέ, which would imply that something had preceded the opening sentence as we have it, no treatise in any tradition opens up quite so *in medias res* as "When their age increases…" It is possible that in the original treatise the words were preceded by a discussion of congenital sterility, but there is a passing mention of this at 636b1 with no indication that the author had dealt with it previously. If there is something missing, it is more likely that the words were preceded by an explanation as to why young males and females just past puberty may not reproduce easily, an explanation which Aristotle may have chosen not to summarize if it had little to say about the fertility of female seed. However, if Aristotle was choosing to summarize only the second part of a treatise, it is a little perverse of him to begin his summary with a phrase looking back to what he had omitted.

We are left then with a conundrum. The phrase προϊούσης δὲ τῆς ἡλικίας does not work well as the conclusion to *HA* IX(VII) and appears to have originated at the beginning of *HA* X, but it does not work well there either.

Now the words προϊούσης τῆς ἡλικίας appear at *GA* II.7, 746b25, in the context of a discussion on sterility following on a short statement about men and women who are sterile from birth:

καὶ γὰρ ἐκ γενετῆς ὅταν πηρωθῶσι τοὺς τόπους τοὺς πρὸς τὴν μίξιν χρησίμους ἄγονοι γίγνονται καὶ γυναῖκες καὶ ἄνδρες ὥστε τὰς μὲν μὴ ἡβᾶν τοὺς δὲ μὴ γενειᾶν ἀλλ' εὐνουχίας διατελεῖν ὄντας.

---

[9] Balme's translation of ὅσοις τῶν παιδίων as "in all babies" masks the contradiction by implying Aristotle is now talking about a different type of convulsion which can attack more than newborns.

τοῖς δὲ προϊούσης τῆς ἡλικίας ταὐτὸν συμβαίνει πάσχειν, ὁτὲ μὲν
δι᾽ εὐτροφίαν τῶν σωμάτων, ταῖς μὲν γὰρ πιοτέραις γιγνομέναις
τοῖς δ᾽ εὐεκτικωτέροις εἰς τὸ σῶμα καταναλίσκεται τὸ περίττωμα
τὸ σπερματικόν, καὶ ταῖς μὲν οὐ γίγνεται καταμήνια τοῖς δὲ
γονή, ὁτὲ δὲ διὰ νόσον οἱ μὲν ὑγρὸν καὶ ψυχρὸν προΐενται,
ταῖς δὲ γυναιξὶν αἱ καθάρσεις φαῦλαι καὶ πλήρεις νοσηματικῶν
περιττωμάτων. πολλοῖς δὲ καὶ πολλαῖς καὶ διὰ πηρώματα τοῦτο
συμβαίνει τὸ πάθος περὶ τὰ μόρια καὶ τοὺς τόπους τοὺς πρὸς
τὴν ὁμιλίαν χρησίμους.

Whenever men and women are stunted from birth in the places
used for copulation they are sterile; as a result, the women do
not attain puberty and the men do not grow a beard but pass
their days as eunuchs; others suffer the same thing as their
age advances, sometimes on account of putting on weight (in
women who become too fat and men who are too well developed the seminal residue is expended on their bodies so that
menses do not develop for the one or semen (*gonê*) for the other),
sometimes on account of disease (the men emit fluid and cold
ejaculate, and the menstrual fluid of the women is poor and
full of diseased residues). But for many men and women, this
condition comes about from deformities in the parts and places
used for copulation.

The cases Aristotle introduces with the words προϊούσης τῆς
ἡλικίας are of individuals who have not been sterile since birth,
and so could refer to those who have already become parents as
well as those who have trouble with procreation at their earliest
attempts. The phrase occurs in nine other places in Aristotle:
Col. 6, 797b28, 798b22 and 31; *GA* V.1, 778a28 and 778b25, 7,
787b6; *HA* IV.10, 537b18; *IA* 710b15, and *Insomn.* 3, 462b9. It is
not common among other classical authors. Prior to Aristotle,
Xenophon uses it once at *Oec.* 7.42.3 and Plato twice at *Phdr.*
279a5 and *Rep.* 498b6. Theophrastus uses it once, Frag. 9, 7.4. No
Hippocratic author uses the phrase. It seems likely that the first
person to link ὑπὲρ τοῦ μὴ γεννᾶν to *HA*, whether Andronicus
himself or a later copyist, aware that the phrase was a favorite
of Aristotle and that he had used it to introduce non-congenital
causes of sterility in the *GA*, appended the phrase to show that,

despite the age gap between convulsive infants and procreating adults, the work was a continuation of the *HA*, adding the δέ in imitation of the introits of Books II, VIII(IX) and IX(VII). With the exception of Book I, which has no connective particle, all other books of *HA* use the particle μὲν οὖν in their opening sentences. The words would be an extremely clumsy bridge, but this is not to say that somebody could not possibly have constructed it in this way.

In addition to questions about the relation of *HA* X to the rest of the *HA*, its authorship has been a matter of dispute. The mere inclusion of a title in a list of Aristotelian works does not guarantee the authenticity of a book bearing that title. The lists themselves are inconsistent, and plainly contain doublets and misplaced entries; and many extant works that were originally attributed to Aristotle, and whose titles appear in the lists (e.g. *Mech.* and *Prob.*), have long been recognized as spurious.[10] This is not to say that Aristotle cannot have written works with these titles, but it does mean that any treatise in our modern corpus bearing a title that can plausibly be identified with one in the ancient lists is not necessarily authentically Aristotelian. The consensus of opinion from the eighteenth century through most of the last century was that *HA* X was spurious.[11] However, in the Introduction to his 1957 translation Tricot suggested that *HA* X could have been an early work of Aristotle,[12] and this suggestion was accepted and elaborated by Balme, the major initiator of the revival of the study of Aristotle's biology in the latter part of the twentieth century. At his death in 1989 Balme left unfinished both a text and translation of books VII–X of the *HA* for the

---

[10] On Aristotelian catalogues, see Moraux 1951, Düring 1957, Gottschalk 1990, Anagnostopoulos 2009.

[11] Aubert and Wimmer 1866, Dittmeyer 1907, Düring 1950, Louis 1964. In his 1619 edition Scaliger took the book to be an early work of Aristotle.

[12] Tricot 1957, pp. 17–18. He cites Robin 1944 as the only dissenter from the "quasi-unanimité" that the work is definitely not by Aristotle, but even then Robin only goes so far as to label the work "douteux" (p. 18).

Loeb Classical Library, and a major new edition of the whole treatise for Cambridge Classical Texts and Commentaries.[13] These were prepared for publication by Gotthelf, another prominent scholar in Aristotelian biology, who was inclined to share Balme's views on the authenticity of *HA* X.[14] Van der Eijk has defended Balme's position,[15] and on the basis of these arguments Mayhew used *HA* X as part of his argument that Aristotle was not sexist.[16]

In contrast I believe that the claim for the Aristotelian origin of the major part of *HA* X is demonstrably false.[17] I will argue that careful analysis of content and style shows that the first five chapters of the treatise are Aristotle's summary of the work of a practicing physician with which Aristotle took issue in what have come down to us as the final two chapters of the treatise. In effect the first five chapters are an extended *endoxon* followed by Aristotle's initial dialectic with its major premise.[18] This would accord with a methodology he recommends in *Topics*

---

[13] Balme 1991, 2002.

[14] Though Gotthelf was not adamant about this (personal communication). He may or may not agree with any point Balme makes in the editions he prepared for publication after Balme's death. The only comments he added in his own right appear in square brackets in the Introductions.

[15] Van der Eijk 1999.

[16] Mayhew 2004.

[17] Föllinger 1996, pp. 143–56, briefly rehearses some of the main arguments against Balme's thesis of the Aristotelian authorship of *HA* X. She places great emphasis on the lack of the εἶδος/ὕλη model in *HA* X (pp. 151–6), citing passages showing this was part of Aristotle's reproductive theory in early treatises such as *Ph.* and parts of *Metaph.*, but it is not clear that Balme could not argue that *HA* X was even earlier. Although it is clear that she thinks the treatise is not by Aristotle, she concludes simply "man gut daran tut, weiterhin Aristoteles' Autorschaft von *HA* X in Zweifel zu ziehen." She does not consider who the author may have been and hence makes no further use of the treatise in her book, which compares the various theories of gender relationship in the classical period and demonstrates the sophistication of Aristotle's arguments compared with earlier theorists.

[18] *Endoxon* was Aristotle's technical term for an opinion on a subject held either by experts or the general public; see below, pp. 41–3.

I.14, 105b12–13 and II.2, 110a10–11.[19] This reading makes the best sense of the transmitted text at several cruces and allows the greatest coherence both within the treatise itself and in its correspondence or lack of it to Aristotelian reproductive theory. Typically Aristotelian expressions in the five chapters of summary coupled with the heavily Aristotelian content and style of the last two chapters led to the whole treatise being included in the Aristotelian Corpus even though, as I shall demonstrate, the theory in the majority of the text is clearly at odds with the fundamental precepts of Aristotle's reproductive theory. I shall therefore refer to the first five chapters of the work as *De non generando* (*Non Gen.*) and the final two chapters as the *Dialectic*. I shall reserve the designation *HA* X for references to the work as a whole, including those made by other scholars.[20]

The work was recognized as apocryphal for the best part of two centuries in large part because many of the hypotheses of *Non Gen.* contradict central ideas to be found elsewhere in the biological works accepted as genuine Aristotle, most notably the claim that a woman contributes seed to conception when sexually aroused in the same way as a man does. In all the biological works accepted as genuine, Aristotle argues that women produce only menses, which, although it is quite often referred to as σπέρμα, *sperma*, is emphatically not the generative equivalent of male seed (which he refers to as both *sperma*, and γονή, *gonê*), and is not tied to sexual arousal. Balme attacked the long-standing belief in this incompatibility, however, and argued that "*GA* does not contradict *HA* X but refines its formulation" (1991, p. 28). This implies that he believes the female reproductive fluid referred to as *sperma* in *HA* X is menses, the work coming at an early point in Aristotle's biological oeuvre

---

[19] See below, pp. 43–8.
[20] My argument requires a convenient designation for each of the two parts of the treatise. That *HA* X is not an apt title for the treatise even if it is seen as a unity is reflected in van der Eijk's 1999 use of quotation marks around the designation "*HA* X."

when he had not yet stripped menses of as many of the powers of seed as he was later to do. It is true that he notes that "in Hist. An. X it [i.e., female *sperma*] is a fluid, without further specification" (1985, p. 197), but immediately prior to this statement he outlines the theory in *GA* which identifies menses as female *sperma* and briefly describes the ways in which menses are parallel to and different from male *sperma*. He concludes: "The general theory is not different, but it is more refined and precise [than that of *HA* X]." It is strongly implied that it is the differentiation of menses as "only nutritive soul" rather than the full analogue of male *sperma* which is the refinement. In arguing in support of Balme's view of *HA* X as an early work of Aristotle, van der Eijk states that the fact that the fluid which forms the female *sperma* of *HA* X is unspecified "need not be a serious problem" in identifying it with menses and concludes: "It seems that '*HA* X' contains no statement that really contradicts the orthodox Aristotelian view that conception takes place when male seed and female menstrual blood meet" (1991, pp. 499–500).

But while it is true that Aristotle does use the term *sperma* to refer to menses in other biological works (often in a qualified way, e.g., οὐ καθαρόν, "impure," *GA* I.20, 728a25, II.3, 737a28), a close reading shows that *Non Gen.* uses the term *sperma* (never qualified) to refer to a female emission <u>in addition</u> to menses, and Aristotle not only does not recognize this possibility anywhere in his biology but categorically denies that any animal can produce two seminal secretions (*GA* I.19, 727a26–30).[21]

---

[21] The ms. reading of *PA* IV.10, 689a12–13, seems to allow that females can produce both menses and *gonê*. After explaining that semen (*gonê*) is discharged via the same passage as the fluid residue (i.e., urine) in males of most blooded animals and all vivipara, Aristotle adds, "And the same is true also of both the menses in females, and the part where they emit semen (*gonê*)," τὸν αὐτὸν δὲ τρόπον καὶ ἐν τοῖς θήλεσι τά τε καταμήνια, καὶ ᾗ προΐενται τὴν γονήν. In a note to the passage Peck comments, "This seems to agree with what Aristotle says on the subject in the *Hist. An.*....", referring to *HA* X. But, as I argue below, pp. 27–9, in *Non Gen.* the author does <u>not</u> think of female *sperma* as being discharged by the same place

A supporter of Balme's could perhaps argue that this denial is not pertinent to *HA* X because the author of that work never claims that menses is a seminal fluid. This is true, but it again leads us to the conclusion that the theory of *GA* is something more than a refinement of that of *HA* X. We cannot discount the possibility that Aristotle changed his mind on the status of menses, but we cannot see the theory of *GA* foreshadowed in *HA* X.

Furthermore, the author of *Non Gen.* has an anatomical understanding of a woman's pudenda which recognizes the clear differentiation of the urethra and the vagina (637a23–8) while in various passages throughout his biological works Aristotle states that in all vivipara without exception male and female use the same part for the discharge of fluid residue and for copulation (*HA* V.5, 541a3–5; *PA* IV.10, 689a; *GA* I.13, 719b29–34 and 18, 726a16–25).[22] If *HA* X is an early work of Aristotle we have to assume that he forgot his earlier knowledge of a woman's anatomy.

---

that discharges the menses, i.e., the cervix. Moreover, what is here said to be true in the case of menses is that, like semen in the male, it is a fluid residue and will be emitted by the same part as urine. In this context the topical adverb ᾗ is redundant, if not confusing. It implies that the place from which *gonê* is discharged in the female is in fact *different from* that from which they discharge menses and urine. I would therefore adopt Platt's emendation for the second part of the sentence, καὶ εἰ προΐενται τὴν γονήν, "And the same is true also of both the menses in females, and, if they emit it, the semen." Here Aristotle is neither affirming nor denying that women emit semen but saying that i_f they did it would be discharged at the same place as the other female fluid residues. The likelihood that this is a hypothetical statement is increased by the use of the term γονή rather than σπέρμα. Although Aristotle does use the latter term to refer to menses, it is not clear that he ever uses the former in this way; see below p. 16, n. 29.

[22] E.g., *PA* IV.10, 689a, "Nature uses the same part for the discharge of the fluid residue and for purposes of copulation similarly in both females and males, in all blooded animals with few exceptions and in all vivipara without exception." καταχρῆται δ' ἡ φύσις τῷ αὐτῷ μορίῳ ἐπί τε τὴν τῆς ὑγρᾶς ἔξοδον περιττώσεως καὶ περὶ τὴν ὀχείαν, ὁμοίως ἔν τε τοῖς θήλεσι καὶ τοῖς ἄρρεσιν, ἔξω τινῶν ὀλίγων πᾶσι τοῖς ἐναίμοις, ἐν δὲ τοῖς ζῳτόκοις πᾶσιν.

Furthermore, if Aristotle was the author of *HA* X and it is an early work, Balme would be forced to argue that although Aristotle had an understanding of the separation of vagina and urethra in the human female in his youth he ignored or forgot about it when developing his metaphysical theories about the relationship between the sexes. Aristotle took the increased specialization of parts in animals to indicate a higher position on the *scala naturae*, so animals with separate passages for the discharge of fluid and solid residue were superior to animals with only a single passage. Recognizing that women have separate passages for the discharge of their two fluid residues (menstrual blood and urine) would have made them superior to men.[23] This would be unusual, perhaps unprecedented, in that Aristotle tried to take account of all empirical evidence when framing his theories, even if only by the expedient of employing vocabulary such as ὡς ἐπὶ τὸ πόλυ, "for the most part."

Other matters of content in *Non Gen.* at odds with Aristotle's theory as expounded in his biological works are the importance of female orgasm, the site in the woman's body where the male and female seminal fluids interact, the action of *pneuma* in drawing *sperma* into the womb, the mechanism which causes multiple births, and the role of heat in the formation of uterine mole. Balme and van der Eijk offer explanations to account for these divergences, but they accept that the statement about multiple births is a complete contradiction of what Aristotle says elsewhere.

Maintaining that *HA* X is an early work of Aristotle ignores the fact that, while it is clear that the extant works of Aristotle were not all written in the same period of his life (indeed what we possess as complete texts often seem to bear the marks of different strata of composition), he evidently on occasion

---

[23] See Dean-Jones 1994, pp. 82–3. If Aristotle thought he had refuted the belief in three passages in women by his dissection of viviparous quadrupeds, he would not consider this a suitable source of knowledge to be used in dialectic; see Bolton 1987, pp. 122–3.

attempted to revise earlier passages as his ideas developed in order to bring them into line with his more developed views;[24] and while such a process was haphazard and frequently left traces of the earlier unmodified opinions, to leave a whole book on generation so much at variance with the exposition of his reproductive theory elsewhere apparently unrevised in any way would be unprecedented. I am, of course, arguing for something which is itself apparently unprecedented: an unacknowledged summary of another author's theories followed by Aristotle's initial reaction to these theories. But in support of my argument I would point to the fact that this coheres with Aristotle's expressed views on how to do philosophy[25] and that it makes the meaning of *Non Gen.* much less opaque if we do not try to make it conform to Aristotle's theory.[26] Moreover, Aristotelian precepts <u>are</u> apparent in the final two chapters and are deployed in a way that <u>undercuts</u> the argument of the first five chapters.

The text was also considered suspect because the style and vocabulary was felt to be un-Aristotelian, demonstrating a general grammatical carelessness and lack of logical sequence deemed uncharacteristic even of Aristotle's admittedly crabbed and terse style. Upholders of Aristotelian authorship acknowledge the stylistic anomalies but maintain that they can be attributed to the early date at which Aristotle wrote the work or to the fact that it is more medical in tone than any extant work, and they point to turns of phrase

[24] E.g., the sudden elevation of the contemplative life over that of the practical at *EN* X.7–8, 1177a11–1179a32; the return to the theory that, in the course of continuous change, there can be a first instant of having departed from the pre-existing state at *Phys.* VIII.8, 262a17–b8, when this had been refuted at VI.5, 235b6–236b18. However, if my explanation about the composition of *HA* X is correct, some of these "unrevised" passages may prove to be embedded *endoxa* also: see below p. 43, n. 81.

[25] See pp. 43–9.

[26] For the impotance of female orgasm, see pp. 19–24; for the site of seminal interaction, see pp. 27–8, 35, and 57–8; for action of *pneuma*, see pp. 27, 30, and 94; for multiple births, see pp. 69–74; for uterine mole, see pp. 58–64.

which could be considered typically Aristotelian. After a very detailed study of the vocabulary and grammar of *HA* X, Rudberg (1911) declared that Aristotelian authorship was impossible ("unmöglich," p. 6) but argued that the style vacillated ("schwanken," p. 24) between the Hippocratics and Aristotle because a Peripatetic Iatrosophist was attempting a synthesis of their theories with the texts in front of him (p. 46). This despite the fact that there is nothing specifically Aristotelian in the first five chapters, nor any indication of his disagreement with much that is written there. The vacillation in style but not in content of the first five chapters can be explained if the theories, vocabulary, and style of a medical text are embedded in a summary written by Aristotle himself.

Non Gen. is no less important a document for being non-Aristotelian. Even embedded in *HA* X, it is a key text for the understanding of developing Greek attitudes to fertility, sterility, and sexual reproduction in general, one which has been insufficiently studied, in part because of the perceived difficulty of the Greek and, prior to Balme's edition, the poor condition of the text, in part because it has been consigned to a backwater of the Aristotelian Corpus, and in part simply because its originality has not been fully appreciated, particularly in regard to its recognition of female sexuality.

Perhaps more importantly, the treatise also gives us unique insight into Aristotle's method. If I am correct, many other problematic passages scattered throughout the Aristotelian Corpus which seem inconsonant with his predominant views could be read as embedded extended *endoxa*.

2 FEMALE *SPERMA* IN *NON GEN.*

(a) Significance of one or two seminal residues

Whether or not female *sperma* in *Non Gen.* is to be identified in some way with menses is really the crux of the matter in deciding between Aristotelian and non-Aristotelian author-ship. In all his other biological works Aristotle is adamant that a female contributes only menses to the conception of a child. He does sometimes use the term *sperma* to refer to menstrual fluid because it is the female's seminal residue, but he makes it clear that it is not equivalent to male semen in transferring form from parent to offspring but merely provides nutritive soul.[27] At *GA* II.3, 737a18–24, he differentiates the *sperma* (not the *gonê*) of the male from περίττωμα τὸ τοῦ θήλεος, the residue of the female, and he goes on to explain (29) that although menses are *sperma*, they are not pure, τὰ καταμήνια σπέρμα οὐ καθαρὸν δέ.[28] He is insistent that no animal can produce two seminal residues. He remarks at *GA* I.19, 727a25–30:

> ἐπεὶ δὲ τοῦτ' ἔστιν ὃ γίγνεται τοῖς θήλεσιν ὡς ἡ γονὴ τοῖς ἄρρεσιν, δύο δ' οὐκ ἐνδέχεται σπερματικὰς ἅμα γίγνεσθαι ἀποκρίσεις, φανερὸν ὅτι τὸ θῆλυ οὐ συμβάλλεται σπέρμα εἰς τὴν γένεσιν. εἰ μὲν γὰρ σπέρμα ἦν τὰ καταμήνια οὐκ ἂν ἦν· νῦν δὲ διὰ τὸ ταῦτα γίγνεσθαι ἐκεῖνο οὐκ ἔστιν.

> Since this [i.e. menses] is that which corresponds in the female to *gonê*[29] in males and because it is not possible for two seminal secretions to be produced in the same creature, it is clear that

---

[27] See, e.g., *GA* II.5, 741a17–32. For detailed, sometimes conflicting, discussions on Aristotle's theory of reproduction, see Dean-Jones 1994, Föllinger 1996, Mayhew 2004, Connell 2016.

[28] See also, e.g., *HA* IX(VII).1, 581b32 and 582a5, residues are excreted τοῖς μὲν ἐν τῷ σπέρματι ταῖς δ' ἐν τοῖς καταμηνίοις.

[29] The term γονή is never used in *HA* X, and it is not clear that Aristotle himself ever refers to the female seminal residue by that term in the rest of his biological works. When he does use the term it is usually explicitly restricted to the male and/or explicitly contrasted with the female seminal residue. The only time the term is unambiguously used to refer to female seminal residue is when Aristotle is discussing theories with which he disagrees, e.g., fertility tests which liken the nature of *gonê* to that of the brain, *GA* II.7, 747a18; see Dean-Jones 2017; see also Empedocles' explanation of the infertility of mules, *GA* II.8, 747b1; mistaken theories of resemblance to parents, *GA* IV.3, 769a34; Democritus' explanation of monstrosities, *GA* IV.4, 769b31. For *PA* IV.10, 689a12–13, see above pp. 11–12, n. 21.

the female does not contribute *sperma* to generation; for if there were *sperma* there would not be menstrual fluid; but as it is, because the latter is formed, the former is not.

Aristotle is here arguing against the theory prevalent in the Hippocratic Corpus[30] that women produced seed in addition to menses. In Hippocratic reproductive theory menstrual fluid gradually built up in the woman's flesh throughout the month, keeping the womb clear for the mingling of male and female seed. Problems arise if the womb is not kept clear of menses, e.g., a woman may not retain her seed because "her menses come more than is fitting, and more moist, with the result that the material from the woman is not taken up for childbearing," τὰ ἐπιμήνια πλείω γίνεται τοῦ προσήκοντος καὶ ὑγρότερα, ὥστε τὸ ἀπὸ τῆς γυναικὸς μὴ ξυλλαμβάνεσθαι πρὸς τὴν τέκνωσιν.[31] If the woman conceived, the menses were used for the nourishment of the growing embryo; if she did not, they were evacuated by being drawn through the womb at the end of the month.[32] Clearly then, menses and female seed are differentiated by the

---

[30] Van der Eijk 2016 puts forward a strong argument that the works contained in the Hippocratic Corpus should not be viewed as standing apart from the rest of ancient Greek medicine. However, as regards gynecology of the fifth and fourth centuries, we have very little outside of the Corpus. We have some later testimonia on Diocles of Carystus' views on infertility (see below, p. 39), but since almost all the evidence for classical Greek medical beliefs about infertility other than those of Aristotle and the author of *Non Gen.* come from the Hippocratic Corpus I shall use the Hippocratic Corpus to represent medical theories of the fifth and fourth centuries. The relationship between the nine or ten treatises that are generally referred to as the Hippocratic gynecological works is very complex. Some treatises presented as a unity are clearly compilations from various authors, others that may have originally been one treatise are presented as two. A substantial amount of material is repeated both within a text and between texts. For a detailed discussion, see Totelin 2009, pp. 9–13. For a discussion of the formation of the Hippocratic Corpus as a whole, see Nutton 2013, pp. 53–71.

[31] *Steril.* 241 (VIII.454.8–9).

[32] See *Nat. Puer.* 15 (VII.492.21–494.20). This is a normative description of the Hippocratic conception of the roles of female seed and menses in gestation. The measures used to address disruptions in this process in the

Hippocratics. *Genit.* 2 (VII.472.16–474.4) might seem to parallel seed in pubescent boys and menses in pubescent girls, attributing both to the opening up of their blood vessels which allows their moisture (τὸ ὑγρόν) to become agitated. However in *Nat. Puer.* 20 (VII.508.6–7), having described the appearance of *gonê* in boys, the same author remarks:

καὶ τῇσι παρθένοισι περὶ τῶν καταμηνίων ωὑτὸς λόγος· ἅμα δὲ ὁδὸς προσγίνεται καὶ τοῖσι καταμηνίοισι καὶ τῇ γονῇ τῇσι παρθένοισι.

And the same account holds true concerning the menses in young girls; a passage appears at the same time for both menses and *gonê* in young girls.[33]

If, then, female *sperma* in *Non Gen.* can be shown to be a seminal fluid produced by women <u>in addition to</u> menses, on this point the treatise can be seen as being in line with the Hippocratic texts and in diametrical opposition to every Aristotelian work on reproduction. Of course, one could still argue that *HA* X was a very early work by Aristotle, but it would be one he would roundly repudiate in later life; we would not expect to find it in completely unrevised form among his later works. If the author of *Non Gen.* does believe women produce <u>both</u> menses <u>and</u> *sperma*, it is far more likely that he was somebody other than Aristotle.

The fact that *Non Gen.* does distinguish between menses and female seed can be obfuscated because although he has technical terms for both (καταμήνια and γυναικεῖα for menses, *sperma* for seed), he on occasion refers to both with generic terms for

major gynecological texts show that it was shared by other Hippocratic authors, see Dean-Jones 1994, pp. 153–60; King 1998, p. 134.

[33] Littré deletes the second occurrence of τοῖσι παρθένοισι, in which case τῇ γονῇ could refer to just the boy's semen, but as the author requires the womb to be empty of menses for conception to occur (ὥστ' ἢν μὲν ἀποκενῶται τοῦ αἵματος ἡ γυνή, λαμβάνει ἐν γαστρί, *Nat. Puer.* 15 (VII.494.15–16)) it is clear that the author does not identify female seed with menses and is referring to two fluids appearing in young girls at the same time.

a fluid: ὑγρότης, which refers to menses at 634a15 and 23 but to female seed at 635a40,[34] and ὑγρόν, which refers to menses at 634a20 but to the mixture of male and female seeds at 636a14.[35] However, a careful reading of the treatise makes it clear that the two fluids (menses and female *sperma*) are produced under different circumstances, have distinctive appearances, and arrive by different paths into the womb.

(b) Circumstances of production

The clearest indication that female *sperma* is distinct from menses in the mind of the author of *Non Gen.* is that he believes it is emitted by the woman at orgasm in either actual intercourse or an erotic dream. A passage at the end of the fourth chapter, 636b13–23, discusses the need for both man and woman to "keep pace," ἰσοδρομῆσαι, with one another if conception is to take place and says there are problems if the man "finishes off quickly," ταχὺ ἐκποιήσῃ, while the woman has hardly started. In context "finishing off" clearly means ejaculation, so the passage makes it clear that in a woman too the emission of *sperma* is something that occurs at the culmination of coition for which she has been previously "excited, prepared and possessed of appropriate thoughts," ὀργῶσα καὶ παρεσκευασμένη εἴη καὶ ἐννοίας ἔχουσα ἐπιτηδείας. Climaxing is also indicated at 634b30 when the author says that women emit *sperma* "whenever they have erotic dreams to completion," ὅταν ἐξονειρώττωσιν αὗται τελέως. In contrast, at *GA* I.19, 727b8–12, Aristotle says:

πολλάκις τὸ θῆλυ συλλαμβάνει οὐ γενομένης αὐτῇ τῆς ἐν τῇ ὁμιλίᾳ ἡδονῆς· καὶ γιγνομένης πάλιν οὐδὲν ἧττον, καὶ ἰσοδρομησάντων[36] τοῦ ἄρρενος καὶ τοῦ θήλεος οὐθὲν γεννᾶται ἐὰν μὴ ἡ τῶν καλουμένων καταμηνίων ἰκμὰς ὑπάρχῃ σύμμετρος.

---

[34] And also to the vaginal lubricant at 635b31. The term refers to the general fluid state of the body in the *Dialectic* at 638b2.

[35] And in the *Dialectic* to general sexual fluids at 638a2 and b34, and to general bodily fluids at 638b20. ὑγρασία at 635b28 refers to the vaginal lubricant.

[36] For the significance of this term in this passage, see below pp. 101–2.

Often the female conceives when she experiences no pleasure in intercourse, and, moreover, when she experiences just as much as the male and she and the male "keep pace" nothing is generated unless there is a proportionate amount of the so-called menses present.

Supporters of Aristotelian authorship have to explain this apparent contradiction. Balme says, "Both *GA* and *HA* X emphasise the need for symmetry between the two contributions, but whereas *HA* X bases this upon simultaneous emission, *GA* bases it upon proportional heat and quantity,"[37] and "In Gener. An, as in Hist. An. X, there is emphasis upon harmony (συμμετρία) in the mingling of male and female contributions. The general theory of Gener. An is not different, but is more refined and precise."[38] This does not address the problem of why Aristotle would choose to negate the importance of ἰσοδρομέω and assert συμμετρία as a different principle if he is merely "refining" his theory. Van der Eijk moots the possibility that the ejaculate the author of *HA* X believes the woman has to emit at climax is in fact the vaginal lubricant which Aristotle says facilitates conception at *GA* II.4, 739a32–5, though he acknowledges the problem presented by *HA* X calling an ejaculate which merely facilitates conception "*sperma.*"[39] In attempting to minimize the importance of sexual arousal as a precondition for the production of female *sperma* in *Non Gen.*, van der Eijk says, "The author of '*HA* X' does not assume ejaculation is necessarily accompanied by pleasure."[40] It is true that the author does not use the term ἡδονή, but it is hard to deny he envisages a strong affective component in the emission of female *sperma*. And given that it is assumed that the man and woman have the ability to slow their sexual process

---

[37] Balme 1991, pp. 28–9.   [38] Balme 1985, p. 197.

[39] Van der Eijk 1999, p. 500. Even Balme admits that *HA* X differentiates the fluid identified in *GA* II.4, 739a32–5, from *sperma*; see below pp. 34–5.

[40] Van der Eijk 1999, p. 500, n. 55. In that case it could not be identified with the moisture Aristotle describes at *GA* II.4, 739a32–5, which is accompanied by pleasure.

to "keep pace" with their partner, this affective component should be observable and mirror that which accompanies male ejaculation.

Menstruation, on the other hand, is a periodic event which should take place at regular intervals regardless of a woman's affective disposition, though the intervals may become more or less frequent if the body, for any reason, becomes more moist or more dry.[41] Furthermore, the release of each fluid has a different effect on the body. *Non Gen.* says that menses are released <u>as a result of</u> the body relaxing, and that after menstruation the womb should be "neither incapacitated nor fatigued," μὴ ἀδύνατος ἀλλ᾽ ἄκοπος,[42] while in a different passage the author says that the emission of *sperma* can <u>cause</u> a woman's body to become enervated and weak because it can be drawn out of the material which the body needs.[43] Finally conception, which requires the emission of *sperma* on the woman's part, is most likely after menstruation has ceased and the uterus has become "empty and dry and thirsty and has no residues" (κεναὶ καὶ ξηραὶ…καὶ διψηραὶ καὶ οὐκ ἔχουσι λείψανα, 635a25). This is in contrast to Aristotle, who says that in order for conception to take place there must be a certain amount of menstrual fluid in the womb.[44] The circumstances of the emission of *sperma* and menses as described in *Non Gen.* give no prima facie reason to equate the two.

Moreover, there are indications that Aristotle's argument against associating the emission of female *sperma* with pleasure are aimed specifically at the formulation of the theory in *Non Gen.* Like the author of *Non Gen.*, the Hippocratics believed that for conception to occur a woman needed to feel pleasure in intercourse and ejaculate *sperma* at orgasm. But unlike *Non Gen.* the Hippocratics show little concern with the timing of female orgasm relative to the male. *Mul.* I.12

---

[41] 634a12–16, 35–8, and 634b1–18 [42] 635a19–20 and 633b24–5.
[43] 635b36–40 and 636b32.
[44] See *GA* I.19, 727b11–12, II.4, 738b8, *HA* IX(VII).2, 582b15.

(VIII.48.15–17) says a woman should feel desire if she is to become pregnant, but this is a general state lasting several days, not a state of climaxing during intercourse. The author of *Genit.* states that:

καὶ ἥδεται, ἐπὴν ἄρξηται μίσγεσθαι, διὰ παντὸς τοῦ χρόνου, μέχρι αὐτῇ μεθιῇ ὁ ἀνήρ· κἢν μὲν ὀργᾷ ἡ γυνὴ μίσγεσθαι, πρόσθεν τοῦ ἀνδρὸς ἀφίει, καὶ τὸ λοιπὸν οὐκ ἔτι ὁμοίως ἥδεται ἡ γυνή· ἢν δὲ μὴ ὀργᾷ, συντελέει τῷ ἀνδρὶ ἡδομένη· καὶ ἔχει οὕτως ὥσπερ εἴ τις ἐπὶ ὕδωρ ζέον ἕτερον ψυχρὸν ἐπιχέει, παύεται τὸ ὕδωρ ζέον· οὕτω, καὶ ἡ γονὴ πεσοῦσα τοῦ ἀνδρὸς ἐς τὰς μήτρας σβέννυσι τὴν θέρμην καὶ τὴν ἡδονὴν τῆς γυναικός. ἐξαΐσσει δὲ ἡ ἡδονὴ καὶ ἡ θέρμη ἅμα τῇ γονῇ πιπτούσῃ ἐς τὰς μήτρας, ἔπειτα λήγει·

She feels pleasure when coition begins, and throughout the entire time until the man releases her. If the woman reaches orgasm during intercourse, she will ejaculate before the man and for the remaining time the woman will no longer feel pleasure in the same way. If she does not reach orgasm she will cease feeling pleasure at the same time as the man. And it is just like what happens if someone pours one lot of cold water into another that is boiling: the water ceases boiling. So, the *gonê* falling from the man into the womb extinguishes the heat and pleasure of the woman. The pleasure and the heat leap up to meet the *gonê* falling into the womb and then subside.[45]

He also uses the analogy of a candle flame flaring up when wine is thrown on it to illustrate the behavior of a woman's heat when it comes into contact with male *gonê*. There may be some problem in conception on this theory if the female failed to emit, but there is no indication the man and woman have to "keep pace" here. The fact that a woman might emit before a man is not said to be a problem, and the analogies suggest that the author believes that if a man reaches orgasm this in itself

---

[45] *Genit.* 4 (VII.474.14–476.8). Rudberg 1911, p. 11, cites this as a similarity between *Non Gen.* and the Hippocratics, but it is so only in that it recognizes the existence of female seed.

might bring a woman to orgasm. The author also believes that women experience a lot less pleasure than men in intercourse anyway (ἧσσον δὲ πολλῷ ἥδεται ἡ γυνὴ τοῦ ἀνδρὸς ἐν τῇ μίξει), so he may not have expected a woman's orgasm to be especially marked. He did not expect the vagina to become lubricated on every occasion that a woman emitted seed.[46] Therefore, the primary sign that a woman had reached orgasm and ejaculated *sperma* was not that she said so, or even that her vagina became lubricated, but that she became pregnant.

Balme cites *Mul.* I.17 (VIII.56.22) as evidence for a Hippocratic belief in simultaneous emission, but in full context (56.20–58.2) this is not so obvious. The statement comes at the end of a description for treatment for an excessively dry or moist womb. Once treatment has been successful the doctor is told to advise women to have intercourse with their husbands, preferably at the end of menstruation. If they do not become pregnant immediately, they should continue having intercourse:

προθυμίην γὰρ σφίσι ποιέει ἡ μελέτη, καὶ ἀναχαλᾶται τὰ φλεβία, καὶ ἢν τὰ ἀπὸ τοῦ ἀνδρὸς ἀπιόντα ὁμορροθῇ κατ᾽ ἴξιν τῷ ἀπὸ τῆς γυναικός, ταχύτερον κυήσει. καὶ γὰρ τόδε αἴτιον ἔστιν ᾗσιν, ἤντε αὐτίκα ἤντ᾽ ἐν ὑστέρῳ χρόνῳ ἀπίῃ.

for the activity will stimulate desire in them, and open up the vessels, and if the material emitted by the man runs together on the same side as that of the woman,[47] she will become pregnant. For this is also a cause (of conception) in women, whether she emits it immediately or at a later time.[48]

The author gives no instruction on how to ensure simultaneity or that there would be any overt sign of it, other than the woman eventually becoming pregnant.[49] In fact, that the woman can

---

[46] See below, p. 31.

[47] That is, into the same "horn" of the womb; see commentary at 635b15–16 & 637a9.

[48] There are problems with the text here and the author's meaning remains unclear, but the passage cannot be used unproblematically as evidence for a belief in the necessity of simultaneous ejaculation.

[49] For a more expansive discussion of this issue, see Dean-Jones 1992.

23

emit her material either immediately or at a (presumably not much) later time seems to exclude the necessity of simultaneity. In his argument at *GA* I.19, 727b7–12, Aristotle appears to be rebutting specifically *Non Gen.*'s explanation as to why, even if there is no other impediment, a man and a woman must emit *sperma* <u>at the same time</u> during coition to assure conception.

(c) Appearance

Supporters of Aristotelian authorship might argue that despite these differences in the circumstances of production, female *sperma* in *Non Gen.* can still be equated with menses if it is a portion of menstrual fluid that is emitted by the body under circumstances of sexual arousal into an empty womb before the body is ready to release the full monthly accumulation in its periodic cycle. Aristotle does not seem to think of the menses as flowing into the womb in a steady stream. At *GA* II.4, 738a12–17, he says the blood first collects in the many fine blood vessels which run from the Great Blood Vessel and the Aorta before it is separated off, ἐκκρίνεται, into the uterus.[50] There is no indication that there is any force, such as sexual arousal, that causes the separating out; in fact, *GA* II.4, 737b26–738a9, argues at length that *sperma*, just like every other residue, is carried to its proper place in the body:

οὐθὲν ἀποβιαζομένου τοῦ πνεύματος, οὐδ' ἄλλης αἰτίας τοιαύτης ἀναγκαζούσης, ὥσπερ τινές φασιν, ἕλκειν τὰ αἰδοῖα φάσκοντες ὥσπερ τὰς σικύας.

without the *pneuma* exerting any force, nor under any compulsion from any other such causes, as some assert, saying the genitals draw them like cupping glasses.

However, such a force seems to be suggested at *GA* III.1, 750b34–751a3:

---

[50] Eventually the amount of blood becomes too much for the fine blood vessels to hold, and that is when menstruation occurs.

ἐπὶ τῶν γυναικῶν τὸ πλησιάζειν τοῖς ἄρρεσι κατασπᾷ τὴν τῶν γυναικεῖων ἀπόκρισιν (ἕλκει γὰρ τὸ ὑγρὸν ἡ ὑστέρα θερμανθεῖσα, καὶ οἱ πόροι ἀναστομοῦνται).

In the case of women, intercourse with males draws down the menstrual secretion (for when it is heated the womb attracts the fluid and the passages open up).

This still seems to envisage the woman's *sperma* remaining in the womb, not mixing with the man's outside the womb as *Non Gen.* insists must happen. In answer to this objection Balme draws attention to a passage at *GA* II.4, 739a26–9, where Aristotle says conception cannot take place unless the menstrual fluid is issuing outside (θύραζε προελθούσης) or there is enough of the residue inside (ἐντὸς ἱκανῆς). But clearly the external appearance of menstrual fluid is simply a sign that there is enough residue within the womb for conception to take place, as is confirmed by a passage at *HA* IX(VII).2, 582b12–17. Nevertheless, let us allow for the moment that at an early stage in his thought Aristotle believed that conception took place when a portion of female *sperma* (i.e., menstrual fluid) was emitted from the womb during intercourse.

If *Non Gen.* does intend to identify a woman's *sperma* as the ejaculation of a proemial part of the menses, we might expect the two fluids to be similar in appearance. The menses, of course, are bloody in appearance (though *Non Gen.* states that the blood can be diluted if the body is particularly moist, 634b17–18, ἐὰν μὲν ὑγρὸν ὑδαρέστερα, ἐὰν δὲ ξηρὸν ἐναιμότερα). However, at 635b1 the author says that the fluid a woman emits when she dreams she has had intercourse with her husband (referred to as *sperma* at 634b35–8, 635b37, and 636b26) should be like the fluid in her vagina after she has had intercourse with her husband (ἡ δ᾽ ὑγρότης ἔστω τοιαύτη οἵα ὅταν πλησιάσῃ τῷ ἀνδρί) and this does not have a blood-like appearance. This would be enough to distinguish menses from female *sperma* were it not for the fact that at the beginning and ending of menstruation *Non Gen.* says that the menses themselves can appear white:

ἄρχονται μὲν ἐκ λευκῶν γαλακτοειδῶν, ἀνόσμων μενουσῶν· τὰ δὲ φοινικᾶ μέν, ἀπολήγονται δὲ λευκότερα ἐσχάτης καταλήξεως.

Menses begin with the milk-like whites, which remain odorless; then they turn red but taper off whiter in color at the very end of the cessation of menstruation.[51]

It could thus be argued that the author of *Non Gen.* believes that the *sperma* emitted by the woman during erotic dreams and coition is menses in the form of "whites," and this is why the fluid in her vagina after both night emissions and intercourse with a man does not have a bloody appearance. But at 634a30–2 "whites" are associated with putrefaction:

ταῖς δ᾽ ὑγιαινούσαις τὰ λευκὰ καὶ σεσημμένα προέρχεται. ταῖς μὲν καὶ ἀρχομένων ταῖς δὲ πλείσταις ληγόντων τῶν καταμηνίων.

In healthy women whites come out in a putrefied state, for some at the beginning of menstruation, but for most when they are tapering off.

Non Gen. never refers to *sperma* as being putrefied. Nor does the author make any connection whatsoever between "whites" and female *sperma*. Therefore in *Non Gen.* both the circumstances of production and the appearance of female *sperma* tell against an identification with menses.

(d) Path into the womb

In *GA* I.19, 726b7–10, Aristotle says that male *sperma* emitted under strain due to excessive intercourse is unconcocted and bloody in nature; so, supporters of Aristotelian authorship could argue, at an early stage in the development of his theory Aristotle may have believed that at the point of orgasm menses were emitted by the uterus in a more concocted state than normal, so that if *HA* X is an early Aristotelian work the difference in appearance, as well as the difference in the circumstances of production, is

[51] 634b18–20.

immaterial in determining authenticity. However, this does not address the objection that in *Non Gen.* there is a difference in the place of emission of the menses and the female *sperma*.

In an extended note on *HA* X.2, Balme states that throughout the treatise Aristotle argues that "the female seed is conveyed in a fluid which the uterus emits during coition into 'the region in front of the uterus'."[52] But *Non Gen.* never says that the <u>womb</u> emits *sperma*; the author always says the <u>woman</u> emits *sperma* (635a34, 636b37, 637a2, 15, 36–7). Furthermore, in explaining why the cervix has to be straight in order for conception to take place the author does not use phrasing that would suggest the uterus was reabsorbing the female contribution <u>back into itself</u>:

εἰς τὸ πρόσθεν γὰρ αὐτῶν καὶ ἡ γυνὴ προῖεται, ὡς δῆλον ὅταν ἐξονειρώττωσιν αὗται τελέως. τότε γὰρ οὗτος ὁ τόπος θεραπείας δεῖται αὐταῖς ὑγρανθεὶς ὥσπερ εἰ ἀνδρὶ συνεγίνετο, ὡς προϊε-μένων ἐνταῦθα καὶ τὸ παρὰ τοῦ ἀνδρός, εἰς τὸν αὐτὸν τόπον καὶ οὐχὶ εἰς τὰς ὑστέρας εἴσω. ἀλλ' ὅταν ἐνταῦθα προϊῶνται, ἐντεῦθεν σπῶσι τῷ πνεύματι, οἷον αἱ ῥῖνες, καὶ αἱ ὑστέραι τὸ σπέρμα. διὸ καὶ παντὶ σχήματι συνοῦσαι κυΐσκονται, ὅτι εἰς τὸ πρόσθεν παντελῶς ἐχούσης γίγνεται καὶ αὐταῖς καὶ τοῖς ἀνδρά-σιν ἡ πρόεσις τοῦ σπέρματος· εἰ δ' εἰς αὐτήν, οὐκ ἂν πάντως συγγενόμεναι συνελάμβανον.

Because it is in fact into the place in front of the uterus that a woman too emits, as is clear whenever they have erotic dreams which reach completion. For then this place needs seeing to by them since it becomes moist, just as if she had had inter-course with a man, since men emit their *sperma* at this place also, into the same place and not into the interior of the uterus. Whenever they emit here, the uterus draws in the *sperma* from this place by means of *pneuma*, just like the nose. For this reason, women become pregnant when they have intercourse in any

[52] Balme 1991, p. 488. Note that this would contradict Aristotle's statement at *GA* II.4, 739b18–20, that if the uterus were to emit seed outside itself it would then have to draw it back in and this would contravene Nature's rule of doing nothing superfluous.

position, because the emission of the *sperma* both by them and by men is in front of the womb, if this is properly positioned. If their emission were into the womb, they would not conceive in any position.[53]

This suggests very strongly that from wherever the female *sperma* is emitted, it is not the womb. If the woman's seed originated within the womb and was emitted through the cervix, it would not always be emitted in the same place as the man emits; it would vary with the divergence of the cervix. Furthermore, if the womb was the <u>source</u> of female *sperma*, the very discussion of emission would be out of place in the contrafactual "If their emission were <u>into</u> the womb they would not conceive in any position." A more appropriate locution would have been "If the woman's *sperma* were to <u>remain</u> in the womb."

Finally at two places the author makes it quite clear that the woman emits her seed in front of the womb by means of a duct separate from the womb. At 636a4–7 in reference to the womb drawing in the *sperma* emitted by a woman during an erotic dream the author says:

πνεύματί τε γὰρ ἕλκει ἡ ὑστέρα τὸ προσελθὸν ἔξωθεν αὐτῇ, ὥσπερ πρότερον εἴρηται. οὐ γὰρ εἰς αὐτὴν προΐεται, ἀλλ᾽ οὗ καὶ ὁ ἀνήρ.

For with *pneuma* the womb draws in what has come towards it from outside, just as was said earlier. For the woman's *sperma* is not emitted into the womb but where the man emits too.

A passage at 637a22–35 describes a καυλός (*kaulos*, "duct") that brings an ἔκπτωσις (*ekptôsis*, "emission") to the area before her womb.[54] In configuration it resembles the passage that runs between the nose and the pharynx except that, whereas the

---

[53] 634b29–39. For the switch from plural to singular to refer to the womb, see below, p. 97. For the need of male and female *spermata* to mingle outside the womb, see below, p. 35.

[54] *HA* III.1, 510b8–9, uses the term καυλός to refer to the cervix. This cannot be what is meant here.

nasal passage has a wider opening towards the exterior air (through which mucus has to pass) and a narrower opening towards the interior (because only *pneuma* should reach the pharynx), the *kaulos* has a narrower opening to the exterior (through which *pneuma* passes[55]) and a wider opening to the interior of the body (through which the *ekptôsis* reaches the area before the womb). To maintain his argument that menses and female *sperma* are basically the same material, even if they are produced at different times and look different, Balme has to argue, contrary to most editors and translators, that *pneuma* is the sole component of the *ekptôsis*.[56] This position is belied by the fact that in describing the *kaulos* the author says women "have a *kaulos*, just as men have a penis, but within the body," ἔχουσι καυλὸν, ὥσπερ καὶ οἱ ἄνδρες τὸ αἰδοῖον, ἀλλ' ἐν τῷ σώματι.[57] Since the <u>configuration</u> of the *kaulos* is likened to the nasal passages, the significance of the reference to the male penis must be its <u>function</u>, i.e., to carry *sperma*. And, as stated above, whereas the passage to the outside is said to be small and narrow so that it only emits *pneuma* (καὶ ἔξω ἔχει πόρον μικρόν τε πάνυ καὶ στενόν, ὅσον πνεύματι ἔξοδον, 637a30–1), the opening in front of the womb is said to be spacious and wide (εὐρύχωρον εὔρουν, 637a32) implying that it carries something in addition to *pneuma*, i.e., *sperma*.

In the treatise as we have it there is no description of the passage of menses through the body into the womb, but it is legitimate to make certain assumptions from the text. At 635a18–22, when describing the state of the uterus before menstruation begins, the author says that it should not open up at the very beginning when only whites are being emitted but when the body sends more fluid. This would imply that the menses do

---

[55] This is not the *pneuma* instrumental in drawing the semen into the womb but the *pneuma* which accompanies the release of *sperma* and causes a sensation of sexual arousal at the site of its emission from the body. The author of *Non Gen.* describes this as being just above the urethra, i.e. the clitoris. For a more detailed discussion of this passage, see notes ad loc.

[56] Balme 1991, pp. 516–17.   [57] 637a22–3.

not flow continually towards the womb over the course of the month, as Aristotle argues, but all at once at a certain point in a woman's cycle, as the Hippocratics believe.[58] That they are not drawn into the womb via the cervix as female *sperma* is hardly needs arguing, but is made clear by the analogy of the womb to eyes, bladder, and intestines at 634a20–7. When they are inflamed, these organs "draw moisture of the type which is naturally secreted into each part," ἕλκουσιν ὑγότητα τοιαύτην ἣ πέφυκεν ἐκκρίνεσθαι εἰς ἕκαστον τόπον (23–4). The sites for the ingress and egress of fluids for each of these organs, and therefore for the womb, are distinct. This accounts for the term ἀποδιδόναι at 634a25, 27, and b8; the womb "passes on" the menses through the cervix after receiving them through another opening.

Non Gen. does not describe the openings whereby menstrual fluid enters the womb from the body, but at 637a18 the author says that hollow structures which draw things without tools either use *pneuma* (as the womb does when drawing in *sperma*) or they have a natural εἴσφυσις (*eisphusis*, "funnel") on top (see notes ad loc.). Given that the author describes the body as actively emitting menses into the uterus (635a22) rather than them being drawn in, it is fair to assume he believed there were "funnels" on the top of the womb. The endings of the oviducts, which may have been seen in the dissection or butchering of animals, would be good candidates to support this belief. In passing references the author of *Non Gen.* uses a generic verb (ἀνοίγεσθαι, *anoigesthai*) for the opening of both the uterus to receive the menses from the body (634a15, 19) and the cervix to discharge them (635a7, 636a31).[59] However, in the passage in which he specifically discusses the action of the womb and

[58] *GA* II.4, 737b28–34 (but see *HA* IX(VII).2, 582b8, where it is stated that for some women the menses flow ἀθρόα and in others κατ᾽ ὀλίγον), *Nat. Puer.* 15 (VII.492.21–494.2), *Mul.* I.2 (VIII.16.3–4). See Dean-Jones 1994, pp. 62–5.

[59] At 634a10 and 636a38 the subject of the verb could be either the womb as a whole or just the cervix or both.

cervix during menstruation he uses the term διαστομοῦσθαι (*diastomousthai*) to refer to the dilation of the cervix (635a9, 15) and ἀναστομοῦσθαι (*anastomousthai*) to refer to the action of the womb itself (635a12, 18, 22). I have translated this latter term as "to expand." The "opening" of the womb "to receive the moisture from the body whenever the body gives it" (δέχεσθαι τὴν ἐκ τοῦ σώματος ὑγρότητα ὅταν τὸ σῶμα διδῷ, 634a15–16) is an expansion that allows it to accommodate the menstrual fluid.

There is no clear point of similarity, then, between menses and female *sperma* in *Non Gen*. They are produced under different circumstances, they look different, and they travel through the body to the womb by different routes.

(e) Female seed and the vaginal lubricant

But perhaps, it could be argued, the female emission that comes to the womb from the outside and is deposited in front of the womb by the *kaulos* is not *sperma* but the vaginal lubricant. The fact that the vagina can become moist during intercourse is recognized in the Hippocratic treatise *Genit.* 4 (VII.474.16–18), but the author attributes this to the womb opening more widely than usual during intercourse and allowing some of the woman's *sperma* to escape. He does not see it as a separate fluid in its own right.[60]

Aristotle refers to the vaginal lubricant at *GA* I.20, 727b3–728a2, where he says:

ὃ δ᾽ οἴονταί τινες σπέρμα συμβάλλεσθαι ἐν τῇ συνουσίᾳ τὸ θῆλυ διὰ τὸ γίνεσθαι παραπλησίαν τε χαρὰν ἐνίοτε αὐταῖς τῇ τῶν ἀρρένων καὶ ἅμα ὑγρὰν ἀπόκρισιν, οὐκ ἔστιν ἡ ὑγρασία αὕτη σπερματικὴ ἀλλὰ τοῦ τόπου ἴδιοις. ἔστι γὰρ τῶν ὑστερῶν ἔκκρισις, καὶ ταῖς μὲν γίγνεται ταῖς δ᾽ οὔ.[61]

---

[60] On the vaginal lubricant, see Dean-Jones 1994, 153–60.
[61] There seems to be something wrong with the Greek here. For ἴδιοις the mss. read ἴδιος ἑκάσταις, "peculiar to the part from which it comes in each individual." It is unclear why the phrase should be modified by a reference

INTRODUCTION

Some think that the female contributes *sperma* during intercourse because sometimes they feel pleasure akin to that of the male and at the same time produce a liquid secretion. This liquid is not seminal but a local sweating. For there is a discharge from the uterus, and it happens in some women but not in others.

At *GA* II.4, 739a20–6, he offers evidence to support his contention that the female secretion during sexual arousal is not seminal:

ὅτι δ' ἡ γιγνομένη ὑγρότης μετὰ τῆς ἡδονῆς τοῖς θήλεσιν οὐδὲν συμβάλλεται εἰς τὸ κύημα εἴρηται πρότερον. μάλιστα δ' ἂν δόξειεν ὅτι καθάπερ τοῖς ἄρρεσι γίγνεται καὶ ταῖς γυναιξὶ νύκτωρ ὃ καλοῦσιν ἐξονειρώττειν. ἀλλὰ τοῦτο σημεῖον οὐθέν· γίγνεται γὰρ καὶ τοῖς νέοις τῶν ἀρρένων τοῖς μέλλουσι μὲν μηθὲν δὲ προϊεμένοις ἢ τοῖς ἔτι προϊεμένοις ἄγονον.

That the fluid which comes with sexual excitement in females contributes nothing to the fetation was stated previously. This might certainly seem to be the case because so-called wet-dreams occur in women at night just as in men; but this signifies nothing, because it happens also in young men who almost emit but end up emitting nothing, and also with those who are still emitting infertile semen.

The fact that this argument does not offer the strongest support to his position is irrelevant for the purposes of this discussion. The passages show that Aristotle believed women could produce a vaginal lubricant when sexually aroused in dreams, but he did not identify this with *sperma*. This is in direct contradiction to *Non Gen.* 634b35–8 (quoted in full above on pp. 27–8), in

to individual women. Aristotle cannot mean the discharge originates in a different place in each woman because he goes on to say it comes from the uterus. For the adjective ἴδιος we might also expect a feminine form to agree with ἡ ὑγρασία αὕτη, though it can be a two-termination adjective. For ἴδιος I read ἴδισις, an unusual word for sweat found only in the Pseudo-Aristotelian *Prob.*, XXXV.4, 965a2 and XXXVIII.3, 966b39, which would parallel the phrase used to refer to the vaginal lubricant at *Non Gen.* 635b19, ἴδρωμα τοῦ τόπου (see below p. 33). The word ἑκάσταις would have been added to explain the referent of the corruption ἴδιος.

which the female fluid produced at climax in erotic dreams is
clearly *sperma*:

εἰς τὸ πρόσθεν παντελῶς ἐχούσης γίγνεται καὶ αὐταῖς καὶ τοῖς
ἀνδράσιν ἡ πρόεσις τοῦ σπέρματος.

The emission of the *sperma* both by them and by men is in front
of the womb if this is properly positioned.

The topic of erotic dreams arises three further times in the
rest of *Non Gen.* at 635a33–b2, 635b32–636a6, and 636b24. The
context of each passage confirms the identification of the fluid
which appears in a woman's vagina after orgasm with *sperma*.[62]

Non Gen. does recognize the vaginal lubricant, but introduces
it later in the treatise as if it had not been previously discussed,
and distinguishes it from *sperma*.[63] At 635b17–31 the author discusses a fluid which the woman produces during coition which
is not seminal, which can in fact even impede conception,
though a certain amount is necessary. It is produced <u>during</u>
intercourse (μεταξὺ, 17) in anticipation, just as saliva is produced at the anticipation of food (πρὸς τὴν φορὰν τῶν σιτίων,
20), not at the culmination (τελέως) of coition as *sperma* is. Nor
can this material be identified with the *ekptôsis* which comes to
the womb from the outside via the *kaulos*. At 635b19 the author
of *Non Gen.* describes the fluid produced during coition as "a
local secretion" (ἵδρωμα τοῦ τόπου), and the analogy to saliva
produced in the mouth clearly precludes its being brought in
elsewhere by a *kaulos*. The analogy with saliva and the mouth is
continued when the author says that when women produce this
fluid they need attention "just as the mouth does from spittle,"

---

[62] See notes ad locc.

[63] Föllinger 1996, p. 150 identifies this fluid with the *sperma* of *HA* X. As
evidence that the treatise is not by Aristotle she says that although the
author is not explicit about the nature of female seed "doch wird an
einer Stelle eine Feuchtigkeit unterschieden, die beim Geschlechtsverkehr
auftrete und eine Art von ἵδρωμα τοῦ τόπου darstelle." The distinction
she sees is with menstrual fluid. She notes that Aristotle recognizes the
existence of such a fluid but simply identifies it as "Vaginalsekret."

ὥσπερ καὶ τὸ στόμα πτύσεως (635b28). πτύσις (*ptusis*) is saliva that has been spat from the mouth; the implication clearly is that the *stoma* of the uterus has ejected the lubricant which is secreted during intercourse.

While *Non Gen.* believes this moistening, although not seminal itself, is a necessary sign for successful conception (ὑγραίνεσθαι in 635b17 is still dependent on δεῖ in 635a33), at *GA* I.19, 727b8–10, Aristotle uses the fact that women often conceive although they have not enjoyed intercourse as evidence that they do not produce seed like a man. On the other hand, at *GA* II.4, 739a26–36, Aristotle states that a female generally feels pleasure before conceiving because in order to conceive her womb has to be open and this allows the emission of a secretion "which is usually accompanied by pleasure in both men and women," μεθ᾽ ἧς εἴωθε γίγνεσθαι καὶ τοῖς ἄρρεσιν ἡ ἡδονὴ καὶ ταῖς γυναιξίν. So, although both authors agree that the vaginal lubricant is a topical secretion and is not seminal, *Non Gen.* considers it a necessary concomitant of conception and Aristotle does not, though it can act as an indicator that conception is more likely.[64]

Balme recognizes that the author of *Non Gen.* makes the distinction between *sperma* and the vaginal lubricant, but he does not recognize that in *Non Gen. sperma* is also different from the menses. He says:

> In *HA* X Arist. does not further identify the female emission [Balme is referring to *sperma* here], though he distinguishes it from a moisture which develops during coition like a "local sweating"... In *GA* however he says generally that the moisture secreted in coition is local only and is not seed...; instead he identifies the female seed with the menses, which he says must be present if a fetus is to develop... The *GA* theory therefore does not radically contradict the *HA* X theory, but refines it.[65]

---

[64] Though at *HA* IX(VII).3, 583a23, Aristotle notes that some women apply oil to the lips of the μήτρα (here probably the cervix) to encourage the male seed to slip out and prevent conception.

[65] Balme 1991, p. 489.

But we have seen that the author of *Non Gen.* does differentiate female *sperma* from menses. The fact that he clearly differentiates it also from the vaginal lubricant means that he believes a woman produces three different fluids in the area of the uterus. It is true that as it stands in D[a] the sentence at 635b28–31 makes it sound as if the woman's only contribution to conception is the vaginal lubricant:

ἀλλ' ἐνίαις τοσαύτη ὑγασία γίνεται ὥστε μὴ δύνασθαι καθαρὸν τὸ τοῦ ἀνδρὸς ἀνασπάσαι διὰ τὴν σύμμιξιν τῆς γιγνομένης ἀπὸ τῆς γυναικὸς ὑγρότητος.

But some women produce so much moisture [referring to the vaginal lubricant] that they are unable to draw up the *sperma* of the man unalloyed on account of the intermingling of the secretion which comes from the woman.

But the entire purport of the rest of the treatise is that the male semen must <u>not</u> be drawn into the womb καθαρόν. It has to be mixed with the female *sperma* outside the womb, so this statement would be problematic however female *sperma* is to be identified. I suspect that after τὸ τοῦ ἀνδρός we should insert καὶ τὸ τῆς γυναικός, which in the context of this passage could easily have been omitted by a copyist who did not fully understand the argument, i.e., that the mixture of male and female *spermata* had to be drawn into the womb without the further admixture of the female lubricant during coition.[66] Whatever it is that the author considers to be female *sperma*, it has to be mixed with the male contribution outside the womb before being drawn in to make a woman pregnant. For the same reason it is clear that at 634b29, 636a12, and 636b16 the singular term τὸ σπέρμα signifies the mixture of male and female *sperma*.

Aristotle may have the specific argument of *Non Gen.* in mind when he asserts that no animal can produce two seminal

---

[66] Unless *Non Gen.*'s author was himself guilty of a careless expression, it is unlikely Aristotle perpetrated this mistake as the *Dialectic* makes it clear that he understands *Non Gen.*'s argument.

residues. He has other arguments against identifying the vaginal lubricant with *sperma*: not all women produce it, it is not necessary for conception, it is a local secretion. This is sufficient argument to counter the identification of the moisture women produce in their vaginas during intercourse, described in *Genit.* 4, as female *gonê*. The assertion that a woman simply cannot have two seminal secretions is only necessary to counter an argument that in addition to menses and this local secretion there exists a fluid produced systemically in coition by all women who become pregnant. *Non Gen.* is the only ancient source that clearly distinguishes female seed from menses <u>and</u> the vaginal lubricant.

(f) Fertility of *sperma* in *Non Gen.*

The timely production of both male and female *sperma* during intercourse is essential to *Non Gen.*'s theory of conception, but beyond this the author does not pay much attention to the fact that the *sperma* itself may be non-fertile, and the acknowledgement that this may be the case is made primarily in the case of the male. Only after four chapters dealing with possible causes of female infertility does the author raise the possibility that the infertility may lie on the male side, and then this is acknowledged in one short phrase:

> ὅσαις δὲ τούτων μηδὲν ἐμπόδιον ᾖ ἀλλ' ἔχουσιν ὃν τρόπον δεῖν εἴρηται ἔχειν, <u>ἂν μὴ ὁ ἀνὴρ αἴτιος ᾖ τῆς ἀτεκνίας</u> ἢ ἀμφότεροι μὲν δύνωνται τεκνοῦσθαι πρὸς ἀλλήλους δὲ μὴ ὦσι σύμμετροι τῷ ἅμα προΐεσθαι ἀλλὰ πολὺ διαφωνῶσιν, ἔσονται τέκνα τούτοις.

> But in the case of women for whom none of these impediments is present but who have the condition we have said they ought to have, <u>if it is not the case that the man is a cause of the infertility</u> or that both are capable of engendering children but are not matched with each other in emitting at the same time but are very discordant, they will have children.[67]

---

[67] 636b6–10.

Non Gen. believed there was a very simple test for male infertility:

τῷ μὲν οὖν εἰδέναι <εἰ> τὰ τοῦ ἀνδρὸς αἴτια ἔστι μὲν καὶ ἄλλα σημεῖα λαβεῖν, ἃ δὲ ῥᾴω μάλιστα <ἂν> φαίνοιτο, πρὸς ἄλλας πλησιάζων καὶ γεννῶν.

And while it is indeed possible to take other signs in ascertaining if the causes lie on the husband's side, it would certainly be apparent more easily if he has intercourse and conceives with other women.[68]

This test assumes that the man is capable of erection and ejaculation—otherwise the source of a couple's infertility would be quite obvious—and so implies that his seed could be infertile. Aristotle mentions a simple test for the fertility of male semen at *GA* II.7, 747a4–23:

εὐλόγως βασανίζεται ταῖς πείραις τό γε τῶν ἀνδρῶν, εἰ ἄγονον, ἐν τῷ ὕδατι· ταχὺ γὰρ διαχεῖται τὸ λεπτὸν καὶ ψυχρὸν ἐπιπολῆς, τὸ δὲ γόνιμον εἰς βυθὸν χωρεῖ· θερμὸν μὲν γὰρ τὸ πεπεμμένον ἐστί, πέπεπται δὲ τὸ συνεστηκὸς καὶ πάχος ἔχον.

It makes good sense to test if the <*sperma*> of men is infertile by examination in water, for the thin and cold *sperma* quickly spreads out on the top of the water, but generative *sperma* sinks to the bottom, because the material which has been concocted is hot, and that which has been condensed and has weight has been concocted.[69]

This test and others like it would be among the ἄλλα σημεῖα referred to at 636b11, many of which would surely, like this, be easier than having the man have sex with different women to see what happened.[70] However, *Non Gen.* is not advocating such

---

[68] 636b10–13.

[69] It is significant here that the male seminal emission is referred to in the neuter, τὸ τοῦ ἀνδρῶν, rather than the feminine ἡ γονή when its fertility is in question.

[70] Flemming 2013, p. 571, n. 23, notes that all reference to male infertility in ancient Greek medical texts either discusses its causation or is diagnostic. There are no suggested therapies. The ancient evidence suggests that men preferred to seek magical remedies for sexual dysfunctions, whether or not

an empirical approach, which would require knowing that the woman was fertile to avoid an infinite regress. A man could most easily be eliminated as the source of a couple's infertility if he has had children by other women (previous wives, slaves, hetairai, prostitutes, all of whom were possible sexual partners for an ancient Greek male), though failing to have such children would not show that he was, in fact, infertile. Having children by different partners is physically possible for women too, but concern over a particular couple's infertility would only arise when the production of legitimate children was at issue, and while it was physically and socially acceptable for a man to have children outside of marriage, unless a woman had given birth to children from a previous marriage this test of her fertility would not be available.[71]

But for both a man and a woman this test fails to address the issue that *sperma* might be fertile at one time but not at another. If Aristotle was not summarizing the entirety of *Non Gen.*, it is possible that the author discussed infertile seed in a later part of the work, where anything he had to say on the lack of potency of seed when ejaculated simultaneously with that of the sexual partner could apply equally to the *spermata* of men and women. If Aristotle's primary interest in *Non Gen.* was the *aporia* of whether women provided generative *sperma* equivalent to male *sperma*, and he was already predisposed to think this was not the case, he may not have bothered summarizing ways to test the fertility of a fluid he considered to be non-existent. On the other hand, even within the wide scope of the Hippocratic Corpus very little is said about male infertility, and when it is touched upon it focuses more on lack of ejaculate or

---

this was driven by a desire for reproduction; see McMahon 1998, Faraone 1999, and Berrey 2014 for why this may have been so.

[71] *Genit.* 7 (VII.478.480–6) refers to women who have borne children of different sexes to different men to demonstrate that both parents provide seed of both sexes. If he is discussing legitimate children here, the women must have remarried after being divorced or widowed.

erectile dysfunction than the possibility of ejaculated but sterile semen (*Genit.* 2 (VII.472.5–16), though n.b. l.13, *Aër.* 21 and 22 (II.74.18–76.2 and 76.12–82.5), *Aph.* V.63 (IV.556.3–7), *Epid.* VII.122 (V.466.23–4), *Prorrh.* II.41 (IX.70.12)). The experience of a largely agricultural culture that seed bears fruit if it meets with the right environment may be part of the reason why women are basically the sole focus of ancient medical concern with infertility.[72]

For the Hippocratics as for Aristotle, the potency of male and female seminal contributions depends primarily on the ratio of heat or coldness they bring relative to the other's contribution.[73] In the classical period the only physician to refer to the possibility of infertile female *sperma* is Diocles, who is recorded by Pseudo-Plutarch as having listed as a possible cause for the failure of a woman who was having regular intercourse to get pregnant that she might have seed "of such a kind that that which brings life is not present in it," τὸ τοιοῦτον ἐν ᾧ τὸ ζωοποιητικὸν οὐκ ἔστιν; he also noted that male seed can be infertile, ἄγονον.[74] Even if it is a clinical text on infertility, it would not be unusual for *Non Gen.* to have hardly anything to say about problems on the male side and nothing at all to say about the fertility of male or female *sperma*.

3 ARISTOTLE'S ENGAGEMENT WITH *NON GEN.* BY *ENDOXON*, *TOPOS*, AND DIALECTIC

(a) Passage following the end of *Non Gen.*

Female *sperma* in *Non Gen.* is then a seminal secretion distinct from the menses. Since this is in conflict with the fundamental principle of Aristotle's theory of reproduction that no animal

---

[72] For the almost exclusive focus of the Hippocratic Corpus on women as the locus of a couple's infertility, see Flemming 2013.

[73] See notes to 636b13.

[74] Diocles fragg. 42b and 43b, van der Eijk 2000, pp. 86–9.

produces two seminal secretions, there is no reason to try to make any other theory expounded in *Non Gen.* conform to those in Aristotle's biological works if it clearly does not, which is not to deny that there may be points of similarity. The dissonance of *Non Gen.* with the rest of Aristotle's reproductive theory might not preclude its being part of Aristotle's juvenalia which for some reason was incorporated into the corpus completely unrevised, but it is far more likely that the author was someone other than Aristotle. Its inclusion in the Aristotelian Corpus is explained by the final two chapters of *HA* X.

But before we get to Chapter 6, immediately following the passage describing the female pudenda and the *kaulos* by which a woman emits *sperma* into the area before her uterus, Bekker's Chapter 5 concludes with a passage the first part of which is one of the most opaque passages in the Aristotelian Corpus. In Balme's text this reads:

ὅ τι συμβάλλεται εἰς τοῦτο ποιεῖ τῶν αὐτῶν παθημάτων ὅτι καὶ ἡ γυνὴ γόνιμον προΐεται. τὰ δ' αὐτὰ αἴτια ταῦτα συμβαίνει. καὶ γὰρ οἷς ἢ νόσου ἢ θανάτου δοκεῖ ἑτέρου τὸ αἴτιον εἶναι, θεωροῦσι τὸ τελευταῖον ἐπὶ τὰς ἀρχάς, ὃ δεῖ ὁρᾶν. τοῖς μὲν γὰρ ταὐτὰ αἴτια τὰ πρῶτα, τοῖς δὲ οὐδέν, τῶν δὲ τὰ μὲν τὰ δ' οὔ. ἀποδίδωσιν οὖν κατὰ λόγον καὶ τὰ ἀποβαίνοντα· καὶ τοῖς μὲν διὰ πάντων συμβαίνει διελθεῖν τῶν αὐτῶν παθημάτων, τοῖς δὲ διὰ πολλῶν οἷς πολλά· τοῖς δὲ δι' ὀλίγων· τοῖς δὲ δι' οὐθενὸς ὅσοις μηδέν.[75]

Balme translates this as follows:

The woman's contribution brings about the same affections to the extent that she too emits a fertile seed. And they are accompanied by these same causes. For those too who believe that an illness or death is due to another thing's cause, examine the final effect back to its beginnings, which is what they need to see. For some things have the same causes in the first place, others do not, and yet others have some that are and some that are not. The effects that they produce, therefore, are also in proportion: in the first case the result is that they go through all the

---

[75] 637a37–b7.

same affections; others, for whom many causes are the same, go through many of the same affections; others go through few; and others, for whom none are the same, go through none.

Balme appends an explanation of the translation arguing that what is being compared here is the conditions that different women undergo after the emission of fertile seed which have been described in the previous five chapters. But not all these conditions have been caused by the emission of fertile seed. Moreover, the first sentence as Balme translates it implies that the woman experiences the same affections as somebody else who is not a woman, "she too," καὶ ἡ γυνή. Balme acknowledges the obscurity of the passage when he remarks after his explanation, "Other edd. have given different interpretations of 637a35–b6, some holding that it is displaced."[76]

The opacity of the passage is explained by the fact that it is at this point that the summary of the medical treatise *Non Gen.* ends and Aristotle begins dealing with it as an *endoxon*.

(b) *Endoxa* in Aristotle

As a general principle, Aristotle stipulated that if observation and demonstrable facts (*phainomena*) seemed to militate against a commonly held belief or the theory of a reputable authority (*endoxon*), a philosopher should not dismiss the *endoxon* out of hand but do the best he could to reconcile *endoxon* and *phainomena*. At *EN* VII.1.5, 1145b2–7, he states the procedure thus:

δεῖ δ', ὥσπερ ἐπὶ τῶν ἄλλων, τιθέντας τὰ φαινόμενα καὶ πρῶτον διαπορήσαντας οὕτω δεικνύναι μάλιστα μὲν πάντα τὰ ἔνδοξα περὶ ταῦτα τὰ πάθη, εἰ δὲ μή, τὰ πλεῖστα καὶ κυριώτατα· ἐὰν γὰρ λύηταί τε τὰ δυσχερῆ καὶ καταλείπηται τὰ ἔνδοξα, δεδειγμένον ἂν εἴη ἱκανῶς.

We must, as in all other cases, set the *phainomena* before us and, after first discussing the difficulties [ἀπορίαι, *aporiai*], go

---

[76] Balme 1991, p. 521.

on to prove, if possible, the truth of all the *endoxa* about these affections or, failing this, of the greater number and the most authoritative; for if we both resolve the difficulties and leave the *endoxa* undisturbed, we shall have proved the case sufficiently.[77]

It is generally agreed that the ensuing discussion of what constitutes pleasure in *EN* VII.2 is the best example of διαπορεῖν (*diaporein*, "puzzling through") authoritative opinions in the light of empirical observation in the Aristotelian Corpus, but how much of the method we can see in the rest of the corpus is a bone of contention. Irwin believes it undergirds all the first principles in Aristotle. Frede believes the procedure as displayed in *EN* VII.2 is the exception rather than the rule. Other scholars fall somewhere between these two poles.[78]

I am arguing that *HA* X was written at a preliminary stage in Aristotle's examination of animal reproduction, when he was still really "puzzling through" the premise that female *sperma* played exactly the same role as male *sperma* in conception. At this stage he does not have his arguments marshaled against this premise as he has when he comes to write the *GA*. Frede argues that the *endoxic* method is most appropriate in the preliminary stage of development of Aristotle's views when he first inspected general assumptions that seem to present *aporiai* when compared with observable data. She states:

> Aristotle may have employed the method for himself whenever he encountered problems of comparable complexity… But, as a matter of fact, in his texts as far as we have them, most of the time he prefers to present his own well-worked out points of view without a detour via a list of "reputable views" and the problems involved in them.[79]

---

[77] Similarly, at *GA* III.10, 760b31–3, Aristotle says that observation (*aisthêsis*) should be trusted more than theories (*logoi*), but as long as *logoi* do not contradict the evidence of the senses they too should be accepted.

[78] See Owen 1961, Irwin 1988, Barnes 1980, Nussbaum 1982, Wians 1992, Smith 1999, Frede 2012.

[79] Frede 2012, p. 212.

Frede notes that the works in which the term *endoxon* occurs most frequently are the dialectical works *Topics* and *On Sophistical Refutations*, where it is used to characterize premises that are suitable for dialectical argument because they hold "a middle position between those [premises] that are obviously true and those that are obviously false."[80] It is obviously true that females have a role to play in reproduction; it is obviously false that every act of intercourse leads to conception. Premises about what the female contribution to conception is (including those positing female *sperma*) hold a middle position. *HA* X may be the only example we have of Aristotle initially coming to grips with an unattested *endoxon*, but it does conform to the method he recommends.[81]

(c) Dialectic and *topoi*

The dialectical argument of classical Greece has a very precise format: it is an interchange between two individuals in which one, the Answerer, defends a premise while the other, the Questioner, tries to lead the Answerer to a conclusion which contradicts the premise he is defending.[82] In the classical

---

[80] Frede 2012, pp. 193–4.

[81] It is also possible that there are dialectical examinations of *endoxa* in Aristotle's works that have gone unrecognized and been mistaken for his own "unrevised" views because they were not explicitly flagged as *endoxa*. Caleb Cohoe (2017) has argued that *De An.* I.4, 408b18–31, is "a dialectical examination of a reputable Platonist position about the intellect." Although the view being examined (that the intellect is separable, operates via a bodily organ, and is indestructible) contradicts what Aristotle says elsewhere about the intellect, it has not previously been recognized as an *endoxon* because Aristotle does not explicitly identify it as such. He puts forward implications of the Platonist view as positive assertions without qualification, but Cohoe argues convincingly that Aristotle would not share these views and only asserts them to engage with them in dialectic. Given the difficulty of inserting new material into a book in the form of a papyrus roll, this theory has an advantage over that supposing that earlier and later theories of Aristotle can appear cheek by jowl.

[82] This is a very adumbrated explanation of dialectic. For a fuller discussion of all the possible permutations, see Bolton 1990, Smith 1999, and Rubinelli 2009.

period dialectical competitions with judges, winners, and losers were held in Athens. Training for these competitions generally involved learning by heart set speeches on various themes that, presumably, were thought to be adaptable for other subjects. In the *Topics*, by contrast, Aristotle formalized the method of dialectical argument in such a way that the student learned the shapes and processes of valid refutations of any type of premise, schemata (*topoi*) which acted as "abstract place-holder(s) for arguments into which content of any sort [could] be inserted."[83] These schemata, *topoi*, of argument could be used in actual competition,[84] or, more commonly, as exercises for students intending to examine logical, ethical, or scientific premises to help them to see the weak points in the arguments of others and to avoid falling into self-contradiction themselves. Aristotle's method requires that the Questioner know in advance the conclusion to which he wants to lead the Answerer, but that he should conceal this conclusion as long as possible, getting the Answerer to concede intermediary premises that should lull him into a false sense of security. The intermediate premises, in Aristotle's terminology, should not be "too close" to the conclusion needed to refute the premise so that the Answerer cannot see where the argument is leading. A great part of the skill of a dialectician is selecting the intermediate premises that will be acceptable to the Answerer yet lead to a conclusion that will contradict his original premise. The defense of the premise, on the Answerer's side, and its refutation, on the Questioner's, are the ἀρχαί (*archai*, origins) of the dialectic. The selection of the target conclusion and the premises intermediate between the original premise and its refutation is facilitated by following the schema of an

---

[83] Levene 2009, p. xviii. Rubinelli 2009, p. 13, describes it as "an argumentative matrix."

[84] In which case Aristotle himself notes some less than valid moves that can be made to increase the chance of victory, though in the main he reserves discussion of these sorts of argument to *On Sophistical Refutations*.

appropriate *topos*. A *topos* has two main parts: an "instruction," usually introduced by a deontic expression, which suggests how to hit upon a premise which can be used to refute the Answerer's premise, and a "law," introduced by γάρ (*gar*, "for") or a similar expression, which "guarantees the reliability of the operations suggested by the instruction."[85]

Any premise that is worthy of dialectic has to be maintained by the majority of people, or the wise, or a majority of the wise, or a professional source. In justifying δόξαι κατὰ τέχνας (*doxai kata technas*, "opinions arising from skills") as sources of premises Aristotle asserts:

θείη γὰρ ἄν τις τὰ δοκοῦντα τοῖς ὑπὲρ τούτων ἐπεσκεμμένοις, οἷον περὶ μὲν τῶν ἐν ἰατρικῇ ὡς ὁ ἰατρός.

A layperson would accept the opinions of those who have examined the subject in question, e.g, on questions of medicine they would hold the same opinions as the doctor. (*Topics* I.10, 104a34–6)

Shortly after this, at *Topics* I.14, 105b12–16, Aristotle explicitly recommends collecting premises for dialectic from written texts. We should expect, then, that medical texts would prove a fertile hunting ground for premises for dialectic.

In competition or pedagogical exercise the sole aim is to successfully defend or refute a premise, regardless of one's own opinions on the matter at hand, but Aristotle also acknowledges *topoi* as useful for scientific investigation—philosophical dialectic—when the aim is to discover the truth or falsity of a premise (*Topics* I.2, 101a34–6). In this case, he says, it is unclear what the role of the Answerer should be:

ἐν δὲ ταῖς διαλεκτικαῖς συνόδοις τοῖς μὴ ἀγῶνος χάριν ἀλλὰ πείρας καὶ σκέψεως τοὺς λόγους ποιουμένοις οὐ διήρθρωταί πω τίνος δεῖ στοχάζεσθαι τὸν ἀποκρινόμενον καὶ ποῖα διδόναι καὶ ποῖα μή, πρὸς τὸ καλῶς ἢ μὴ καλῶς φυλάττειν τὴν θέσιν

---

[85] Rubinelli 2009, p. 14.

But in dialectical collaborations between those who engage in arguments not for the sake of competition, but for testing and inquiry, it has never been articulated what the Answerer must aim at or what type of answers he should and should not give, with a view to defending his premise in a good way or a bad way. (*Topics* VIII.4, 159a32–6)

Aristotle then proceeds to delineate how an Answerer should answer in these circumstances. As in the other forms of dialectic, he should still try to answer in the persona of the individual who first put forward the premise, whether he himself agrees with it or not, but he must not accept any premise that is "unacceptable without qualification," ἁπλῶς ἄδοξον, nor reject a premise that is "acceptable without qualification," ἔνδοξος ἁπλῶς (*Topics* VIII.5, 159a39–b36). If this is to be differentiated from the behavior of the Answerer in the other forms of dialectic it would seem that it requires the Answerer to try to the best of his ability to answer according to the world view of the individual who first posited the premise, but to be readier to concede when that world view cannot withstand the contradictions being drawn from accepted premises. Similarly, in pursuit of the truth the Questioner would have to be readier to concede if the *topos* was unable to produce the refutation of the premise.[86] In this scenario there seems to be less need to conceal the course of the argument, so the intermediate premises will be fewer and more pointed. It is closer to the procedure for the examination of *endoxa* in light of *phainomena* proposed at *EN* VII.1.5, 1145b1–7, though still framed more as an attempt to refute than to reconcile because the method begins by examining the *aporiai* of authoritative opinions. It is only after these have been "puzzled through" that a reconciliation can be attempted.

---

[86] This would not, of course, entail the truth of the premise; it may simply indicate a poorly chosen *topos*.

Devious intermediate premises are clearly not needed at all if the Answerer and the Questioner are the same person.[87] *Topics* VIII.1, 155b10–16, says:

τῷ δὲ φιλοσόφῳ καὶ ζητοῦντι καθ᾽ ἑαυτὸν οὐδὲν μέλει, ἐὰν ἀληθῆ μὲν ᾖ καὶ γνώριμα δι᾽ ὧν ὁ συλλογισμός, μὴ θῇ δ᾽ αὐτὰ ὁ ἀποκρινόμενος διὰ τὸ σύνεγγυς εἶναι τοῦ ἐξ ἀρχῆς καὶ προορᾶν τὸ συμβησόμενον, ἀλλ᾽ ἴσως κἂν σπουδάσειεν ὅτι μάλιστα γνώριμα καὶ σύνεγγυς εἶναι τὰ ἀξιώματα· ἐκ τούτων γὰρ οἱ ἐπιστημονικοὶ συλλογισμοί.

To the philosopher searching by himself it is of no account if <the premises> from which the deduction proceeds are true and intelligible but the Answerer does not concede them because of their being close to the *archê* <of the Questioner, i.e. the refutation of the Answerer's premise> and he sees the result <of conceding>. Instead the philosopher would probably be quite anxious that the premises be as intelligible and close to the *archê* as possible, for scientific deductions derive from these.

Clearly solitary, philosophical dialectic has this important difference from the competitive and pedagogical variety, but it is still a form of dialectic. The philosopher does not have to lull the suspicions of an actual interlocutor, but he must still try to produce the refutation of an authority's premise by means of intermediary premises to which the authority would have to concede.[88] As Bolton states, when involved in solo dialectic, Aristotle "is alone responsible for the proper presentation of the opponent's position, with whatever resources for defense the latter may involve."[89]

---

[87] "A skilled practitioner could dispense with the need for a partner and explore the consequences of a set of views alone," Smith 1997, p. xv.

[88] Robin Smith says of the *Topics* that although it, "disavows any pretensions to scientific precision, there are strong echoes of its procedures in Aristotle's own scientific works," Smith 1999, p. xi.

[89] Bolton 1990, p. 199.

My argument requires the further step of assuming that this solitary dialectic could take written form, much as a modern scholar or student might take notes on a text, including their adumbrated objections to it, in preparation for a later, more polished argument. The strongest evidence that this is in fact what occurred is the format of *HA* X itself, but also, in the same passage where he discusses collecting premises from written works, Aristotle outlines some written preparations the dialectician should make for later argument, written or oral. He says a dialectician should "make diagrams[90] about each kind of thing, putting them down separately" τὰς δὲ διαγραφὰς ποιεῖσθαι περὶ ἑκάστου γένους, ὑποτιθέντας χωρίς, and also that he should "note down (Pickard-Cambridge "put them down," Smith "make marginal notes") the opinions of each <authority>, for example, that Empedocles said that the elements of bodies were four" παρασημαίνεσθαι δὲ καὶ τὰς ἑκάστων δόξας, οἷον ὅτι Ἐμπεδοκλῆς τέτταρα ἔφησε τῶν σωμάτων στοιχεῖα εἶναι. Admittedly, this is not describing the preliminary working through of an objection to a premise in writing, but it does show that Aristotle expected philosophers to use writing in the early stages of their study of a topic, and it may be the former practice to which he is alluding at *Top.* II.2, 110a10–11, with the use of the reflexive pronoun: Ἔτι τὸ πρόβλημα πρότασιν ἑαυτῷ ποιούμενον ἐνίστασθαι· ἡ γὰρ ἔνστασις ἔσται ἐπιχείρημα πρὸς τὴν θέσιν, "And then, making the problem into a proposition for himself, a man should form an objection to it: for the objection will be an attack upon the premise."[91]

---

[90] διαγραφή is a term Aristotle used to refer to diagrams in his anatomical works (e.g., *HA* I.17, 497a32, IV.1, 525a9) but could also refer to tables such as that at *EE* II.2, 1220b37–1221a14, which is called a διαγραφή at 1228a28.

[91] That preliminary notes were made with the intention that they would be used in a more polished version for publication in some way has been argued particularly in the case of Thucydides. Prentice 1930 argued that much of the *Histories* is formed from notes which Thucydides had written down on

(d) The *topos* following the *endoxon*

Keeping all this in mind, I read the passage at the end of *Non Gen.* 5 as a premise drawn from the *endoxon* of *Non Gen.*, that women provide generative seed equivalent to male semen,[92] followed by the *archê* of the refutation, that uterine mole is a disease, not the beginning of life, and the *topos*, that the same causes should give the same results. I translate:

> Whatever is contributed to this (i.e., the mixture of fluids in the area before the uterus), he (i.e., the author[93]) makes the cause[94] of the same experiences (i.e., excitement and lassitude) <in women as in men> because <he believes> that the woman too is emitting a generative fluid. And it follows that these things (i.e., male and female seminal emissions) are the same causes <in reproduction>. And, in fact, those to whom it (i.e., female *sperma*) also seems to be the cause of something else, either disease or death, are not[95] examining the conclusion with a view to their initial premises, which they ought to keep in view. Because for some experiences all[96] the causes are the same, in others none, and of others some causes are the same and others are not. And so they produce affections in proportion. In some con-

---

single sheets as "rough sketches" or "notes for future composition" which were put in order by a later editor. He states, "much in this book, as it has come down to us, must be regarded merely as tentative or experimental" p. 126. Dorandi 1991 denies that individual sheets were used, but argues that authors composed by excerpting notes they had written on continuous papyrus rolls.

[92] Balme 1985, p. 197, says: "The conclusion that the female contributes seed is clearly the purpose of the whole argument." It is indeed the reason Aristotle chose this text as an *endoxon*, but is an assumption behind the text, not a conclusion towards which either the author of *Non Gen.* or Aristotle is working.

[93] When referring to an opponent in a dialectical exchange, Aristotle often simply uses a third person singular verb for which the reader has to supply the subject; see Smith 1999, p. xxvii.

[94] Inserting τὸ αἴτιον before τῶν αὐτῶν παθημάτων; see commentary at 637a36.

[95] Accepting Barnes' insertion of οὐ, see commentary at 637a38.

[96] For πρῶτα read πάντα; see commentary at 637b2.

ditions they (i.e., sufferers of a condition) go through all the
same experiences, in those conditions which have many causes
the same they go through many of the same experiences, in
others they go through few, and in those conditions which
have no causes the same they go through none of the same
experiences.[97]

The passage opens with a formulation of the premise on which
Non Gen. is based—that a woman emits fertile *sperma* like a
man—and the empirical *phainomenon* that the author of *Non
Gen.* cited in support of the premise—that men and women
experience the same affections after orgasm. The opening of
the passage ("Whatever it is...") indicates that the status of the
fluid is the issue up for dialectical discussion. In the persona of
the Answerer, Aristotle then states the natural consequence of
the belief that the fluid the woman emits parallels male semen:
that the male and female orgasmic ejaculates play the same
role in generation. This is the premise that he will defend, as
Answerer, and attempt to refute, as Questioner. He then ellip-
tically refers to a *phainomenon* that supporters of the premise
adduce as evidence for their position: that the woman's ejaculate, unmingled with the man's, is the cause of something else
(this "something else" will prove to be uterine mole). This other
condition, though, is a disease or death, and it is here Aristotle
locates an *aporia* in their argument on the basis of which he
gives the instruction for the *topos*: examine this argument, that
female *sperma* is generative, *gonimon*, γόνιμον, like the male's, on
the basis of the premise that it is also a source of a diseased
or fatal affection. The reference to αἴτια (*aitia*, causes) in the
statement of the premise and the supporting *phainomenon* suggests that the instruction on how best to go about refuting the
premise is to show that the theory does not cohere with a basic

---

[97] Words in parentheses explicate the referents of pronouns, etc. Words in
angled brackets fill in ellipses in the Greek. See the commentary on this
passage for a detailed explanation of its grammatical structure.

law of cause and effect.[98] The role which Bolton believes *endoxa* and dialectic play in the *GA* is particularly relevant here.

> The role which the examination of pangenesis plays in Aristotle's discussion of sperma deserves close attention since this examination is entirely dialectical in character. Aristotle undertakes to show that the denial of this received doctrine "is more apparent" (722a1–2) than the doctrine itself. To do this he argues against the received doctrine solely by reference to other *endoxa*—either by appealing to obvious commonly accepted views to show that the arguments cited to support this doctrine are without force (as at 722a2ff.); or by showing that the doctrine has consequences which anybody will admit are "plainly impossible" or "absurd" (as at 722b6–30, 723b9ff.). Aristotle's arguments presume no technical information or theory. They rely on nothing which Aristotle could not expect to be much more widely accepted and, indeed, "more apparent" than the premise and assumptions on which the doctrine of pangenesis is based.[99]

That the fundamental law of cause and effect is the basis of the instruction in 637a37–b1 is confirmed by the statement of the law that will guarantee the valid refutation of the premise if the instruction is followed: the degree of similarity between any two conditions depends on the number of causes the two conditions have in common. This is a variant of a *topos* about cause and effect that is listed not in the *Topics* itself, but in *Rhet.* II.23.17, 1399b5–6: ἄλλος ἐκ τοῦ τὸ συμβαῖνον ἐὰν ᾖ ταὐτόν, ὅτι καὶ ἐξ ὧν συμβαίνει ταῦτά, "Another <*topos*>: <argue> from the fact that if the outcome is the same, those things from which

---

[98] Rubinelli 2009, p. 15, notes that not all *topoi* are fully articulated, but that what is missing is easily inferred. The tendency to be elliptical in a work directed at others is exacerbated to the point of sphinxicity when Aristotle is penning a "note to self." Bolton 1990, pp. 204–9, argues that to ensure success a counter-argument must proceed from a premise that is "more *endoxon*" than the premise under examination. This would be another way to characterize the *topos* here.

[99] Bolton 1987, pp. 154–5.

the outcome results are the same."[100] Aristotle acknowledges some similarity in the condition men and women experience after orgasm, but he does not think they are exactly the same because he does not think the fluids they emit at orgasm are equivalent. In the attempt to refute the identity of the causal status of a man's and a woman's ejaculate two *phainomena* will be canvassed in the ensuing argument: the similarity between the sexual response in females of different species and the similarity or lack of it between wind-eggs in birds and uterine mole in women.

The conclusion to which he is aiming, as Questioner, is that the condition of uterine mole in women is a diseased, sometimes fatal, condition which is not comparable to the normal physiological production of wind-eggs in birds. This means that in women there is no condition comparable to that of wind-eggs. If wind-eggs are caused by the fluid a hen emits when sexually excited and a woman does not exhibit the same affection after emitting at the culmination of an erotic dream and drawing the ejaculate into her uterus, this ejaculate cannot be the same *aition* in reproduction as the hen's emission in sexual excitement.[101] This is sufficient, on the basis of the Answerer's premises, to refute the contention that the woman's ejaculate plays the same causal role in reproduction as the man's semen.

So, I argue that *HA* X is best understood as being composed of Aristotle's summary of a written medical treatise ὑπὲρ τοῦ μὴ γεννᾶν, *On Failure to Reproduce* (or an excerpt thereof) which he is using as an *endoxon* to provide the premise that a woman's ejaculate at orgasm is equivalent to male semen. Because of the way the argument unfolds in Chapters 6 and 7, I believe he is employing the method outlined in *Topics* to refute this premise, but is doing so at some time before he has fully formulated his

---

[100] The relation of this chapter to *Rhetoric* as a whole is contested.
[101] In his biological works Aristotle equates unfertilized eggs with a woman's menstrual fluid, e.g., *GA* II.3, 737a28–34, III.1, 750b11–16.

own theory on reproduction, and so is still at the stage of "puzzling through" the *aporiai* of the *endoxon*.

4 CHAPTERS 6 AND 7[102]

(a) Launching of *Dialectic* with animal exempla

In *Non Gen.* the author made use of examples from non-human animals in only one passage, that which used multiple births to illustrate the fact that the conception of a single child does not necessarily utilize all the seminal fluid produced from a man and a woman (636b39–637a15). This argument was needed to show why the failure of the uterus to draw in the man's and woman's emission in its entirety did not in and of itself signal infertility. Recourse to the animal exemplum was forced upon the author because multiple births are not frequent in humans, probably even less so in antiquity than today, and in antiquity superfetation—the conception of a second child when a woman is already pregnant from a previous act of intercourse—was considered to be a viable cause of twinning, the most common form of human multiple birth.[103] Litter-bearing animals were the simplest way to illustrate the point that there was more material in one emission of seed than was needed for the conception of a child and that therefore a woman did not have to draw in all the fluid emitted during intercourse to become pregnant. Were Chapter 6 simply a continuation of the treatise by the same author, then, the opening words, φανερὰ δὲ τὰ ζῷά ἐστιν ὅταν ὀχευθῆναι δέηται, "Female animals make it clear

---

[102] For a more detailed discussion of the language and stages of the argument in these chapters, see notes ad loc.

[103] *GA* IV.5, 773a33–774a17; *HA* IX(VII).4, 585a3–23. Elsewhere Aristotle associates superfetation with animals other than humans: *HA* V.9, 542b32; VI.11, 566a15; 33, 579b32. Hippocratic authors believed superfetation was possible but that it usually resulted in the death of at least one of the fetuses, e.g., *Superf.* 1 (VIII.476.1–12); *Epid.* V.11 (V.210.12–212.4); *Vict.* I.31 (VI.506.8–13). Superfetation is also common as a cause of mythological twins, e.g., Castor and Pollux, Heracles and Iphicles.

when they need mating," would be excessively abrupt. The discontinuity is explained when we read the words as the launching of the *Dialectic* that Aristotle has just outlined in a *topos*.

Because Aristotle is engaging in dialectic with himself he does not need to pose the intermediate premises in the form of questions to which he appends a yes or no in the persona of the Answerer. If he believes the Answerer would accept the premise without qualification, he can state it as accepted. The train of Aristotle's thought here has been missed because the *Dialectic* at the end of *HA* X displays all the shortcomings Keyt identifies in Aristotle's "informal argument."

> It is not always clear where in the text a particular argument begins or ends. Nor is it always clear what a particular argument is meant to establish. Important premises are presupposed. Those that are furnished are at crucial spots loosely expressed. The order of steps is often unclear.[104]

The first premise supposed to support the existence of *sperma* in women is that, like women, female animals feel sexual desire. The *phainomenon* used to support this is that hens, and other female animals, pursue males. It is reasonable to think that this is a premise that the author of *Non Gen.* would accept. (It is possible that in a competitive context an experienced dialectician, seeing the trajectory of the argument leading to the fact that women do not lay wind-eggs, might object that the premise was too close to the Questioner's *archê*, but this is not a concern in the philosophical use of dialectic.) Aristotle then states the law that the *topos* said was to be applied, making it specific for this premise:

> εἰ δὴ ταὐτὰ πάθη πᾶσι τοῖς ζῴοις φαίνεται ὄντα περὶ τὴν συνουσίαν, δῆλον ὅτι καὶ ταὐτὰ τὰ αἴτια συνβαίνοντα.

> So, if the same affections are apparent in all animals in respect to intercourse it is clear that the same causes are indeed occurring. (637b9–11)

---

[104] Keyt 2017, p. 123.

Again, it can be assumed that the author of *Non Gen.* would readily concede this.

(b) Wind-eggs

The next premise is that the desire for intercourse in birds is caused by a desire to emit, not just to receive. As supporting *phainomena* Aristotle first adduces the case of hens that lay eggs even when they have not mated with a cock. These eggs are called ὑπηνέμια, wind-eggs. Wind-eggs were of particular interest to Aristotle in establishing the differences in the male and female contributions to conception, and he referred to them often in his biological works, e.g., *HA* V.1, 539a30–b2, VI.2, 559b20–560a20, *GA* I.21, 730a5–8, II.3, 737a30–3, II.5, 741a15–32, III.1, 750b3–751a25, III.7, 757b1–30. Aristotle argues that the fact that wind-eggs do not develop into animals but can go bad demonstrates that the female can only pass on nutritive soul to her seminal residue and that the sentient soul of a living being has to be provided by the male. In an extended discussion of wind-eggs at *GA* III.1, 750b3–751a24, Aristotle explains that the avian equivalent of menses is drawn down into the bird's uterus during treading by the male. In birds that produce a lot of this residue simply hearing or smelling a male causes them to become pregnant with wind-eggs. The *GA* passage says that birds need only a small stimulus (μικρὰ...κίνησις) to cause them to emit *sperma*, while the *Dialectic* says that hens can produce wind-eggs if the male is not present (ἐὰν γὰρ μὴ παρῇ ἄρρην, 637b14).

In support of the Answerer's premise Aristotle also relates an anecdote of a woman who caught grasshoppers while they were ἔτι ἀπαλάς, "still tender," i.e. young, and kept them to see what would happen. When they had grown they became pregnant spontaneously, αὐξηθεῖσαι αὐτόματοι ἔγκυοι.[105] The production

---

[105] Aristotle rejects this assertion at *HA* V.28, 555b18–556a7 and *GA* II.5, 741a33–5. See below pp. 67–8.

of wind-eggs in hens and spontaneous pregnancy in grasshoppers shows that females do emit something when they feel a desire for coition, so Aristotle comments, "From these things it becomes clear that every female contributes to the *sperma*, even if this is seen to come about in just one type of animal," ἐκ δὴ τούτων δῆλον ὅτι συμβάλλεται εἰς τὸ σπέρμα πᾶν τὸ θῆλυ, εἴ γε καὶ ἐφ᾽ ἑνὸς γένους φαίνεται τοῦτο γιγνόμενον.[106] This statement would clearly be acceptable to the author of *Non Gen.*

The *Dialectic* proceeds on the Answerer's assumption that the appropriate human female parallel for the hen bird's emission (which has been tied to sexual excitement) is the emission women have when reaching climax in an erotic dream. The *phainomenon* that supported this in *Non Gen.* (though it was not argued for explicitly) is that the emission leaves women in the same state of lassitude as men experience after orgasm. But semen is clearly a man's contribution to reproduction, so an obvious objection to the claim that the woman's lassitude results from the same cause as the man's is that a woman's ejaculate alone never results in the condition of a viable pregnancy, which one would expect if her ejaculate played the same role in reproduction as a man's. In the guise of the Answerer Aristotle anticipates and responds to this objection by saying that the man's semen, too, does not produce an offspring unless it harmonizes, συναρμοσθῇ, with the woman's contribution.[107] Aristotle then states *Non Gen.*'s conclusion from this evidence: if conception is to take place there must be an emission of *sperma* by both the man and the woman.[108] All ancient theorists agreed that human reproduction was sexual, and in fact this formulation of reproduction would not be out of place in Aristotle's

---

[106] 637b18–20.
[107] Bolton 1990, p. 204, commenting on *Top.* VIII.1, 156b18–20, says, "Sometimes the questioner will aid the answerer, in order to gain his confidence, by bringing objections against his own premises." Aristotle is here not trying to gain anybody's confidence, but rather presenting the best defense he believes the Answerer could muster.
[108] 637b31–2.

biological works as long as the πρόεσις (*proesis*, ejaculate) on the female's part was not associated with sexual excitement and her *sperma* was not taken to be equivalent to the male's as a reproductive cause. These are the conclusions drawn, however, by *Non Gen.* Aristotle has not yet refuted these, but the dialectic is proceeding towards the conclusion he wants following the *topos* of cause and effect.

Aristotle then proceeds to ask why, if a woman's sexual excitement is the same affection as that of birds, neither she nor other animals such as horses and sheep produce wind-eggs. In the spirit of philosophical dialectic, using a premise derived from *Non Gen.* itself, Aristotle proffers the possibility that female birds produce wind-eggs because they emit directly into their womb rather than in front of it, as *Non Gen.* says women do:

> ἢ ὅτι ἡ μὲν ὄρνις εἰς τὴν ὑστέραν προΐεται, καὶ οὐκ ἔστιν ἔξω τόπος εἰς ὃν ἀφίησιν οὐδὲ ὁ ἄρρην;

> Is this because the bird emits into the womb and there is not any external place into which even the male discharges?[109]

The "puzzling through" the *aporia* of the lack of a human equivalent to wind-eggs is still proceeding along the principles of dialectic, but now assumes the vocabulary used in the *Prob.*[110] This may be because Aristotle is unsure that the Answerer would proffer this as a response to the question posed.

Aristotle then elucidates the reasoning behind this suggestion. Perhaps female quadrupeds do not produce anything like wind-eggs because they ejaculate into the area before the womb where their *sperma* mingles with other fluids and unlike the emission of female birds does not enter the womb.[111] This answer to the conundrum requires that among quadrupeds the

---

[109] 637b35–37.

[110] For some observations on the similarity in vocabulary between *HA* X and *Prob.*, see below, p. 101.

[111] At *HA* V.5, 541a25–6, Aristotle mentions that at breeding time both male and female quadrupeds produce a secretion around their genitalia.

female emission is not drawn into the womb unless it is mixed with the male contribution. This would explain why, if their ejaculate at orgasm is *sperma*, nothing similar to a wind-egg is ever constituted from it in an unmixed state, including, in women, after an erotic dream.[112] In birds, on the other hand, the female's ejaculate does enter her womb and there concocts a body ὅμοιον τὰ ἄλλα πλὴν οὐ ζῷον· διότι δεῖ ἐξ ἀμφοῖν τὸ ζῷον εἶναι, "similar in other respects except that it is not a living animal, because the living thing must come out of both."[113] Here, of course, the statement is asserting the necessity of the male contribution, which has never been in doubt in either *Non Gen.*'s or Aristotle's reproductive theory. Here Aristotle is allowing the Answerer to proffer wind-eggs as evidence that the female contribution to conception is equivalent to the male, which Aristotle argues against roundly in the *GA*. However, he has still not refuted the premise of *Non Gen.* on the basis of premises that would be acceptable to the author himself.

(c) Uterine mole as parallel to wind-eggs

This is achieved in Chapter 7, which begins with the phrase ἔστι δ' ἐνστῆναι, "It is possible to object."[114] Here Aristotle argues that emitting in front of the womb rather than directly into it would not be a sufficient explanation for why women do not produce wind-eggs. First, that the womb does draw in their emission is shown by women's testimony that they do wake up dry after ejaculating in an erotic dream. And then, if their wombs can draw in the mingled *sperma* of male and female from this place, there is no reason they should not draw in the woman's unmingled *sperma*. Why then (and again Aristotle here

---

[112] The condition *Non Gen.* calls "wind-pregnancy" (ἐξανεμοῦσθαι), which is discussed at 636a9–28, involves the mingled male and female sperma; see below p. 64.

[113] 638a4–5.

[114] An ἔνστασις is a technical term Aristotle uses for an objection to a premise; cf. *APr.* II.26, 69a37.

uses the format of a direct question) do women and other animals not produce wind-eggs? If birds and women share the αἴτιον of γόνιμον σπέρμα and in both cases it can enter the womb unmixed with male *sperma*, it should produce the same effect.

In the guise of the Answerer Aristotle replies that it does: women produce uterine moles, the equivalent of wind-eggs.[115] The case history that Aristotle proceeds to report begins by suggesting that the reason this condition is not generally recognized as a "wind-egg" is that although it is caused by the woman's seed being drawn into her womb after an erotic dream without being mingled with a man's, before the condition is recognized, an act of intercourse intervenes and women think an actual pregnancy has occurred as a result of this, συγγενομένης τῷ ἀνδρὶ καὶ δοξάσης συλλαβεῖν,[116] the implication being that they are wrong in this assumption. But even as he is relating the case history, the Answerer implicitly acknowledges that mole is a rare pathological event, not a common physiological occurrence like a bird's wind-eggs. The woman does not "give birth" to the mole until she becomes seriously ill, and some women never "give birth" to the mole at all.

Here the focus of the examination shifts a little, from using wind-eggs as evidence for the generative power of a woman's *sperma* to considering the causes of mole generally. Aristotle entertains the possibility that moles occur when an exceptionally hot womb draws in and holds unmixed *sperma*. For the purposes of arguing for female *sperma*, to this point the unmixed *sperma* under discussion has been assumed to be female, but logically, of course, by *Non Gen.*'s assumption that male and female *sperma* are equivalent and need to be mixed outside the

---

[115] A uterine mole was conceived to be a very hard, discrete, fleshy mass which could cause symptoms very similar to pregnancy and which a woman could pass after many years. The condition was also recognized by Hippocratic authors; see notes ad loc. and Dean-Jones 2019.
[116] 638a11–12.

womb, this unmixed *sperma*, in the case of both wind-eggs and mole, could just as well be male.

πότερον δὲ διὰ θερμότητα γίνεται τὸ πάθος τοῦτο, ὅταν τύχῃ ἡ ὑστέρα θερμὴ καὶ ξηρὰ οὖσα καὶ διὰ ταῦτα σπαστικὴ πρὸς αὑτήν, καὶ οὕτως ὥστ᾽ ἔστιν ἀνελέσθαι καὶ φυλάξαι πρὸς αὑτήν; οὕτω γὰρ ἐχούσαις, ἐὰν μὴ μεμιγμένον ᾖ τὸ ἀπ᾽ ἀμφοῖν, ἀλλ᾽ ὥσπερ τὸ ὑπηνέμιον ἐνδέξαιτο ἀπὸ θατέρου, τότε γίνεται ἡ καλουμένη μύλη, οὔτε ζῷον, διὰ τὸ μὴ παρ᾽ ἀμφοῖν, οὔτ᾽ ἄψυχον, διὰ τὸ ἔμψυχον ληφθὲν εἶναι, ὥσπερ τὰ ὑπηνέμια.

A further question then is, does this condition arise because of heat, whenever the womb happens to be hot and dry and for this reason is disposed to draw <material> into itself, and is so hot and dry that it is able to hold onto it and keep it within itself? For when the uterus is in this condition, if the *sperma* from both parents is not mixed but were to be received from one of the two as is the case of the wind-egg, then the so-called mole is generated, neither an animal—since it is not from both of them—nor is it without soul because it was taken up with some soul in it, just like wind-eggs.[117]

It is significant that in the rest of the discussion of mole or wind-eggs in *HA* there is no differentiation made between male and female contribution, an essential element in the explanation of both phenomena in *GA*. Balme 1991, p. 532, believes the term ἔμψυχον refers to the nutritive soul, but in this *Dialectic* Aristotle is trying to account for the mole in terms of the *endoxon* of *Non Gen.*, in which male and female *sperma* are equally ἔμψυχον. This would be the only reference in the whole of *HA* X to the asymmetry between male and female contributions that we see in *GA*. Either Aristotle is very carefully keeping all the observations and theories of *GA* out of consideration here, or he is writing at a time they are still developing.

In the *Dialectic* Aristotle does not explicitly reject heat as the cause of mole but in *GA* he roundly dismisses it as a possibility:

---

[117] 638a18–26.

"it is not due to heat, as some say," οὐ διὰ θερμότητα, ὥσπερ τινές φασιν.[118] He does, however, assert that heat is the cause of wind-eggs, because the bird's womb is close to her diaphragm, "because the area around the diaphragm is hot, <the eggs> are brought to completion as regards size, but in respect of generation they are incomplete," διὰ τὸ τὸν τόπον εἶναι θερμὸν τὸν πρὸς τῷ διαζώματι τελειοῦται τοῖς μεγέθεσιν, πρὸς δὲ τὴν γένεσιν ἀτελῆ.[119] Wind-eggs and uterine mole are not put in juxtaposition at all in GA, but it is possible that it was his consideration of the various theories about mole that influenced Aristotle's explanation of wind-eggs.

Not only is mole differentiated from wind-eggs by the rarity of the condition, it is also chronic; it can last for years, in the illustrative case cited by Aristotle relieved only by a bad case of dysentery. Again, trying to account for this discrepancy under the theory that the two conditions share at least some of the same causes (i.e., that their basic cause is unmixed *sperma*), Aristotle explains that the bird's womb opens naturally as it becomes full of eggs and once open has to emit them all. This is true whether or not the eggs have been fertilized.[120] As contrast Aristotle argues that insofar as a mole is not a living being it is inert, and because it never develops the need for more or different nourishment it can remain in a woman's womb until

---

[118] GA IV.7, 776a2. Van der Eijk 1999, p. 500, notes that the text of HA X "toys" with the idea of heat as a cause of mole rather than accepting it outright.

[119] See also GA III.1, 750b14–16, GA I.3, 717a2–3. GA I.8, 718b16–32, explains why birds have to have a womb close to their diaphragm. Their eggs have to have a hard shell for protection after they are laid, and heat is necessary to produce that. Neither vivipara nor ovipara that are very prolific need this protection to ensure some offspring. But avian wind-eggs, like the seminal residue of all other female animals, including the menstrual fluid of women, are only alive insofar as they provide nutritive soul to the offspring.

[120] Laying eggs is not equivalent to giving birth. As with the birth of vivipara, chicks hatch when they have developed to the point where the nourishment inside the egg will no longer support them, GA III.2, 752b16–754a16.

she herself dies. Even when the mole reaches a considerable size, εὐμεγέθη, it does not cause the woman's womb to open as wind-eggs do the bird's because if it were size itself that caused parturition in humans a woman's womb could never bring a fetus to full-term.

Without explicitly rejecting heat as the cause of mole, Aristotle goes on to consider whether the condition could be caused by the womb being too warm to let go of the *sperma* once it has taken it up but too cold to concoct properly:

πότερον δ᾿ ὥσπερ εἴρηται, διὰ θερμότητα γίνεται τὸ πάθος ἢ μᾶλλον δι᾿ ὑγρότητα, ὅτι καὶ ἔστι τὸ πλήρωμα οἷον μύει ὅταν μὴ οὕτως ᾖ ψυχρὰ ἡ ὑστέρα ὥστε ἀφεῖναι, μηδ᾿ οὕτω θερμὴ ὥστε πέψαι;

But does the condition come about through heat, as has been said, or rather through fluid (because it is in fact the fullness which closes <the *stoma*>), whenever the womb is not so cold as to discharge it, and not so hot as to concoct?[121]

The term ὑγρότης is vague but has to mean the mingled male and female *sperma*, however they are to be identified, because if there was enough heat in the womb the fluid would be concocted, and if the concoction is to produce something beyond a mole it must be a fetus. When the illustrative case used in the *Dialectic* of a woman developing mole after intercourse with her husband is repeated almost verbatim at *GA* IV.7, 775b27–34,[122] Aristotle introduces the condition as one that occurs during pregnancy, γίνεται δέ τισι τοῦτο τὸ πάθος κυούσαις, and at 776a2–4 he identifies a mole as a κύημα ("fetation"), that is the initial conceptus formed from <u>both</u> male semen and female menses.[123] The

---

[121] 638b1–4.

[122] It is possible Aristotle copied this history from *HA* X or in both cases from an otherwise unknown medical text.

[123] *GA* I.20, 728b34; see Peck 1942, pp. lxii–lxiii. Unusually at *GA* III.1, 750b10 and 13, Aristotle uses the term κύημα for wind-eggs, but it is clear that he is not using it in this sense in *GA* IV.7 for he goes on to say that "Nature is unable to complete her work and to bring the process of formation to it's

Dialectic's consideration of cold as an alternative to heat in the causation of mole approaches that of *GA*, but it continues to talk of cold as the environment of the womb itself whereas in *GA* the lack of heat is inherent in the κύημα, a result of an excess of menstrual fluid compared with the heat carried by the male semen; see notes ad loc.

The *Dialectic*, 638b10–15, then proceeds to explain the chronic nature of mole first by the extreme nature of the uterus itself (ὑστέραι ἀκρόταται) and then by saying that the mole does not move like the embryo (ἔμβρυον) because it is not alive and so does not cause labor. But embryos were known to move much earlier in a normal pregnancy without causing labor, and even though some Hippocratics believed labor was caused by the fetus fighting its way out of the womb looking for more appropriate nourishment, Aristotle believes labor is the natural result of the vessels in the umbilical cord collapsing.[124] Again, we do not see the mature theory of the *GA* anywhere in *HA* X.

Although Aristotle refers to the lack of heat as a cause of mole in the *GA*, he does not give many details on the process of its formation. At 775b37 he says he has discussed the mole in the *Prob*. It may be that the questions raised in the *Dialectic* were the basis for a *Problêma* on the mole, but no such discussion is found in the extant *Prob*. Given the incomplete and inconclusive nature of the remarks in the *Dialectic*, which are not as definitive as those in the *GA*, it is unlikely that the *GA* is referring back to this passage, so we should assume that Aristotle elaborated the suggestions he puts forward in the *Dialectic* elsewhere. This might explain why Aristotle does not explicitly state the

consummation" ἔοικε γὰρ ἡ φύσις ἀδυνατεῖν καὶ οὐ δύνασθαι τελειῶσαι οὐδ' ἐπιθεῖναι τῇ γενέσει πέρας. Such language would be entirely unnecessary if there had been no male contribution because the process of reproduction would never have started. In Aristotle's reproductive theory as stated in his biological works, a mole could not develop from menses alone because the *archê* of a woman could not get hot enough to concoct her seminal residue into flesh, nor could it develop from male semen alone because male semen does not contribute material to the new animal.

[124] See Dean-Jones 1994, pp. 211–12.

conclusion of the *Dialectic* (i.e., the claim that a woman's *sperma* parallels a man's in fertility is false) in *HA* X. At this stage in his thought he has reached an impasse as to what exactly the uterine mole is and he leaves that for a full-blown treatment in a *Problêma* on another day.[125]

The chapter, and treatise, ends by explaining that in fact mole is a rare condition anyway,[126] and that most cases of false pregnancy have nothing to do with seed retained in the womb but are rather the result of a confluence of body fluids in the area between the womb and the belly. Returning to the language of the *Topos* (δι' ὁμοιότητα...τὸ πάθος πάσχουσιν, 638b15), Aristotle argues that because mole and this *pathos* share some symptoms, many doctors do not differentiate between the two but immediately jump to the conclusion that the woman is suffering from mole although a simple examination of the womb would show this not to be the case. The author of *Non Gen.* does not raise the issue of uterine mole, but Aristotle's explanation of the *pathos* caused by a confluence of fluids is directed against the condition "wind-pregnancy" (ἐξανεμοῦσθαι), which *Non Gen.* discussed at 636a9–28, and attributed to the failure of mingled male and female *sperma* to develop. Aristotle's discussion of uterine mole, then, is directed both at *Non Gen.*'s assumption that female *sperma* is as γόνιμον as a male's and that once conception had taken place the κύημα could fall out of the womb without being noticed.

(d) Treatment of the subject matter in Chapters 6 and 7 in the rest of *HA* and *GA*

Wind-eggs and mole are not the only *phainomena* discussed in Aristotelian biological works that appear in the *Dialectic*. The

---

[125] Smith 1999, p. 51, says, "Aristotle does not say the <dialectic> will provide us with a *proof* of anything but only says that it will help us to see what is true or false."

[126] Which may have been one of the arguments he used against its being considered equivalent to wind-eggs in the eventual *Problêma*.

estrus cycle and its relation to mammalian fertility is dealt with at, e.g., *HA* VI.18, 572b30–573a31, and *GA* II.8, 748b20–9, though Aristotle mistakenly assimilated it to the menstrual cycle.[127] At *HA* V.5, 541a25–6, he mentions that at breeding time both male and female quadrupeds produce a secretion around their genitalia. The *Dialectic* mirrors not only Aristotelian subject matter but also Aristotelian language. For example, wind-eggs are described as ἔμψυχον (*empsuchon*, ensouled) but not as an animal. There are frequent references to concoction and residues. There is even a mention of viviparous animals, ὅσα ζωοφορεῖ (*hosa zoophorei*).[128] After bringing his medical treatise to completion why should Aristotle, if he were the author of *Non Gen.*, suddenly revert to philosophical mode to undercut himself? Far simpler to assume he is examining a medical treatise authored by somebody else.

Now it is of course *prima facie* possible that the *Dialectic* was appended to *Non Gen.* by Theophrastus or any one of a number of Peripatetics who were familiar with Aristotle's dialectical methods and biological works, but in that case there are a number of strange omissions in the argument. A fundamental argument in the *GA* is that no animal can produce two seminal residues and that as the female seminal residue is menstrual fluid she cannot also produce seed.[129] Any student of Aristotle familiar with his biological works would surely have lodged this objection against the argument of *Non Gen.* And the possible value of wind-eggs as support for the theory of *Non Gen.* could have been dismissed much more cleanly by one familiar with Aristotle's theory that because the womb of birds is placed high in their body—by the diaphragm—the female's seminal residue is subject to more concoction than that of other female animals whose womb is lower in the body. That birds have their diaphragm near to their womb is noted at *HA* III.1, 510b20–34,

---

[127] See Dean-Jones 1994, pp. 91–2, 187, 229.
[128] For a discussion of these and similar points, see below, pp. 98–108.
[129] *GA* I.19, 727a25–30.

but no connection is made between this fact and wind-eggs until *GA* I.8, 718b18–28 and III.1, 750b14–17. Furthermore, why would a Peripatetic familiar with the *GA* have even mooted the possibility of heat as a cause of the mole in the face of the categorical denial of *GA* IV.7, 776a2–4, or put forward only as a possibility the explanation of mole offered there? It is true that the treatment of mole in *GA* is very terse, but the reference to the discussion of the condition in the *Problêmata* shows that there was also a more extended discussion available that would have made the inconclusive musings of the *Dialectic* even more pointless if it had been written subsequent to *GA*.

From the arguments advanced in the *Dialectic* it would seem that the author knew the *HA*, or at least parts of it, but was unfamiliar with the *GA*. The most reasonable explanation for why an author so well versed in Aristotelian biology and dialectic would be unfamiliar with the *GA* is that it had not yet been written at the time the *Dialectic* was being composed.[130] In these circumstances it seems that the most likely identity for the author of the *Dialectic* is Aristotle himself. Why then does the anecdote about the woman who was delivered of a mole by dysentery, told at *GA* IV.7, 775b26–34, appear virtually verbatim in the *Dialectic* at 638a10–18? The simplest answer is that the passage was not copied from *GA* to the *Dialectic* but vice versa. This would explain the only variant between the passage in the *Dialectic* and *GA*. After the attack of dysentery, the *Dialectic* explains, the woman "gave birth to a lump of flesh of considerable size (σάρκα εὐμεγέθη)," while *GA* simply says that she produced "a lump of flesh (σάρκα)" without any reference to its size. In the *Dialectic* Aristotle originally introduces the case of the mole in the persona of the Answerer trying to support the claim that the female ejaculate could cause an affection like wind-egg. In that context he would want to make the

---

[130] I do not accept Balme's arguments (Balme 1987) for the priority of the *GA* to the entirety of the *HA*, though I accept that the *HA* was constantly updated by Aristotle and his students; see Lennox 1996, pp. 244–6.

mole resemble an embryo as closely as possible, just as wind-eggs are the same size, or close to the same size, as fertilized eggs. He may also have been differentiating uterine mole from "wind-pregnancy," where the withered *sperma*, mingled from the male and female contributions, falls away from the woman unnoticed because of its smallness, μικρότητα, 636a15. When Aristotle came to use the anecdote in his account of reproduction in *GA*, the size of the mass was irrelevant.

A similar point could be made about the reference to parthenogenesis in grasshoppers which Aristotle uses in the first remarks of the *Dialectic*. He discussed the generation of grasshoppers at *HA* V.28, 555b18–556a7, opening with the words, "Grasshoppers copulate in the same way as other insects."[131] Nothing is said about the possibility of parthenogenesis in grasshoppers either in this passage, in the rest of the *HA* or, indeed, in the rest of the Aristotelian Corpus. At *GA* II.5, 741a33–5, Aristotle remarks: "If there is any class of animal which is female and has no separate male, it is possible that this generates offspring from itself. This has not so far been reliably (ἀξιοπίστως) observed." The adverb here may be used to dismiss the testimony of, among others, the female τις at the *Dialectic* 637b17 who was the source for the story about parthenogenetic grasshoppers. This *endoxon* was included in the *Dialectic* as further support that what a woman emitted at orgasm played the same causal role in reproduction as a man's semen, so it may have been introduced simply as a premise which the hypothetical Answerer would concede; but in a philosophic dialectic—a search for truth—there is no need to use any premise which is known, or strongly suspected, to be false. At the time of composing the *Dialectic* Aristotle may still have been in two

---

[131] Not all insects copulate, *GA* I.16, 721a9–10, but in those that do most do so by the male mounting the female and the female inserting part of herself into him, *GA* I.18, 723b19–25, *HA* V.8, 541b35–542a18, which is what Aristotle describes in the case of grasshoppers. Although some insects are produced by spontaneous generation, *GA* III.9, 758a30 and b8, none are said to reproduce parthenogenetically.

minds about the reliability of the *endoxon*. This could explain his more forceful language when he finally came to reject it. The statement "Grasshoppers copulate in the same way as other insects" is a more pointed introduction to the reproductive habits of that insect than the more normal καί (*kai*, also) or ὁμοίως (*homoiôs*, likewise) or τὸν εἰρημένον τρόπον (*ton eirêmenon tropon*, in the manner already described) which he uses to introduce the reproductive habits of other insect species. It is perhaps meant as a flat rejection of the folk belief in parthenogenetic grasshoppers which was allowed some credence in the *Dialectic*.[132]

In the *Dialectic*, Aristotle includes quadrupeds as well as women in the first part of his discussion about wind-eggs. In Chapter 7, however, the focus is totally on women and no mention is made of any other animal. The discussion of uterine mole in *GA* IV.7 ends at 776a8–14 by explaining that no viviparous quadruped suffers from uterine mole because no other animal produces the excess of menstrual fluid that women do. Here again we see evidence that the *Dialectic* of *HA* X was written before the fuller consideration of uterine mole in a *Problêma* and the *GA*.

5 ARISTOTLE'S OBJECTIONS TO *NON GEN.*'S VERSION OF PANGENESIS

Furthermore, while the *Dialectic* shows no knowledge of the *GA*, we have seen that in the *GA* Aristotle shows he is fully cognizant of specific arguments—not just general theories about female *sperma*—put forward in *Non Gen.*, notably his statement at *GA* I.19, 727a25–30, that it is impossible for any creature to produce two seminal secretions and his explicit remark at *GA* I.19, 727b8–12, that conception need not take place even if the

---

[132] As a repository of observed facts *HA* was under constant revision, so material would continue to be added and corrected after the composition of *GA*.

male and female "keep pace."[133] The same is true of *Non Gen.*'s arguments for a particular version of pangenesis.

Pangenesis is the belief that resemblance of offspring to parents is caused by *sperma* being formed from material from every part of a parent's body mingling with *sperma* from all the parts of the other parent's body. The features of the resultant offspring resemble the parts which each parent provided the most or strongest *sperma*. So, a child could have its father's nose but its mother's eyes. The fact that a child could resemble its mother as much as its father was perhaps the main reason for a belief in female *sperma* and so, as Bolton argues, Aristotle "thinks that to undermine this theory will be to undermine the dominant received basis for believing that <u>both</u> sexes contribute to generation by emitting *sperma*."[134]

Of all the apparent discrepancies between *Non Gen.* and *GA*, van der Eijk, 1999, p. 501, believes that the only one that cannot be reconciled with *GA* is *Non Gen.*'s explanation of multiple birth—that it is caused by a single secretion of *sperma* from the entire body (pangenesis) being separated into different places in the womb, 637a9—with Aristotle's flat denial of this fact at *GA* IV.4, 771b27–33.[135] Balme notes this as a problem, 1985, p. 198, but offers no solution. In Balme 1991, p. 513, in a note on 637a9 he comments "This argument is *corrected* (my italics) and further developed at *GA* 771b27–772a37", which is simply an admission that the two views cannot be reconciled.

---

[133] See above, pp. 19–24.   [134] Bolton 1987, p. 154.

[135] Aristotle introduces the section on pangenesis with wording slightly more reminiscent of *Non Gen.* than of the Hippocratic treatise *Genit. GA* I.17, 721b11–12, reads (φασί τινες) ἀπὸ παντὸς ἀπιέναι τοῦ σώματος. Here the infinitive is inserted between the noun and its modifying adjective, as is the verb at *Non Gen.* 637a12–13, ἀπὸ παντὸς ἔρχεται τὸ σπέρμα τοῦ σώματος. Although the term τὸ σπέρμα does not appear in the *GA* sentence, it is the term Aristotle uses throughout the passage. In the Hippocratic treatise *Genit.*, on the other hand, the author uses the term γονή and does not break up the noun/adjective phrase: τὴν δὲ γονήν φημι ἀποκρίνεσθαι ἀπὸ παντὸς τοῦ σώματος, *Genit.* 3 (VII.474.5); see also *Genit.* 8 (VII.480.7–8).

Non Gen. is not the only treatise to argue that pockets in the womb cause multiple births. This is also stated in, e.g., *Vict.* I.30 (VI.504.14–22). However, at the beginning of his arguments Aristotle states:

διόπερ ἐπισκεπτέον, ἐπειδή φασί τινες ἀπὸ παντὸς ἀπιέναι τοῦ σώματος, περὶ τούτου πῶς ἔχει πρῶτον. ἔστι δὲ σχεδόν, οἷς ἄν τις χρήσαιτο τεκμηρίοις ὡς ἀφ' ἑκάστου τῶν μορίων ἀπιόντος τοῦ σπέρματος, τέτταρα.

Since some people say that <*sperma*> comes from the whole body, first of all, we need to examine what the case is about this. Basically, there are four types of evidence which someone might use to support the claim that *sperma* originates in each of the parts of the body.[136]

The first thing to note here is that Aristotle considers claims that the *sperma* comes from the whole body to be equivalent to claims that it comes from each of the parts of the body. Among Hippocratic authors too, when pangenesis is mentioned specifically, the origin of the seed in the parts of the body is always emphasized, e.g., *Aër.* 14 (II.60.1–2), ὁ γὰρ γόνος πανταχόθεν ἔρχεται τοῦ σώματος, ἀπό τε τῶν ὑγιηρῶν ὑγιηρός, ἀπό τε τῶν νοσερῶν νοσερός: "For the seed comes from all over the body, healthy seed from healthy parts, diseased seed from diseased parts."[137] Similarly *Vict.* I.7 (VI.480.11), in a context which is most likely to refer to conception, says ἀνάγκη δὲ τὰ μέρεα ἔχειν πάντα τὰ ἐσιόντα, "It is necessary that the stuff which enters has all the parts." In the same vein *Genit.* 8 (VII.480.7–9) says:

καὶ †ἐν αὐτῆφι τῇ γονῇ† ἐξέρχεται καὶ τῆς γυναικὸς καὶ τοῦ ἀνδρὸς ἀπὸ παντὸς τοῦ σώματος, καὶ ἀπὸ τῶν ἀσθενέων ἀσθενὴς καὶ ἀπὸ τῶν ἰσχυρῶν ἰσχυρή.

---

[136] *GA* I.17, 721b 11–14.
[137] See also *Morb. Sacr.* 5 (VI.364.19–20), ὁ γόνος ἔρχεται πάντοθεν τοῦ σώματος, ἀπό τε τῶν ὑγιηρῶν ὑγιηρός, ἀπό τε τῶν νοσερῶν νοσερός. It is generally recognized that *Aër.* and *Morb. Sacr.* are very closely related, some believe from the same author.

The seed comes from the whole body of both the woman and the man, both weak seed from the weak parts and strong seed from the strong parts.

The passage goes on to explain that the child will resemble the parent who has contributed seed from the greater number of parts:

ὁκότερος δ᾽ ἂν πλέον ξυμβάληται ἐς τὸ ἐοικέναι καὶ ἀπὸ πλεόνων χωρίων τοῦ σώματος, κείνῳ τὰ πλείονα ἔοικε.

Whichever parent has contributed more to the likeness and from more parts of the body, to that parent the child bears a greater resemblance. (*Genit.* 8 (VII.480.16–18))[138]

This implies that just as the seed was assembled part by part it can be distributed part by part.

Much of Aristotle's criticism of pangenesis in *GA* I.18, 722a1–724a14, focuses on the argument that the *sperma* is drawn from the parts of the body. In particular, he asks how the parts of the body could live in the *sperma* if they were sundered from one another (722b18–30). It is impossible, he says, for parts to become connected in the right places if they are separated from the parts of the parent piecemeal. Nor does the intense pleasure felt in intercourse give evidence for pangenesis, as some argue. If this were so, the pleasure should be felt in each of the parts contributing *sperma*, and in some before others,[139] but in fact it is felt at the end of intercourse (723b33–724a4).

---

[138] The author of *Genit.* recognized at least one of the problems inherent in claiming that seed was drawn from the parts of the body. In explaining how children can resemble their parents in features which their parents no longer possessed when they engendered their children, he remarks that the deformed animal contains τὸν ἀριθμὸν πάντα, "the entire number," of the healthy animal (*Genit.* 11 (VII.484.15)). This would imply that the author did not think that seed was drawn from the parts of the body at each act of intercourse, but still indicates that parts of the *gonê* were thought to correspond to parts of the body.

[139] Because *sperma* from the nose would have further to travel before ejaculation than *sperma* from the hips.

INTRODUCTION

The author of *Non Gen.* subscribes to the theory of pangenesis, but in a way that is not susceptible to these criticisms. In explaining why it is that all the *sperma* produced by a man and a woman at orgasm does not have to be used up in the formation of a new individual, he introduces the phenomenon of multiple births in other animals. The point he is making is that no particular part of the *sperma* corresponds to any particular body part, so being formed from only a portion of the *sperma* will not leave an individual lacking in anything.[140] *Non Gen.* 637a10–13 reads:

εἰ πολλὰ ἀπὸ μιᾶς ὀχείας γίνεται, ὅπερ φαίνεται ἐπὶ τῶν ὑῶν καὶ τῶν διδύμων ἐνίοτε γινόμενον, δῆλον ὅτι ἀπὸ παντὸς ἔρχεται τὸ σπέρμα τοῦ σώματος ἀλλ ἐφ᾽ ἑκάστου εἴδους ἐμερίζετο. ἀπὸ παντὸς μὲν γὰρ ἐνδέχεται ἀποχωρισθῆναι, καὶ τὸ πᾶν εἰς πολλά. ὥστε ἅμα καὶ κατὰ μέρος ἀδύνατον.

If many young come from one coupling, which is clear in the case of pigs and sometimes in the case of twins in humans, it is clear that the *sperma* comes from the whole body but is parceled out in respect of each individual. For of course it is possible for an individual to be separated off from all the *sperma* and for all the *sperma* to separate into many individuals. So that it is impossible at the same time for *sperma* to be separated off from the body part by part.[141]

He is thus disputing the argument on which Aristotle focuses much of his criticism of pangenesis.

Aristotle returns to the issue of the *sperma* being separated from the body ἀπὸ παντός at *GA* I.20, 729a4–7, beginning with a sentence very close in vocabulary and structure to *Non Gen.* 637a10–11, but followed by the diametrically opposite conclusion:

[140] For a discussion of the Anaxagorean overtones of this idea, see notes ad loc.
[141] See notes ad loc. for arguments as to why the οὐκ in l.12 should be excluded.

72

ἀπὸ μιᾶς γὰρ ὀχείας πλείω γίνεται ἐν τοῖς πλείω δυναμένοις
γεννᾶν ἑνός. ᾗ καὶ δῆλον ὅτι οὐκ ἀπὸ παντὸς ἔρχεται ἡ γονή. οὔτε
γὰρ ἂν κεχωρισμένα ἀπὸ τοῦ αὐτοῦ μέρους εὐθὺς ἀπεκρίνετο
οὔτε ἅμα ἐλθόντα εἰς τὰς ὑστέρας ἐκεῖ διεχωρίζετο.

More <than one> young come from one coupling in those animals which are able to produce more than one. And in this it
is clear that the *gonê* does not come from the whole body. For
neither would pluralities of stuff be separated off from the same
part at one and the same time nor, having entered the uterus
together, would they be divided up there.

In this passage Aristotle is reading *Non Gen.*'s claim that *sperma*
is not separated off κατὰ μέρος, part by part, in a temporal
sense. He argues that if *sperma* that came from one body was to
engender ten different bodies, even if it was separated off at one
moment from the body as a cohesive whole, there would have
to be enough *sperma* from each body part to replicate itself ten
times. But these ten discrete emissions from each part could not
occur at the single moment of ejaculation of cohesive *sperma*
from the whole body. Nor, if the *sperma* entered the uterus as a
unity, could it be divided up there into ten discrete unities. This
repeats the argument at *GA* I.18, 723b 9–16:

ἔτι ἀπὸ μιᾶς συνουσίας καὶ τῶν ζῴων ἔνια γεννᾷ πολλά, τὰ δὲ
φυτὰ καὶ παντάπασιν· δῆλον γὰρ ὅτι ἀπὸ μιᾶς κινήσεως τὸν
ἐπέτειον πάντα φέρει καρπόν· καίτοι πῶς δυνατὸν εἰ ἀπὸ παντὸς
ἀπεκρίνετο τὸ σπέρμα; μίαν γὰρ ἀπόκρισιν ἀπὸ μιᾶς ἀναγκαῖον
γίγνεσθαι συνουσίας καὶ μιᾶς διακρίσεως. ἐν δὲ ταῖς ὑστέραις
χωρίζεσθαι ἀδύνατον· ἤδη γὰρ ὥσπερ ἀπὸ νέου φυτοῦ ἢ ζῴου,
οὐ σπέρματος εἴη ἡ διαχώρισις.

Furthermore, even some animals engender multiple offspring
from one act of intercourse, and plants do, in fact, do this uni-
versally. For it is clear that these produce the fruit of an entire
season from one instigation. And yet, how is this possible if
the *sperma* is separated off from the whole body? For one secretion must come from one act of intercourse and one instance
of separation. And it is impossible that it be divided up in the

uterus. For at that point it would already be just like a division of a young plant or animal, not of *sperma*.

The language here is not as reminiscent of *Non Gen.* as that at *GA* I.20, 729a4–7, but it is clearly addressing the same argument, and it is an argument expressed only in *Non Gen.* among extant texts.

It is admittedly difficult to understand what could be meant by saying something came from the whole of a thing without also in some way coming from all its parts. We may be seeing another attempt at making sense of this idea at *GA* IV.3, 769a26–b3, where, in disputing the explanation for resemblance to parents given by pangeneticists, Aristotle says one such theory is somewhat better than the others, though he also says it "is unclear and tortuous in many points," οὐ σαφὴς μὲν καὶ πλασματίας ἐστὶ πολλαχῇ. This is one that takes the *gonê* to be a unity, albeit one formed from many things, τὴν γονὴν μίαν οὖσαν οἷον πανσπερμίαν εἶναί τινα πολλῶν, where a large number of juices had been blended into one fluid, κεράσειε πολλοὺς χυμοὺς εἰς ἓν ὑγρόν.

Like Aristotle's arguments against two seminal secretions and the need for the woman to keep pace with the man in order to conceive, his objections to the version of pangenesis stipulating a single secretion of *sperma* from the whole body are aimed most clearly at *Non Gen.*

Throughout the *HA*, although Aristotle refers to various informants—individuals, groups of lay people, and specialists—and often gives conflicting explanations on certain topics,[142] when

---

[142] E.g., I.11, 492a14, Alcman is mistaken to say we can breathe through our ears; II.14, 505b20–1, "Some say… (τινὲς φασιν)" the fish called the ship-brake has feet, but it does not; IV.7, 532b18–25, refers to the expertise of experienced fishermen; V.30, 556b16, refers to the knowledge of farmers; VI.13, 568a4–10, invokes knowledge about the Black Sea by the inhabitants of the seaboard; VI.32, 579b28–9, cites hunters on female hyenas; VIII(IX).1, 608b28–610a14, the sorts of things one can learn from diviners.

discussing human reproduction in *HA* IX(VII) he never indicates the sources for his information nor any alternate theories, apart from correcting women who believe they have been pregnant for longer than eleven months, *HA* IX(VII).4, 584b19–25. In the *GA*, however, he does refer to a variety of theories for different reproductive phenomena. It would seem that although Aristotle consulted many different authorities when compiling the information in the *HA*, he did not seek out *endoxa* on reproduction until he came to compile the *GA*, or at least he did not include references to *endoxa* on the subject in the *HA*. In gathering *endoxa* for the *GA*, *Non Gen.* was one of the treatises Aristotle consulted, considered, and finally rejected on several points, most importantly that female *sperma* played the same role in reproduction as the male. The philosophical dialectic he had with this *endoxon* helped shape his later more polished discussions, with an intermediary discussion on the uterine mole in his *Problêmata*. If this hypothesis is correct, we can assume that this was not an isolated exercise on Aristotle's part and he did in fact practice the method outlined in the *Topics*. It may be that Aristotle destroyed or simply failed to retain all other such preliminary studies. If so, we will probably never know if this was preserved accidentally or if *Non Gen.* had some particular resonance for him.[143] It may be also that similar *endoxa* are embedded in other Aristotelian works, explained as early, unrevised theories, but it is beyond the scope of this study to seek them out.

6 THE MEDICAL NATURE OF *NON GEN.*

(a) Audience of *Non Gen.*

We saw above, p. 45, that written medical texts would furnish Aristotle with *endoxa*, and it has been generally accepted that

---

[143] Of course, it is possible that *Non Gen.* is one of his own early works on reproduction, though for reasons enumerated above, pp. 11–14, I find this unlikely. I think it is more likely that it is a work of his physician father Nicomachus, but this is unprovable.

the material in *HA* X has been heavily influenced by medical writers. Following Rose, Rudberg characterizes *HA* X as an attempted synthesis of Aristotelian and Hippocratic theories by a Peripatetic Iatrosophist (p. 46). Louis characterizes the author as "un médecin, riche d'une longue expérience et d'une solide culture, et dont le vocabulaire a un caractère technique très prononcé" who "connait bien les oeuvres d'Aristote."[144] Balme disputed the "iatric" nature of *HA* X, but van der Eijk, in arguing in support of Balme's thesis of Aristotelian authorship, calls this a "hardly defensible reading" of the text and instead draws attention to the "diagnostic" character of the treatise and says it is not "a biological but...a predominantly medical work intended to provide instructions as to how to deal with an important practical problem."[145] This raises the question of the audience of the original treatise. Van der Eijk states that we do not have to assume it was meant for a professional medical readership, but it is hard to know who else could be assumed to be literate who would be called in to deal with a woman's infertility apart from doctors (and perhaps midwives).[146] There are several indications in *Non Gen.* that it was not written to be used by the infertile couple themselves.

The clinical nature of the treatise is made clear in the second sentence, where the author says "first, in the case of the female, it is necessary to observe (δεῖ θεωρεῖν) how things stand with the uterus, what state it is in, so that if the cause is located here it can be treated (τυγχάνωσι θεραπείας)."[147] The author continues by saying that if the womb is in good condition,

---

[144] Louis 1969, p. 153.

[145] Balme 1985, p. 194; van der Eijk 1999, pp. 496–7. By and large the Hippocratics were concerned with infertility, a condition they appeared to think was largely tractable, rather than sterility. Aristotle acknowledges congenital sterility in both men and women at *HA* IX(VII).1, 581b21–3; see Flemming 2013.

[146] Soranus *Gyn.* I.2.5–6 assumes that some midwives at least will be literate, though there is no evidence of this for the earlier period.

[147] For possible clinical indications of the opening sentence, see below p. 110.

"they may direct their attention (ποιῶνται τὴν ἐπιμέλειαν) to one of the other two causes." The third person verb form suggests that the subjects of this verb are different from the audience to whom the impersonal δεῖ θεωρεῖν was directed. Besides the condition of the uterus, the other two possible causes of infertility canvassed by the author are the male's contribution to conception and the failure of the man and the woman to "keep pace" with one another during intercourse. The latter of these two possibilities is quite clearly an area in which the attention of the sexual partners themselves is more appropriate than medical therapy. As to ascertaining if the man is infertile, at 636b12–13 the author acknowledges that while "it is indeed possible to take other signs (ἔστι μὲν καὶ ἄλλα σημεῖα λαβεῖν)" it "would certainly be apparent more easily if he has intercourse and conceives with other women (ῥᾷω μάλιστα φαίνοιτο πρὸς ἄλλας πλησιάζων καὶ γεννῶν)," and this again is something that would be more evident to the man himself rather than the observations of a doctor. It would seem then that the subjects of ποιῶνται are the couple who are trying to conceive, on whose shoulders the responsibility for ascertaining the cause of their infertility will fall if the woman's uterus seems to be in working order. The third person indicates that these are not the primary audience of the treatise, and we can assume that the impersonal instruction δεῖ θεωρεῖν, and similarly the impersonal form σκεπτέον at 634b26, is being given to physicians.[148] At 635b31–2 the pronoun in the phrase τοσόνδε δεῖ κατανοεῖν, which either limits how much the one inquiring should inquire about or justifies the detail of the inquiry, further indicates that the audience of the treatise is not the infertile couple themselves.[149]

Some observations may have been made by the woman herself. In Chapter 2 the author discusses the observations that

---

[148] Scot translates the impersonal, the passive, and third person plural verb forms in this sentence as first person plural (*debemus considerare, medicabimur eam <matricem>, intendemus medicinari*).

[149] See also comments on ἂν ἀπορήσῃ at 635a24.

indicate that the cervix has opened in the right way, including tactile observations. At 635a8 this is expressed using a passive participle, "the cervix will be softer to the touch (θιγγανόμενον ἔσται τὸ στόμα μαλακώτερον)."[150] In the Hippocratic Corpus this sort of observation is made sometimes by the doctor himself, sometimes by the woman and sometimes by a third party, a midwife.[151] In this text there is no indication that an intermediary is present, and if my argument that the use of ποιῶνται at 633b18 shows that the impersonal instructions in the rest of the text are directed at physicians is correct, it seems preferable to assume that this instruction too is aimed at a doctor. Clearly, however, there are times when the doctor would have to depend on a woman's testimony. One of the signs that tell that there is no growth on the *stoma* is that the womb opens and closes in the right way when a woman is having sex with her husband (636a39). The fact that it is not specifically stated that the doctor needs the woman to inform him in this case does not mean that the target audience is not a doctor.

(b) Lack of therapy and pathology

Although *Non Gen.* is a clinical text, in the five chapters we have it does not concern itself with therapy beyond identifying what conditions need, and would respond to, treatment, though this is a matter of great concern for the author.[152] This is in contrast to the Hippocratic gynecology, which often lists multiple treatments for the same complaints. In relation to the focus of the Hippocratic gynecology on infertility Flemming states "the main reason for all this discussion is treatment."[153] The lack of therapy could be taken as an indication that the work was

---

[150] Unfortunately there are textual difficulties in the other two passages where the touching of the cervix occurs in *HA* X; see notes to 635a13 and 638b31.
[151] See note on 635a8 and Dean-Jones 1994, pp. 35–6.
[152] Van der Eijk 1999, p. 496.
[153] Flemming 2013, p. 573.

not intended for a medical audience if it were not for the fact
that many treatises of the Hippocratic Corpus do not contain
directions for treatment. This is especially true of treatises that
are particularly concerned with signs such as *Prog.* and *Prorrh.
II*, and among which *Non Gen.* could perhaps be counted.[154] The
assumption would be that once the condition was identified a
professional would know the sort of treatment it required. On
the other hand, the concern the author shows with nosology
and the need or otherwise for treatment, not to mention the fact
that this is a gynecological text, aligns it with treatises that do
suggest therapies for the conditions they outline, such as *Mul.* I
and II, *Morb.* I and II, *Aff.*, and *Int.* It must be added, though,
that these texts also describe the pathology that patients suffer in the disease conditions they identify, very often involving
phlegm or bile, and there is very little sign of this in *Non Gen.*
The only indication that the woman might be subjectively suffering something other than failure to conceive is at 634a27–30
in the discussion of putrefied menses when the author says:

> ἐὰν δ' ἀνόμοια καὶ σεσημμένα μᾶλλον ἢ οἷα ταῖς ὑγιαινούσαις
> προέρχεται, τοῦτο μὲν ἤδη πάθος καὶ ἐπίδηλον γίνεται· ἀνάγκη
> γὰρ καὶ πόνους τινὰς ἐπισημαίνειν ἐχούσης ὡς οὐ δεῖ.

> But if the fluid is dissimilar and more putrefied than that which
> is emitted by healthy women, at this time it is already a con-
> dition and it is becoming evident. For some suffering must be
> indicating that the womb is not as it should be.

Other than this, the implication of *Non Gen.* is that the woman
undergoing diagnostics is functioning in general as a healthy
person. Here, for example, is what the author has to say about
a woman whose cervix is not properly aligned:

> ἐὰν δὲ μὴ εἰς ὀρθὸν βλέπωσιν αἱ ὑστέραι ἀλλ' ἢ πρὸς τὰ ἰσχία ἢ
> πρὸς τὴν ὀσφὺν ἢ πρὸς τὸ ὑπογάστριον, ἀδύνατον συλλαβεῖν
> διὰ τὴν προειρημένην αἰτίαν, ὅτι ἀνελέσθαι οὐκ ἂν δύναιντο
> τὸ σπέρμα. ἐὰν μὲν οὖν ἰσχυρῶς τῇ φύσει οὕτως ἔχωσιν ἢ ὑπὸ

---

[154] Van der Eijk 1999, p. 496, n. 33.

νόσου, ἀνίατον τὸ πάθος· ἐὰν δ' ᾖ ῥῆγμα ἢ φύσει ἢ ὑπὸ τῆς νόσου διὰ φλεγμασίαν συσπασάσης, ἐπὶ θάτερα αὐτῇ τὸ πάθος.

But if the uterus is not looking straight but either towards the hips or towards the tailbone or towards the underbelly it cannot conceive on account of the reason already mentioned, that it cannot take up the *sperma*. If the uterus is firmly established in this state either by nature or by disease, the condition is incurable. But if there is a rupture either naturally or as a result of a disease which contracts the womb through inflammation, the condition tends the opposite way for the woman.[155]

Obliquity of the cervix is a common problem in the Hippocratic gynecology, one which involves suffering on the woman's part, and often dealt with at great length.[156] Here is a fairly typical shorter example:

ἢν παραλοξαίνωνται αἱ μῆτραι, καὶ τὸ στόμα αὐτῶν λοξὸν γίνηται, τὰ ἐπιμήνια αὐτῇ τοτὲ μὲν κρύπτεται, τοτὲ δὲ προφανέντα οἴχεται, καὶ οὐχ ὅμοια γίνεται, ἀλλὰ κακίω τε καὶ ἐλάσσω ἢ πρὸ τοῦ, καὶ ἡ γονὴ οὐκ ἐγγίνεται τούτου τοῦ χρόνου, καὶ ὀδύνη ἴσχει τὴν νείαιραν γαστέρα καὶ τὰς ἰξύας καὶ τὴν ὀσφῦν καὶ τὸ ἰσχίον, καὶ ἐφελκοῦνται. ὁκόταν ὧδε ἔχῃ, φάρμακον χρὴ πῖσαι ἐλατήριον, καὶ λούειν θερμῷ, καὶ πυριῆν· ὁκόταν δὲ νεοπυρίητος ἢ νεόλουτος ᾖ, τὸν δάκτυλον ἐσαφάσσουσα, ἀπορθούτω καὶ παρευθυνέτω τὸ στόμα τῶν μητρέων, καὶ ὑποθυμιήσθω τὰ εὐώδεα, καὶ τῶν ποτημάτων δίδου πειρεύμενος ὅ τι ἂν μάλιστα προσδέχηται· σιτίοισι δὲ χρήσθω μαλθακοῖσι, καὶ σκόροδα ἐσθιέτω ὠμὰ καὶ ἑφθά· καὶ τῷ ἀνδρὶ συνευδέτω καὶ ἐπὶ τοῦ ὑγιέος ἰσχίου κατακείσθω· τὸ δὲ ἕτερον πυριήσθω. ἡ δὲ νοῦσος δυσαπάλλακτος.

If a woman's uterus shifts to an oblique position, with its mouth at an angle, her menses will at one time be absent, and at another time reappear, only to be lost again; they are no longer normal, but worse in quality and less in amount than before. The woman does not become pregnant during this time, pain occupies her lower abdomen, hips and tailbone, and ulceration

---

[155] 634b39–635a5.   [156] E.g., *Mul.* II.133 (VIII.280.12–302.12).

occurs. When the case is such, as purge have the patient drink squirting cucumber juice, bathe her in hot water, and apply a vapor bath. When she has just been bathed or received a vapor bath, have her—by inserting her finger—straighten and widen the mouth of her uterus, and foment herself below with fragrant substances; give beverages you know by experience will be most acceptable. Have the patient employ mild foods, and eat garlic both raw and boiled. She should sleep with her husband, lie on the healthy hip, and apply vapor baths to the other one. The disease is difficult to get rid of.[157]

It may be that *Non Gen.* originally contained disease symptoms and therapies but Aristotle did not bother to summarize them because he considered them irrelevant for the purposes of the *endoxon.* Or it may be that in summarizing a medical text he thought it pointless to include any discussion of therapy anyway. At *EN* X.9, 1181b5–6, he states that men cannot become physicians from handbooks because the courses of treatment described for different types of people "seem to be useful for experienced men, but useless for the inexperienced" τοῖς μὲν ἐμπείροις ὠφέλιμα εἶναι δοκεῖ, τοῖς δ' ἀνεπιστήμοσιν ἀχρεῖα. Whether Aristotle deliberately omitted this material, or whether the original treatise was intended to be primarily semiotic for causes of sterility in otherwise healthy women, the lack of therapy cannot be used to argue against the clinical nature of *Non Gen.*

(c) Similar conditions in the Hippocratic Corpus

Almost all of the issues that *Non Gen.* raises as impeding conception are mirrored in the Hippocratic gynecology, though as with the case of the misaligned cervix in *Nat. Mul.* 40 they usually also involve pathology and therapy: e.g. too scanty or too frequent menstruation, *Mul.* I.4–6 (VIII.24.20–30.22); putrefied menses, *Mul.* I.2 (VIII.18.19–20.11); misalignment of the *stoma, Mul.* I.10 and 13 (VIII.40.12–42.8 and 50.19–52.5), *Nat. Mul.* 7

---

[157] *Nat. Mul.* 40 (VII.384.4–16), trans. Potter 2012, pp. 272–4, adapted.

(VII.320.18), *Steril.* 213 (VIII.408.4–5); dilation of *stoma*, *Mul.* I.13 (VIII.50.13–19–52.5–7), *Nat. Mul.* 13 and 45 (VII.330.12–13 and 390.1–4), *Steril.* 241 (VIII.454.6–456.6); lack of attraction in womb, *Steril.* 213 (VIII.408.19–410.2); a hard *stoma*, *Mul.* II.156–8 (VIII.330.19–336.21), *Nat. Mul.* 39 (VII.382.15–19); lack of elasticity in the womb, *Genit.* 9 (VII.482.3–22); a form of "wind-pregnancy," *Mul.* II.179 (VIII.362.3–15); ulceration of the uterus, *Mul.* I.3 and 63 (VIII.24.10–13 and 126.20–13.21), *Nat. Mul.* 55 (VII.396.14), *Steril.* 213 (VIII.410.6–15).[158]

There is an important condition, though, regarding which *Non Gen.* might seem to have a different opinion from other gynecological texts of the period, that is uterine displacement, the so-called "Wandering Womb." This is the belief that the womb could be displaced to other parts of the body, from the brain to the feet, causing a wide variety of ailments which are discussed in many passages in the gynecology, e.g., *Mul.* I.7 (VIII.32.1–34.5), *Mul.* II.123–53 (VIII.266.11–328.14), *Nat. Mul.* 3–6 and 47–9 (VII.314.14–320.17 and 390.23–392.20), *Steril.* 247 and 248 (VIII.460.3–462.15).[159] Even Plato, at *Ti.* 91b–d, attests a belief in the womb's ability to relocate or issue forth from the body if it is desirous of reproducing. At *GA* I.13, 720a11–13, Aristotle dismisses this possibility in a few words:

Ἐπεὶ οὖν δεῖ καὶ τοὺς τῶν ἀρρένων πόρους τοὺς σπερματικοὺς ἐρηρεῖσθαι καὶ μὴ πλανᾶσθαι καὶ τοῖς θήλεσι τὰς ὑστέρας.

Since, therefore, the seminal passages in males must indeed be anchored in place and not roam around, so also must be the uterus in females.[160]

---

[158] Rudberg 1911, pp. 12–17, has a more detailed list of parallel passages. I am not arguing, as Rudberg was, that the author of *Non Gen.* was aiming at a synthesis of Hippocratic theories. I simply aim to demonstrate that many of his concerns fit in with the mainstream in fifth- and fourth-century BCE Greek medical thinking. A full examination of the relationship of *Non Gen.* to the Hippocratic gynecology is for another study.

[159] See Hanson 1991, pp. 81–7; Dean-Jones 1994, pp. 69–77; King 1998, p. 36 and pp. 222–4.

[160] At *HA* III.4, 515a2–5, Aristotle notes the attachment of the uterus to blood vessels.

Other than this Aristotle makes no reference to uterine displacement. Balme 1985, p. 198, sees this as a similarity with *HA* X and uses it as part of the argument for Aristotelian authorship. He also argues that the common view that "the uterus moves about casually and is merely a receptacle within which the male seed develops" was "strangely ignored in *GA*" because Aristotle had refuted it in *HA* X.[161] However, the only refutation of the "Wandering Womb" in *Non Gen.* occurs at 634a2 when the author states:

> δεῖ δὴ τὴν ἔχουσαν καλῶς ὑστέραν πρῶτον μὲν τῷ τόπῳ μὴ ἐν ἄλλῳ καὶ ἄλλῳ εἶναι ἀλλ᾽ ὁμοίως τῇ θέσει.

> Indeed, the womb which is in a good condition should not first be in one place and then in another but should remain in the same position.

The modality and the fact that the statement is restricted to healthy wombs leans more to a belief in the possibility of displacement than otherwise. The statement is too enigmatic to be conclusive, but it is possible that once again we are looking at the results of Aristotle's selection in his summarizing. He does not need dialectical arguments to refute the "Wandering Womb." This would be best achieved in his *Dissections.*

(d) Lack of concern with blocked passages

To a large extent then, the author of *Non Gen.* saw the same sorts of conditions hampering conception as the authors of the Hippocratic Corpus. These authors can differ among themselves. For example, *Nat. Puer.* 12 (VII.486.2) and *Mul.* II.162 (VIII.338.15–16) appear to advocate activity to promote mingling of male and female seed after coition; *Mul.* I.11 (VIII.46.14) and *Steril.* 220 (VIII.424.16–21) quietude. One author appears to recognize uterine contractions as part of labor pains, *Mul.* I.34 (VIII.80.3–5), but is unique in this. But the gynecological

---

[161] Balme 1991, p. 29.

treatises are to a great extent uniform in their approach to the female body and problems of infertility.[162] We have seen that *Non Gen.* differs from the other Hippocratic works that evince a belief in female seed in distinguishing it from both menses and the vaginal lubricant. The author's belief that female *sperma* is deposited at the mouth of the womb by a *kaulos* which mirrors the function of a penis leads to his omitting any reference to one of the major causes of failure to conceive recognized in the Hippocratic Corpus—the blockage of a woman's passages.

The Hippocratics believed that the flow of a woman's seed to her womb could be impeded by the congestion of the passages in her body.[163] *Steril.* 213 (VIII.412.13) identifies one cause for failure to conceive as the passages in a woman's body being filled with blood so that they cannot receive the seed, αἱ γὰρ φλέβες τοῦ αἵματος πλήρεις ἐοῦσαι τὴν γονὴν οὐ δέχονται. The γονή in question is clearly the woman's because the man's γονή is received by the womb, not the passages of a woman's body. There were those who argued that the *sperma* was drawn from all over the body during sexual intercourse, citing as proof the pleasurable warmth and tingling felt all over the body just prior to ejaculation.[164] Others believed that *sperma* was drawn from the body at an earlier point and stored in the brain ready for rapid deployment to the genitals.[165] Evidence for passages connecting the head to the womb came from the fact that at puberty, when the fertile *sperma* began to appear in the genital area, hair also began to grow there, and as men begin to engage in sex, hair grows on their chins and chests, areas in which the

---

[162] See Flemming 2013.

[163] For more on female infertility and the treatments for it in Hippocratic medicine, see Hanson 1991 pp. 81–7; Dean-Jones 1992; Demand 1994, pp. 17–18; King 1998, pp. 140–1; Flemming 2013.

[164] *Genit.* 1 (VII.470.7–8).

[165] *Aër.* 22 (II.76.12–82.5), *Nat. Puer.* 20 (VII.506.13–510.17), Diocles 41a and b (van der Eijk 2000, pp. 84–7). *Nat. Mul.* 10 (VII.326.4–5) suggests a belief in this when the author identifies a non-irritant white flux emanating from the uterus as originating in the brain.

sperma settled on its way down the body from brain to genitals. The theory did not need to concern itself with the relative
lack of body hair in women; it merely stated that women had
weaker *sperma* and less of it, and did not become as agitated
during sex as men. Whatever the assumed origin of the *sperma*,
one of the first steps a Hippocratic would take in treating a
woman for infertility would be to fumigate her to make sure her
passages were open so that her *sperma* could reach her womb
and mingle with the man's.

When fumigation was diagnostic and its efficacy depended
on the doctor ascertaining what he could smell on the woman's
breath or hair, he had to ensure that the smell could not reach
his nose by any route other than through the woman's body.
Most commonly the doctor was instructed simply to insert in
the woman's vagina a strong-smelling pessary or suppository
soaked in some aromatic substance. The pessaries were left in
the vagina for an extended period of time (sometimes a day,[166]
sometimes overnight,[167] but often unspecified) for the duration
of which the woman was told to keep still; then the doctor tested
to see if he could smell the substance on the woman's breath or,
sometimes, on a linen cloth which had been wrapped around
her hair at the beginning of the procedure.[168] If he could smell
the substance, any problem the woman had in conceiving did
not come from the blockage of her passages. If her breath or
hair was odorless, however, there was some obstruction that
needed to be removed before conception could take place. This
diagnostic test for infertility is mentioned by Aristotle at *GA*
II.7, 747a7–14. Sometimes a doctor adopted a more elaborate
procedure of fumigation which necessitated sitting a woman
over aromatic ingredients which were heated to give off a
vapor. In these cases the doctor is directed to wrap the woman

---

[166] *Mul.* I.75 (VIII.162.3).
[167] *Steril.* 214 and 219 (VIII. 414.20–1 and 424.4–6); *Nat. Mul.* 96 (VII.412.19–
20).
[168] *Mul.* I.78 (VIII.178.15–17).

in a cloak, again to trap all the vapor.[169] In one case the doctor is instructed to order the woman to keep her mouth closed.[170] A more invasive way to ensure that the odor could only go upwards through the woman was to lead the smoke from the fumigation directly into the woman's body. This could be done by covering the vessel in which the fumigation was placed with the top half of a gourd, the tapering end of which had been trimmed to fit into the woman's vagina.[171] A yet more invasive strategy was to lead the vapor directly into the womb by means of a reed inserted into the cervix.[172]

Hippocratic gynecology is filled with references to this type of practice and the conditions that could necessitate it. *Non Gen.*, at least as we have it, does not discuss therapy, but if it did there would be no need for this sort of procedure because while the author believed the *sperma* was drawn from a woman's body, he did not believe that the passages through which it passed were connected to the womb or involved with the conveying of menstrual blood. The καυλός through which female seed was deposited before the womb was a dedicated *iter*.[173]

It is particularly this latter point which may account for Aristotle's use of the treatise as an *endoxon* for dialectic. Other medical writers assume that a woman contributes *sperma* like a man to conception, but it could easily be argued that their therapies for infertility focused more on establishing regular healthy menstruation, and this could be squared quite easily with a belief that menses was a woman's only contribution to

---

[169] *Aph.* V 59 (IV.554.3–6); *Mul.* I 51 (VIII.110.9); *Mul.* II 114, 126, 134 and 146 (VIII.246.17–18, 272.5, 302.20–1 and 322.11); *Nat. Mul.* 34 (VII.374.16).

[170] *Mul.* II 126 (VIII.272.7).

[171] *Loc.* 47 (VI.346.13–15); *Nat. Mul.* 61 (VII.398.19–400.2); *Steril* 222 (VIII.430.17–19). See E. Craik, *Places in Man* (Oxford 1998), pp. 226–7.

[172] *Steril* 221 and 230 (VIII.428.4–6 and 440.11).

[173] Though it should be noted that fumigations from each of these procedures except the last could permeate through the body to the head if this *iter* itself ramified throughout the body. However, as it is said to carry only the *ekptôsis* and *pneuma*, it is not clear what would block it, and in the Hippocratic Corpus no therapy is ever directed at the *kaulos*.

conception. *Non Gen.*'s insistence that female *sperma* was essential to conception, different from menses, was more of a challenge. Aristotle does not address *Non Gen.*'s description of the anatomy of the *kaulos* because once he has dispensed with the possibility of a third female seminal secretion in addition to menses and the vaginal lubricant he has no need to argue against a dedicated path for its delivery, and once again the non-existence of such a path would be best demonstrated by dissection.

(e) Organization

Non Gen. also differs from many treatises in the Hippocratic Corpus, especially the gynecology, in the extent of its organization. This is in part due to the fact that many of the gynecological treatises are compilations.[174] *Genit.* & *Nat. Puer.* and *Sept./ Oct.* seem to be single-authored and are more cohesive because their subject matter lends itself to a natural progression. *Mul.* I. has a rough progression in that the first nine chapters deal with menstrual disorders and the next fifteen with causes of infertility.[175] Much of the material in these first twenty-four chapters is rehearsed briefly in the first chapter of *Steril.* (chapter 213), and it is this material that corresponds most closely to that of *Non Gen.* However, in *Non Gen.*, the conditions are presented as if they should be considered in a particular order. Chapter 2 opens with a reference back to Chapter 1, καὶ πρῶτον ταῦτα σκεπτέον εἰ καλῶς ἔχει, μετὰ δὲ ταῦτα... Chapter 3 begins with a reference to Chapter 2, περὶ μὲν οὖν τὸ στόμα τῶν ὑστερῶν ἐκ τούτων ἡ σκέψις ἐστίν... Chapter 4 is introduced as an addendum, κωλύονται δὲ καί..., listing a few remaining conditions that could cause infertility before the author summarizes all the previous chapters and introduces his theory of ἰσοδρομῆσαι,

---

[174] See above, p. 17, n. 30.

[175] He then progresses to problems during pregnancy (chapters 25–34), during lochial bleeding (35–41), postpartum problems (42–56), general uterine problems (57–73), and a long list of therapies (74–109), but there is no clear organizing principle within these sections.

ὅσαις δὲ τούτων μηδὲν ἐμπόδιον ἦ ἀλλ' ἔχουσιν ὃν τρόπον δεῖν εἴρηται ἔχειν... Chapter 5 covers a number of conditions which a couple might think signal infertility but do not.[176]

In both *Mul.* I and *Steril.* (and *Mul.* II and *Nat. Mul.* where there is overlap) the authors present the conditions from a much more pathological viewpoint. As presented in *Non Gen.*, the woman could be suffering most of the conditions described without any obvious health problems other than infertility. The author needs this to be the case, because although he has ordered his text as if every other possible cause needed to be eliminated before the issue of the simultaneous emission of *sperma* was broached, in actual practice one would assume that this would be one of the first questions he would ask of an apparently healthy woman who was trying and failing to conceive. If the woman answered that yes, she and her husband were climaxing together, it would be then that the author would turn to other possible causes without having to abandon his theory of ἰσοδρομῆσαι; simultaneity would be necessary but not sufficient. One can imagine, though, that often the answer would be that no, she and her husband did not have simultaneous orgasms. Even with the best will in the world on all sides, this circumstance would not be easily tractable. This fact, compounded by all the other reasons the author gives for why a healthy woman might not conceive, could be deployed to explain why a woman remained infertile even under expert treatment.

It is intriguing to compare *Non Gen.* to the organization Leith sees in the group of medical papyri known as "medical cate-chisms" which deal with disease entities and are organized in a question and answer format.[177] He notes that these proceed under five headings: definition, cause, signs, differentiation, and therapy. The earliest of these medical catechisms dates to the second century BCE (though most of them are later, falling in the second and third centuries CE), and Leith traces the origin

---

[176] Of course, the chapter breaks are not original to the text.
[177] Leith 2009.

of this format to the Aristotelian methodology outlined in the *Topics* and the *Posterior Analytics*, though he does not believe they are related directly to the Aristotelian dialectical method.[178]

In looking for parallels to this organization in earlier medical literature Leith notes that in the Hippocratic Corpus "there does not appear to be a conception of disease which would be fully capable of being described in terms of these various topics."[179] Diocles of Carystus wrote a treatise *Pathos, Aitia, Therapeia* which promises a separation in the discussion of disease, cause, and therapy in a non-Hippocratic way, and the longest fragment we have from that work, frag. 109 (quoted by Galen), does indeed list the signs of a form of melancholia before describing the causes, though, in the extant fragment, it does not define the disease.[180]

Non Gen. is not as clearly organized as the medical catechisms, but like Diocles' work it does show more organization than the Hippocratic treatises. The treatise opens with a bald statement of the three broad <u>causes</u> of a couple's failure to reproduce, but follows this immediately with a <u>definition</u> of a sort, though more of the healthy womb than the diseased one. The author says "a womb is healthy which does not cause pain and satisfactorily carries out its proper function, and after its functions is neither incapacitated nor fatigued." The author then proceeds to outline the information that can be gleaned about the health of the womb from <u>signs</u> given by its menstrual discharges. After this he lists <u>different</u> ways in which the womb can be unhealthy with signs from the state of the *stoma*, a woman's night emissions, etc. As has been noted, there are no sections on therapy, but this could be attributable to the specifically semiotic nature

---

[178] Leith 2009, pp. 112–16. In this he is following the lead of Mansfeld 1990 and 1992 and Runia 1999, who identified Aristotle's method as the model for Aetius' *Placita*. It should be noted that Leith does not consider the medical questions in the *Problêmata* to be comparable to the method in the medical papyri because the questions in the *Problêmata* differ in scope, structure, content, and purpose from the headings in the papyri, p. 117, n. 23.

[179] Leith 2009, p. 117.   [180] Ibid.

of the original treatise or to Aristotle's lack of interest in engaging with that part of the treatise.

This arrangement of material is not so methodical as to be derived from a dialectical form, but it suggests that medical treatises of the second half of the fourth century BCE were becoming more logically organized without the influence of the Lyceum and were perhaps another influence on the development of the medical catechism.

7 STYLE

(a) Scholarly opinions

That *Non Gen.* was originally a treatise written by somebody other than Aristotle at a date prior to that of *GA* and summarized by him as an *endoxon* for a dialectic on female *sperma* has been established on the basis of content alone. It is difficult, and may be impossible, to come to any definitive conclusions about how similar or dissimilar the style of *HA* X is to the rest of Aristotle's oeuvre. Scaliger thought its diction and style were entirely Aristotelian, "dicendi ratio et stilus ipse…omnino illius est,"[181] while Spengel rejected it out of hand, saying that parts of it were completely alien not only to Aristotle but to the Greek language, "aut a graeca lingua aut ab Aristotelis dictione omnino aliena."[182] Rudberg believed not only the theories but also the style of *HA* X vacillated between Hippocrates and Aristotle, "Auch Ausdrücke und formelhafte Wendungen erinnern bald an Hippokrates, bald an Aristoteles,"[183] and both he and Louis generate lists of lexical and other disparities between the treatise and other works of Aristotle.[184] But these do not necessarily carry much weight either for those supporting or

---

[181] Rudberg 1911, p. 2.
[182] He goes so far as to argue that *HA* X is a back translation from Guil.'s mid-thirteenth-century Latin translation (see Louis 1969, p. 152, n. 1).
[183] Rudberg 1911, p. 24.
[184] Rudberg 1911, pp. 26–46; Louis 1964, pp. 151–2.

those challenging Aristotelian authorship. Balme remarks "almost every treatise of Aristotle in its extant form exhibits a quota of idiosyncratic lexeis, while the occasional lapse into popular syntax...is seen in major treatises whose authenticity cannot be doubted without doubting most of Aristotle," and in lodging her objections to Balme's thesis, Föllinger states that she agrees with these comments.[185] Of course, if my hypothesis is correct this farrago of diction is what we might expect and it might seem to render moot any discussion of style. We simply say the bits that look Aristotelian in the first five chapters are Aristotle's own phrasing in the summarization and the bits that are not are the original words of *Non Gen*. To some extent this is true, but there are still important points to be made.

(b) Aristotle as summarizer

The first is to ratify the conclusion made on the basis of the content of the *Dialectic* that Aristotle himself and not some later Peripatetic is the summarizer of *Non Gen*. A survey of vocabulary alone will not suffice as it was the medley of vocabulary which led Rudberg to assert the treatise was the work of a "Kompilator" synthesizing Hippocratic and Aristotelian theories. However, embedded within the non-Aristotelian vocabulary and theories we find apparently innocuous expressions that are exclusively, or almost exclusively, Aristotelian.[186] These include:

- λέγεται δὲ καί...ἀλλὰ μὴν, 633b25...27. This locution is used by Aristotle 27 times to introduce statements that may seem a little outlandish, e.g., that bears' guts grow together during hibernation (*HA* VII(VIII).17, 600b9), that a swarm of bees will carry the king bee if he grows tired (*HA* VIII(IX).40,

---

[185] Balme 1985, p. 193; Föllinger 1996, p. 147. Van der Eijk, 1999, p. 499, agrees that arguments on style are inconclusive.
[186] Unless noted, the expressions occur in works generally considered to be genuinely by Aristotle.

624a29), that a young horse committed suicide after being tricked into mating with his mother (*HA* VIII(IX).47, 631a1). The speed of dolphins is introduced with this clause at *HA* VIII(IX).48, 631a20 and is explicitly said to be ἄπιστα. Rudberg claims that λέγεται with the accusative and infinitive, while common in Attic, is not frequent in Aristotle,[187] but this is not the case, at least with the formulation λέγεται δὲ καὶ. ἀλλὰ μὴν is also one of Aristotle's favorite phrases; see Bonitz 1955, p. 33. It appears 13 times in the *GA*, often to introduce objections to some theory that Aristotle thinks is clearly mistaken, e.g., at I.18, 722a35, it is used after Aristotle states that if *sperma* is drawn from parts of a body it must be drawn from the elements not the assemblage. He then immediately adds ἀλλὰ μὴν ἄνευ γε ταύτης οὐκ ἂν εἴη ὅμοια, "But surely, without this <the assemblage> they <the parts> would not be similar <to the parent>." Sometimes Aristotle has already distanced himself from the theory under discussion by explicitly attributing it to somebody else. At *GA* IV.1, 764a23–5, after declaring Democritus' statement about sexual differentiation in the embryo superior to Empedocles', he adds: "But surely, if heat and coldness were the cause of the difference in the parts, this ought to have been said by those who hold the former <theory> (i.e., Empedocles')" ἀλλὰ μὴν κἂν εἰ τῶν μορίων τῆς διαφορᾶς αἴτιον ἡ θερμότης καὶ ἡ ψυχρότης, τοῦτο λεκτέον ἦν τοῖς ἐκείνως λέγουσιν. At *Non Gen.* 633b25, ἀλλὰ μὴν[188] introduces the objection to the statement introduced by λέγεται δὲ καὶ. It should be noted that despite ἀλλὰ μὴν being so prevalent in the *GA* and many other treatises of Aristotle[189] it does not appear at all in the first nine books of the *HA* and in Book X only here, if my emendation is accepted, and at 637b11 in Chapter 6. The

---

[187] Rudberg 1911, p. 37.
[188] See commentary ad loc. for support of this reading.
[189] E.g., 11 times in *De an.*, and 73 times in *Met.* It does not appear at all in *Ath. Pol.*

possible significance of this will be dealt with in the notes ad loc.

- ἐστι δ᾽ ὥσπερ...οὕτω καὶ...ὁμοίως δὲ καὶ, 633b18, 23, 30. Aristotle uses ἐστι δ᾽ (or δὲ) ὥσπερ 9 times in addition to this occurrence. The only author who uses this phrase before Aristotle is Xenophon, at *Eq.* 4.2. Theophrastus uses it 5 times. Other than that, the expression is not used again until the first century BCE. Moreover of the 9 other times Aristotle uses the phrase it is followed 3 times by either οὕτω καὶ, ὁμοίως δὲ καὶ, or both, as in this text. Theophrastus does not use these terms after ἐστι δὲ ὥσπερ.

- ἐκ τῶνδε φανερόν, 634a5. This phrase is not used by anybody before Aristotle, who uses it 12 times in his corpus in addition to here. Speusippus uses it once, Theophrastus twice, and thereafter it is used only by commentators on Aristotle. It is used here to refer to the movement of the uterus towards the opening of the vaginal canal to aid conception and its withdrawal afterwards. Aristotle recognizes this phenomenon elsewhere in his biology.

- ἀνάγκη γὰρ καὶ, 634a29. This expression occurs only 9 times before the first century BCE, once in the Hippocratic *Morb. Sacr.* and 8 times in Aristotle, including here and once in *Aud.* In this passage Aristotle is acknowledging that one of the causes of sterility in women, putrefied menses, will have been preceded by other pathological signs which he does not detail but which would have been listed in most other gynecological texts of the period.

- τε γὰρ, 636a4. τε γὰρ without an answering τε or καί is a very uncommon juxtaposition of particles. It is generally emended away. It appears most frequently in Aristotle, of which Denniston allows five cases to be certain (*APo.* I.9, 75b41, *De an.* I.2, 405a4, *PA* III.1, 661b29, *Pol.* VI.2, 1318b33, and VII.13, 1333a2). It is used at 636a4 in the very un-Aristotelian argument that both the womb and the woman's whole body can draw in by *pneuma* the *sperma* she emits at the culmination of erotic dreams.

- ὥσπερ πρότερον εἴρηται, 636a5. Apart from this occurrence, this locution appears only at *Poet.* 7, 1450b13, Theophrastus *HP* I.22, and Asclepius' commentary on Aristotle's *Metaphysics*.[190] This is a reference back to 634b34, where it is asserted that the uterus draws in *sperma* by *pneuma*, like the nostrils, something Aristotle denies at *GA* II.4, 739b9–20.

- σημεῖον δὲ καὶ 636a37. Other than here, this phrase appears 17 times in the Aristotelian Corpus (including once in the spurious *Problêmata*) and 12 times in Theophrastus. Other than a couple of uses in the first century BCE it is not used again until the Aristotelian commentators of the second century CE. Here it is used to discuss signs that show the *stoma* does not have growths upon it, with which Aristotle would probably agree.

- εἴπερ γὰρ καὶ, 636b15. Other than one use by Antiphon, nobody uses this expression before Aristotle. In the Aristotelian Corpus it appears here and 3 other times. It is not used again before the first century CE. Here it is used after a definitive statement that failure to keep pace with one's partner during intercourse means a couple will be infertile. This is one of the tenets of *Non Gen.* that Aristotle expressly argues against in *GA*. After the definitive positive statement, the phrase εἴπερ γὰρ καὶ introduces the woman's contribution to the *sperma*, which has not been doubted in the treatise up to this point, as a hypothetical.

There are probably other exclusively Aristotelian expressions scattered throughout the first five chapters of *HA* X, but these are enough to show that only Aristotle could have been the author of those chapters, and that Aristotelian expressions frequently occur in relation to content to which he would not himself assent.[191]

---

[190] It is also restored in a papyrus fragment of the fourth century CE biblical commentator Didymus Caecus.

[191] In modern Bayesian analysis of literary style, "function words" such as these expressions are often used in attributing disputed works to authors.

Continuing to leave specific examples of vocabulary to one side, it is much more difficult to identify seemingly innocuous expressions or phrases that Aristotle must have borrowed from another author to suggest where he was copying *Non Gen.*'s words verbatim, but there are some possibilities. Rudberg discusses fifty places in the text of *HA* X which he believes show grammatical anomalies.[192] These include issues such as Ionic forms, free exchange of singular for plural, anacolutha, variation between present and gnomic aorist, unusual word order, use of plural verb with neuter plural subjects, prolepsis, periphrasis, omission of ἄν, and present indicative after ἐάν. Balme remarks "every breach of classical rules in *HA* X can be paralleled <in Aristotle>,"[193] but we are discussing fifty apparent solecisms in a very short treatise vs. the whole of the rest of Aristotle's corpus. Forty-three of the alleged transgressions occur in the eight Bekker columns that comprise *Non Gen.* and only seven in the three that make up the *topos* and *Dialectic.* This discrepancy, calculated as it is in the work of a scholar who had no concept of a division in the treatise, buttresses my claim that there is a difference in original authorship between the two parts of the treatise. I list some of the more significant discrepancies here.

- θεραπείας δέονται, 634a11. This phrase (or δέονται θεραπείας) occurs 3 more times in *Non Gen.*, at 634a34, 634b7, and 635b26, and once in the *Dialectic* at 637b29, where Aristotle appears to be paraphrasing the passage around 635b26.[194] The phrase

---

Function words "are words with very little contextual meaning... The logic behind using function words is that writers do not necessarily think about the way they use these words. Rather these words flow unconsciously from the mind to the paper. Therefore, the usage of function words should be invariant under changes of topic," Peng and Hengartner 2002, p. 176.

[192] Rudberg 1911, pp. 33–40. Louis 1969, p. 151, n. 6. cites six examples of "constructions insolites," none of them in the *Dialectic.*

[193] Balme 1989, p. 27.

[194] The phrase is restored in a fragment of the fourth-century BCE orator Hyperides.

does not appear again until Galen, after which it becomes a common phrase in medical and pseudo-medical writing.

- σημαίνουσι δεόμεναι, 634a21. Although σημαίνω is a very common verb in Aristotle, it is never used in this middle sense where the subject of the verb is also the subject of the participle. In fact, this is one of the usages that Spengel considers completely alien to the Greek language, but as Rudberg says, it is not difficult to understand what is meant and there is a similar construction in Xenophon's *Hell.* 6.2.34.[195]

- (τὰ καταμήνια) μεταβάλλωσι, 634b1. It is not unheard of for Aristotle to use a plural verb with a neuter plural subject, but within the confines of *HA* X this occurs almost exclusively in *Non Gen.*, and particularly in this passage on menstruation in health and sickness (ἄρχονται, b18, ἀπολήγονται, b20, ἔχουσιν, b24), but also in the passage discussing σπάσμα (γίνονται, 636a29).[196] The neuter plural subject περιττώματα takes a plural verb in the *Dialectic* at 638b22 (ὦσιν) and b24 (ἐπισπῶνται) in a passage that returns to the clinical nature of *Non Gen.*

- ἡ γυνὴ προΐεται...ἐξονειρώττωσιν...αὐταῖς...συνεγίνετο...προΐωνται, 634b30–2. This rapid switching between singular and plural in reference to a woman occurs in the same passage as the four examples of neuter plural subjects governing plural verb forms. A similar rapid switch is seen at 634a39 (τὰς εὐφυεῖς) and 634b1 (προσεξαμαρτάνῃ αὕτη).

- τῷ μὲν μὴ εὐθὺς ἀνεστομῶσθαι, 635a18–19. This is just one of a number of strange uses of the articular infinitive in *Non Gen.* See also 635a23, τοῦ μὴ εὐθὺς συμπίπτειν, 636b13, τοῦ δὲ πρὸς ἄλλους μὴ συνδρόμως ἔχειν. Elsewhere in the treatise, as is more common in the rest of the Aristotelian Corpus, Aristotle introduces the genitive of the articular infinitive by the term σημεῖον (ἐστι), e.g., 636a26, 32, and 37.

- In ancient Greek the womb could be referred to either by the singular or plural of the word ὑστέρα without any

---

[195] Rudberg 1911, p. 38.
[196] And perhaps also at 637a18 if Scaliger's conjecture ἕλκονται is accepted, as it is by most editors.

difference or nuance of meaning. Both the medical authors and Aristotle can alternate between the two in the same paragraph. In *HA* I–IX Aristotle uses the singular almost twice as often as the plural and in the *GA* he uses the singular form 76 times and the plural 54. In *Non Gen.* the singular is used 19 times, the plural 16 times. However, in three extended passages in which the womb is under discussion but the noun itself does not appear (634a4–12, 17–21; 635b5–14) the author of *Non Gen.* uses plural forms of verbs and adjectives throughout. In contrast, when the actual term ὑστέρα is absent he uses a singular form to refer to the womb on only two brief occasions, 634b38 (ἐχούσης) and 635b15–16 (θιγγανομένης...αὐτῆς). In the *Dialectic*, on the other hand, the singular form of the word is used 14 times, the plural only twice, once when Aristotle is paraphrasing *Non Gen.* Chapter 5 (637a15–17), and once in what is possibly a genuinely plural context (638b6). In addition a plural participle is used at 638a22 to refer to the womb (ἐχούσαις). The preference in the *Dialectic* clearly differs from that in *Non Gen.* and in showing a decided preference for the singular form is more in line with the rest of the *HA* and *GA*.[197] Moreover, there is no passage in either the *HA* or *GA* involving an extended discussion of the womb that omits the actual noun as there is in *Non Gen.* 634a4–12, 17–21, and 635b5–14. Rather, Aristotle often seems to repeat the term excessively when it would have been perhaps more natural to use a pronoun, e.g., *GA* II.7, 745b26, 31, 33, 34, and 35; III.2, 754a1, 4, 5, and 7; III.3, 754b10, 13, 14, 17, 18, 26, 28, 30, and 32. The same tendency can be seen in the *Dialectic* at 637b35–638a2 and 638a26–35.

- In *HA* IX(VII).2, 582b24 and *GA* II.4, 739a31 Aristotle refers to the descent of the uterus down the vaginal canal that is

---

[197] Although, as I say, there is no difference in nuance between the two terms in Greek, I have translated the plural form as "uterus" and the singular as "womb" to mark this preferential difference in the two parts of the treatise.

necessary if the uterus is to draw in the male semen. In both passages he uses, not surprisingly, the term καταβαίνω. *Non Gen.* also discusses this phenomenon in 634a3 but uses the phrase γίγνεσθαι τὸ πορρώτερον. The return of the uterus to its original position in the *HA* IX(VII) passage is explained as ἀπέρχονται πάλιν εἰς τὸν ἄνω τόπον τὸν οἰκεῖον, but in *Non Gen.* as ἐπανιέναι πορρωτέρω.[198] The use of πορρωτέρω is reminiscent of the Hippocratic use of πρόσω at *Mul.* I.2 (VIII.14.14 and 20) to describe the *stoma* moving down the vagina.

It is hard to say conclusively that any of these traits derive from the original *Non Gen.* Some or all of them could be the result of Aristotle paying less attention to standard grammar because he was summarizing for himself.[199] Clusterings of anomalies, such as neuter plural verbs with neuter plural subjects, are perhaps more significant, especially if they coincide with non-Aristotelian vocabulary.

(c) Vocabulary

Rudberg's list covering vocabulary, grammar, and stylistics runs to twenty pages. Most of his comments are on vocabulary, and Louis, too, remarks, "c'est essentiellement son

---

[198] See commentary ad loc. for a discussion of the same term being used to signify opposite directions.

[199] It may seem anachronistic to imagine Aristotle taking notes for himself, but the language of *Top.* I.14, 105b12–17, suggests something along these lines. "One should also collect premises from written works, and create outlines about each type, putting them down independent of one another, e.g., about good or about animal (and about every type of good), starting from what it is. One should also make note of the opinions of each authority, e.g., that Empedocles said that the elements of bodies were four in number" ἐκλέγειν δὲ χρὴ καὶ ἐκ τῶν γεγραμμένων λόγων, τὰς δὲ διαγραφὰς ποιεῖσθαι περὶ ἑκάστου γένους ὑποτιθέντας χωρίς, οἷον περὶ ἀγαθοῦ ἢ περὶ ζῴου, καὶ περὶ ἀγαθοῦ παντός, ἀρξάμενον ἀπὸ τοῦ τί ἐστιν. παρασημαίνεσθαι δὲ καὶ τὰς ἑκάστων δόξας, οἷον ὅτι Ἐμπεδοκλῆς τέτταρα ἔφησε τῶν σωμάτων στοιχεῖα εἶναι.

vocabulaire qui se distingue de celui d'Aristote."²⁰⁰ His list is shorter than Rudberg's, contains very few words not included by Rudberg, and is not categorized, so I shall use Rudberg's list in my survey. In the following comparisons it should be taken into account that *Non Gen.* is nearly three times as long as the *Dialectic*.

a) Absolute *hapax legomena*

Of 6 *hapax legomena* found nowhere else in Greek, 5 occur in *Non Gen.* and 1 in the *Dialectic* (ἀφυγραίνεσθαι, 637b29). The *hapax* in *Non Gen.* sometimes fulfill a clear medical need: διαθιγγάνεσθαι (634a9) expresses the excessive nature of the contact; διαστομοῦσθαι (635a9 and 15) differentiates the "opening up" of the cervix from the "opening up" of the uterus; ἵδρωμα (635b19) refers to a bodily exudate similar, but not identical, to sweat; or they are unobjectionable compounds: προσσπαστικός (635a25, b3, 636a7); σπερμοποιεῖν (636b34).²⁰¹

b) Aristotelian *hapax legomena*

Of words which may be common elsewhere in Attic but are *hapax* for Aristotle, 14 are in *Non Gen.* and 7 in the *Dialectic*. Many of these are medical terms, e.g., ἄνοσμος, 634b19, ἐφυγραίνεσθαι, 635b35 and 636a2, πεπλανημένως, 634a13 and 17, φλεγματικός, 634a26. This is equally true of most of the Aristotelian *hapax* in the *Dialectic*, e.g., ἀνόσως, 635b39, ἐπιφλεγμαίνειν, 638a33, εὐσταλής, 638b31. One particularly interesting *hapax* in the *Dialectic* is ἐπιμηνίων referring to menses at 638b17, notably in a context describing a medical condition which many doctors mistakenly identify as mole. Aristotle discusses menstruation a lot in his biological works and he almost always refers to it as καταμήνια, as he does throughout most of *HA* X. The Hippocratics use both καταμήνια and ἐπιμήνια with

---

roughly equal frequency. As van der Eijk remarks (1999, p. 493) in arguing for Aristotelian authorship for the whole treatise, the occurrence of more medical language than is normal for an Aristotelian treatise could be accounted for by "the possibility that Aristotle, within another, more specialized and technical framework, may have gone into far greater medical detail." The occurrence of expressly medical vocabulary then does not in and of itself suggest that Aristotle was summarizing rather than composing *Non Gen.*, though the appearance of the *hapax* ἐπιμήνια in a medical context in the *Dialectic* is suggestive.

(c) Rare words in Aristotle

Of the thirty words which Rudberg classifies as rare elsewhere in Aristotle only four occur in the *Dialectic*, and all could be taken to have medical import, ἐξονειρωγμῷ (637b27 and 28), ἀσθενήματος (638a37), πλήρωμα (638b2) (which occurs in *Non Gen.* (636a30)), and σχέσις in the sense of cessation of menses (638b17). The latter two words occur in the Hippocratic Corpus, as do about half of the other "rare" words. However, there are some less specialized words in *Non Gen.* which argue for summarization of another author rather than free composition of a medical text by Aristotle.

- One of the most suggestive is not included in Rudberg's list. In addition to καταμήνια and ἐπιμήνια the Hippocratics use the term τὰ γυναικεῖα for menses. This term occurs 4 times in *Non Gen.*, at 634b12, 635a8 and 14, and 636a39. Elsewhere in Aristotle it occurs 4 times in the space of one Bekker page at *HA* IX(VII).1–2, 582a10 and 34, b20 and 24. It also occurs in *PA* II.2, 648a31 when Aristotle is discussing the theories of Parmenides and Empedocles. In *GA* it is only used in the genitive to modify another noun, τῆς τῶν γυναικείων περιττώσεως at *GA* II.4, 739a27, and τὴν τῶν γυναικείων ἀπόκρισιν at *GA* III.1, 751a1. Given that καταμήνια, his preferred word for menses, is a bona fide medical term, it seems unlikely that Aristotle would use τὰ γυναικεῖα in free composition.

- When discussing spasm in infants at *HA* IX(VII).12, 588a3 and 11, Aristotle uses the form σπασμός, the form also used at *Metr.* II.8, 366b26. The only other treatise in the Aristotelian Corpus which uses the form σπάσμα is the Pseudo-Aristotelian *Problêmata*, which uses it once but also uses σπασμός twice. The Hippocratics also overwhelmingly favor the masculine term over the neuter, so this is not simply a question of preferring medical terminology.

- Both the Hippocratics and Aristotle have a variety of words for pain, ἀλγηδών, ἄλγημα, ἄλγος, ἀνία, λύπη, ὀδύνη, πόνος. ὀδύνη is by far the most common in the Hippocratic Corpus, followed by πόνος, with ἄλγημα running a distant third. The least common of these in Aristotle is ἄλγημα, which, other than in *Non Gen.* at 635a12 (and twice in the *Problêmata*), occurs only in *HA* III.3, 512b18 and 25, when Aristotle is quoting almost verbatim a passage from the Hippocratic *Nat. Hom.* ὀδύνη and πόνος, on the other hand, both well established as medical words for pain, are relatively common in the Aristotelian Corpus. Again, it seems unlikely that Aristotle would use the word ἄλγημα if he were composing a treatise from scratch, even if it were a medical treatise.

- At *Non Gen.* 5, 636b17, 20, and 23 the author uses the very unusual word ἰσοδρομῆσαι to explain that in order for conception to take place the woman and man must "keep pace" with each other in their love-making. The only time Aristotle uses the word in his biological works is at *GA* I.19, 727b10, when he denies that the male and female "keeping pace" with one another has anything to do with whether or not the female gets pregnant. The only other time the word is used in the Aristotelian canon is in works generally agreed to be spurious: *de Mundo* 399a8, when the text is discussing planets which have an annual cycle like the sun rather than a monthly one like the moon, and twice in the *Problêmata* at XVI.3, 913a38 and XVI.12, 915b10, both occurrences discussing why when bodies of unequal weight are thrown the heavier part moves in a straight line but the lighter part revolves. When Aristotle wishes to discuss complementarity in male and female contributions to conception, he uses the term and concept of συμμετρία, e.g., *GA* I.19, 727b10, IV.2, 767a16, IV.4, 772a17. When he does use a term to refer to fluid streams flowing together, it recalls the language of *Mul.* I.17 (VIII.56.22), ὁμόρρους, at *GA* III.11, 763b3.

The upshot of this is that apart from the second category, about four-fifths of the non-Aristotelian vocabulary occurs in the less than three-quarters of the treatise comprised by *Non Gen.* Of itself this is not significant. What is significant is that while much of this vocabulary seems to be of a medical nature, certain terms are used where there are medical terms available more in line with Aristotle's own usage and the rare terms often appear elsewhere in his oeuvre in contexts which suggest he is transmitting the theory of others.

While not rare terms in Aristotle, the deployment of the terms προίημι and ἀφίημι in *HA* X is worthy of note. When referring to the emission of *sperma* in both male and female *Non Gen.* always uses the verb προίημι; the author reserves the verb ἀφίημι for the discharge of menses, flatulences, and the results of unsuccessful conceptions (634a17, b5, 9, 635a20, b4, 5, 636a14, 636b5). In the rest of *HA* and *GA* Aristotle prefers προίημι to ἀφίημι for the emission of male *sperma*, but it is unclear that he ever uses the term for the emission of female *sperma*, apart from a reference at *GA* II.8, 748a22, to menses in horses and another at *GA* III.1, 751a19, to the behavior of humans and quadrupeds in heat, ὀργῶντα, and as we have seen (above pp. 36 and 57, n. 111), it is not clear that Aristotle actually equates this emission with a female's seminal contribution. In the rest of his biological works Aristotle uses ἀφίημι for the emission of *sperma* when it can refer equally to male and female, e.g., *HA* I.3, 489a9, 11; IX(VII).2, 583a5, though he does occasionally use the term specifically for the emission of male *sperma*, e.g., *HA* IX(VII).2, 583a5; *GA* I.4, 717b12; I.15, 720b30; IV.4, 772a10.

In the *Dialectic*, ἀφίημι is used of the male seminal emission at
637b36 and of the seminal emission of female birds at 637b14
and 15, though this may not be very significant since Aristotle
would equate this with a woman's menses. *Non Gen.*'s use of
προίημι and ἀφίημι then differs from that of Aristotle in the rest
of his biology and in the *Dialectic*.

It is impossible for any single lexical item to be certain
that Aristotle could not have used it, or used it that way, in
independent composition. However, the cumulative effect of
vocabulary choices, especially when combined with the discrepancies between the first five and last two chapters, suggests that a great deal of the diction of *HA* X originates in
the work of another author, just as Aristotle uses γονή to refer
to female seed when discussing the theories of Democritus
and Empedocles (see above, pp. 11–12, n. 21 and p. 16, n. 29).
Gershenson and Greenberg have argued that *Phys.* I.3, 186a32–
187a11, is an attempt to meet the Eleatics on their own terms
after Aristotle has already demolished their theories from his
own perspective. They say that among other differences the
argument in this passage "employs a different basic vocabulary," one that reflects Eleatic usage.[202]

There are a couple of terms in *Non Gen.*, though, that resonate
as Aristotelian technical terms: περίττωμα at 634b8 and εἶδος at
637a13.[203] Aristotle uses the term περίττωμα to signify any "useful residue" which is concocted from the surplus of nourishment after the body has derived what it needs. περίττωμα is not
found in the medical writings of the Hippocratic Corpus, but it
does appear in two fragments of the fifth–fourth-century BCE

---

[202] Gershenson and Greenberg 1962, p. 143. Much in Gershenson and
Greenberg's description of the latter passage reads as if Aristotle were
using an Eleatic text as an *endoxon* for a dialectic, though not first laying out
the *endoxon* before engaging with the *aporiai* Aristotle believes it presents.

[203] περίττωμα also occurs in the *Dialectic* at 638b20 and 26, also in the
context of the cessation of the menses because they are being "spent,"
καταναλίσκεσθαι, elsewhere.

historian and physician Ctesias,²⁰⁴ and it is likely to have had a non-technical meaning before Aristotle adopted it. εἶδος, of course, is a very common Greek word. Its use at 637a13 at first blush may seem to have a technical Aristotelian connotation in that it is used in accounting for multiple offspring resulting from one act of intercourse, which in *GA* IV.4, 771a17–772b11, Aristotle attributes to the father's *gonê* having the ability to instantiate several *archai* in the female seminal matter because of its level of heat relative to the amount of material.²⁰⁵ Assuming for the sake of argument that Aristotle would use the term εἶδος to signify the individual form of each offspring (rather than the species form), 637a13 would still not be a very precise way of deploying the term. In Aristotelian terms εἶδος + ὕλη, *hylê*, matter, produces an individual. εἶδος itself is not an individual. Saying that the homogenized *sperma* was "parcelled out in the case of each form," ἐφ᾿ ἑκάστου εἴδους ἐμερίζετο, suggests that the parceling out is what produced the forms, whereas in Aristotle's theory it is the instantiation of a form which parcels out the appropriate amount of matter. In *Non Gen.* εἶδος seems to be used with the non-technical sense of the separate body of each fetus. In their analysis of the "Eleatic" vocabulary of *Phys.* I.3, 186a32–187a11, Gershenson and Greenberg point out that certain terms that might be considered technical vocabulary in Aristotelian contexts are used without specialized meaning, e.g., συμβεβηκός. Whether περίττωμα and εἶδος originated in *Non Gen.* or were Aristotle's paraphrase of other terms, they cannot be used to argue for original Aristotelian authorship of *Non Gen.*²⁰⁶

---

²⁰⁴ The term also appears frequently in testimonia to the Presocratics and pseudo-Hippocratic writings.

²⁰⁵ In this passage Aristotle refers to the individuals as ἔμβρυα, ζῷα, or κυήματα, never εἴδη.

²⁰⁶ *Non Gen.* is more in line with Aristotelian usage than Hippocratic in preferring *sperma* over *gonê* and avoiding the term μήτρα/μήτραι for womb. Given the consistency of this usage throughout *Non Gen.*, it is more likely to have been the choice of the original author than a paraphrase of Aristotle's.

A third term which might be thought of as "Aristotelian" is πάθος, and Balme treats it as one by defining it in a note to 634a3 as "a condition that is not always present but occurs naturally, and may or may not be morbid."[207] But in this broad definition it is hardly restricted to Aristotle, and it is not surprising that it occurs in reference to both morbid and non-morbid conditions in *Non Gen.*, though its morbid sense is more common: morbid: 634a26 (inflammation), 28 (putrefied menses), 36, 38, and 40 (irregular menses), 635a3 and 5 (oblique *stoma*), 636a11, 13, and 24 (wind-pregnancy), 636b6 (closed *stoma*), 634a3 and 635b5 (necessity for a lack of πάθος in normal functioning); non-morbid: 635b18 and 26 (vaginal lubricant), 635b31 (good conditions for conception), 636a21 and 637a6 (pregnancy). In the *Dialectic* the only non-morbid use is for sexual excitement at 637b9; all other uses refer to uterine mole, 638a10, 18, 19, 36, 638b2, 4, 16, 18, 32.[208]

---

[207] Balme 1991, p. 479.

[208] The term occurs 18 times in *Non Gen.* and 10 times in the *Dialectic*. In the *Dialectic* at 637b25 we find the term παθήματα, the only appearance of the term in the *HA*, to refer to the relaxation and loss of strength women feel after a nocturnal emission, but the term appears nowhere in *Non Gen.* Bonitz 1870, p. 554, says that there was no discernible difference between Aristotelian usage of πάθημα and πάθος except that he prefers πάθος in every number and case except genitive plural, "inter πάθημα et πάθος non esse certum significationis discrimen, sed eadem fere ui et sensus uarietate utrumque nomen, saepius alterum, alterum rarius usurpari...nomen πάθημα raro ab Ar usurpatur, quantum memini ubique numero plurali..., ac pluralis quidem numeri longe frequentissimus est genetiuus," so the occurrence of παθημάτων in the *topos* at 637a36 and 637b4 is not significant as it is preferred over παθῶν by both Aristotle (51 occurrences to 43) and the Hippocratics (15 to 4). In the Aristotelian Corpus παθήματα is used 10 times and πάθη 246 times. In the *HA* πάθη appears at III.12, 519a3, and VIII(IX).49, 631b5 (in both cases in reference to non-morbid states), and in *Non Gen.* at 636a21, and in the *Dialectic* at 637b9. In the Hippocratic Corpus παθήματα (22 occurrences) is clearly preferred to πάθη (4 occurrences). Aristotle may have used παθήματα at 637b25 because in the context of the *Dialectic* πάθος was so closely tied to the morbid condition of uterine mole.

(d) Stylistics

Rudberg complains of a general lack of coherence and logical ordering in the treatise.[209] Some of this may be due to the summary nature of the text, but much of it derives, I think, from a failure to understand the relationship of the last two chapters to the first five. The first five chapters themselves follow quite a clear ordering, discussed above, pp. 87–90, and shown in the outline of the structure of the treatise on pp. 114–23.[210]

The author of *Non Gen.* does use frequent repetitions, as both Rudberg and Louis remark.[211] This is sometimes manifest as a tendency to restate a positive assertion in its negative formation, e.g., 634a12–13 τὰ καταμήνια γίνεσθαι καλῶς, τοῦτο δ' ἐστὶ δι' ἴσων χρόνων καὶ μὴ πεπλανημένως, "As regards normal menstruation: this is at regular intervals and not erratically." The author also repeats specific phrases, e.g., θεραπείας δεῖσθαι (634a11, 21, 34, b7, 11, 31; 635a36, b26; 637b29), ὑγιαίνοντος τοῦ σώματος 634a13, 18, b2, 6), but it is easy to see that these are formulaic phrases that recur because of the technical nature of the treatise.

However, some of the phrases that Rudberg flags as repetitions are in fact important progressions in the argument, e.g., he lists as examples of repetition six references to night emissions in women (634b30, 635a33–b4, 635b32–636a9, 636b24, 637b27–32, and 638a5–9) The first occurrence is used as evidence that women emit their seed in front of the womb, the second that women are sometimes dry after waking from an erotic dream but become moist later in the day when the womb releases the seed it had drawn in, the third that women are sometimes weaker, sometimes stronger after releasing seed in an erotic dream, the fourth as an explanation as to why women are sometimes more vigorous in these circumstances. The final

---

[209] Rudberg 1911, p. 34.

[210] And see above pp. 88–9 for a discussion of the possible similarity to medical catechisms in organization

[211] Rudberg 1911, p. 41; Louis 1969, p. 151.

two passages are Aristotle's discussion of and objections to the theory of *Non Gen.* Night emissions are not particularly important in the rest of Aristotle or in the Hippocratic Corpus.

Rudberg also notes the author's predilection for prolepsis, especially involving the indirect question construction, e.g., 633b15, 635b6, and 637b6.[212] Each of these involve a leading verb introducing signs that reveal a situation: θεωρεῖν, ἀποδηλοῖ, and φανερά...ἐστιν. This coheres fairly well with Smyth's statement that prolepsis "is especially common after verbs of saying, seeing, hearing, knowing, fearing, effecting" (2182a). Other examples are τῷ τόπῳ, 634a1, οἷον αἱ ῥῖνες, 634b34, and πέφυκε οὕτως, 637a21. The choice would then seem to be one of stylistics rather than, as Rudberg implies, the result of poor grammar, and significantly, examples of prolepsis cluster in *Non Gen.* as opposed to the *Dialectic.*

Rudberg spends considerable time discussing the author's attempts at euphony and avoidance of hiatus, which he says is unusual for Aristotle except in the more revised works.[213] He notes examples in the first five chapters at 633b15, 29; 634a3, 8, 9; 634b27, 38; 635a17, 26; 635b25, 33; 636a18, 37; 636b14, 17; 637a5, 12, 13, 18; and in the last two at 637b22, 35, and 638a27. His conclusion is that the effort is not fully carried out, shows no more than traces, and is not consistent. In reference to Jaeger's use of avoidance of hiatus by Diocles to demonstrate Aristotelian influence, von Staden commented "Diocles' inconsistent deployment of a stylistic device that is so widely shared by Greek writers of the late fifth and fourth century B.C. hardly constitutes proof of 'Aristotelianisms' in Diocles' prose."[214] This shows how little value should be placed on these sorts of argument for purposes of determining a specific author or the date of a treatise. More significant for my purposes is that nineteen of Rudberg's twenty-two examples fall within the chapters comprising *Non Gen.* and only three in the *Dialectic,* so

---

[212] Rudberg 1911, p. 37.   [213] Ibid., pp. 43–5.
[214] Von Staden 1992, pp. 234–5.

there may be some significance in the distribution of hiatus avoidance in this one small text.

As Balme says, the unpolished nature of Aristotelian prose does not lend itself to easy decisions over what could or could not be genuine, and on stylistic grounds alone it would be hard to come to any conclusion on whether *HA* X is authentic. However, the discrepancy between the first five and the last two chapters in expression, vocabulary, and style goes to support my thesis that we are dealing with two separate authors, of which the latter exhibits fewer anomalies with general Aristotelian style.

(e) Date

To act as an *endoxon* for Aristotle before he wrote *GA*, *Non Gen.* had to have been written at the latest some time early in the third quarter of the fourth century BCE. Even those who believe *HA* X is post-Aristotelian do not date it much later than Aristotle's time.[215] Rudberg and Louis believe it was most likely written in the Peripatos around the time of Strato (end fourth–early third centuries BCE),[216] and, as has been noted, Föllinger agrees with Balme and van der Eijk that issues of style are inconclusive and therefore do not eliminate the possibility it was written during Aristotle's lifetime. The sophistication of the arguments against pangenesis from parts of the body and the general organization of the treatise suggest that it was later than the Hippocratic gynecology, as does its title, ὑπὲρ τοῦ μὴ γεννᾶν. Of the sixty to seventy treatises in the Hippocratic Corpus, περί appears in the title of forty-eight, ὑπέρ in none. Apart from one occurrence in the fifth century (Herodotus IV.8), ὑπέρ in the sense "concerning" does not occur till the fourth century BCE and

---

[215] Some words that are thought of as late occur in at least one other text of the fifth and fourth centuries BCE: e.g. καταλήξεως, 634b20, is used by Aeschylus at *Ag.* 1479 and *Cho.* 1075; κατασκελετεύεται, 636a15, by Isocrates at 15.268; συνδρόμως by Aeschylus at *Ag.* 1184.

[216] Rudberg 1911, p. 45; Louis 1969, pp. 153–4.

is generally considered a later usage. However, Stevens cites three examples in Plato, forty-five in Demosthenes, and sixteen in Aristotle himself. As he states, "we might expect there to be some period when a usage such as ὑπέρ c. gen. = 'concerning' was beginning to appear; and...its occurrence before Aristotle is clearly established."[217] It is not firmly established, however, much before Aristotle, so some time in the third quarter of the fourth century BCE seems a reasonable date for the composition of *Non Gen.*

8 THE OPENING WORDS OF *HA* X[218]

Because of the abruptness with which many ancient medical treatises end, the final words of *Non Gen.* before the introduction of the *topos* ("Similarly, women have the passage to the place in front of the uterus larger and more spacious than the one to the outside," ὁμοίως δὲ καὶ αἱ γυναῖκες μείζω τὸν εἰς τὸ ἔμπροσθεν τῶν ὑστερῶν πόρον ἔχουσι καὶ εὐρυχωρότερον τοῦ ἔξω[219]) do not mean that we are missing any sizable section of the treatise, though the greater organization that *Non Gen.* displays in comparison with many medical texts might lead us to expect a more rounded conclusion. The title of the treatise would also lead us to expect a continuation beyond the problems of conception into those of pregnancy and parturition, as in *Mul.* I and II, *Steril.* and *Nat. Mul.* If the original *Non Gen.* focused solely on conception rather than the entire process of reproduction, we might have expected a title such as ὑπὲρ τοῦ μὴ συλλαμβάνειν.

Something of the same ambiguity has been seen to hover over the beginning of *HA* X, προϊούσης δὲ τῆς ἡλικίας, "But as this time of life proceeds." This would imply that something had preceded the text which Aristotle chose not to summarize,

---

[217] Stevens 1936, p. 208.
[218] For the ms. tradition of the *HA*, see above pp. xii–xvi and Balme 2002, pp. 1–48. Here I include only material relevant to my argument.
[219] 637a34–5.

but the pattern of the mss.' inclusion or omission of these words provides strong reasons for believing that they were not originally part of *Non Gen.*; see above pp. 2–8. So, unless the phrase indicates that we have lost the first part of the treatise, the original opening words of *Non Gen.* would have been, "If a man and a woman fail to reproduce after having intercourse with one another…", Ἀνδρὶ καὶ γυναικί τοῦ μὴ γεννᾶν ἀλλήλοις συνόντας. This phrase appears in the predicate position with τὸ αἴτιον. The effect is subtle, but it shows that the author is primarily concerned with the clinical situation that would confront a physician who had to deal with actual patients, rather than a purely theoretical discussion of the causes of infertility: "if a man and a woman fail to reproduce after having intercourse with one another, the cause is sometimes attributable to…" as opposed to "the cause of a man and a woman failing to reproduce after having intercourse with one another is sometimes attributable to…"[220] Although much of the clinical material contained in *Non Gen.* was irrelevant for the purposes of Aristotle's dialectic with the text on the *aporia* of the fertility of female *sperma*, it could also act as an *endoxon* for other aspects of reproductive theory that he could deal with more summarily later in the *GA*, so Aristotle summarized the text *in toto*.

---

[220] In his Latin translation, *Procedente autem etate uiro et mulieri non generandi inuicem conuenientes causa aliquando quidem in ambobus est aliquando autem in altero solum*, Guil. may have been trying to capture the force of the Greek word order by postponing *causa* to the same position in the Latin. At the end of Book IX(VII) the scribe of Gᵃ adds a remark in Greek noting that a tenth book of the *HA* has been discovered in Latin of which the opening words are ἡ τοῦ μὴ γεννᾶν τῷ ἀνδρὶ καὶ τῇ γυναικὶ συνερχομένοις μετ' ἀλλήλων αἰτία ποτὲ ἐν ἀμφοῖν ποτὲ δ'ἐν θατέρῳ μόνον ἐστιν. The variations from the Greek of the mss. can be explained if they are a back translation from Guil.'s Latin. The scribe of Gᵃ took the position of *causa* in the Latin translation to indicate that the preceding phrase was in the attributive position and consequently produced a Greek translation which would fit more closely with a primarily theoretical interest in infertility. Latin lacks a definite article, so this translation is grammatically sound.

TEXT AND CRITICAL APPARATUS

SIGLA

Dᵃ   Vaticanus gr. 262, fourteenth century

Apographa quae coniecturas praebent

Sᶜ   Taurinensis C I 9 (56), early fifteenth century
 Lᶜ   Ambrosianus I.56 sup., early fifteenth century
 Gᵃ   Marcianus gr. 212, early fifteenth century
 Q   Marcianus gr. 200, fifteenth century
  Fᵃ Marcianus gr. 207, fifteenth century
   Xᶜ Laurentianus 87.27, fifteenth century
Rᶜ   Utinensis VI, I, second half fifteenth century
Vᶜ   Neapolitanus III D 5 (289), late fifteenth century

Orib.   Oribasius: *Lib. Incert.* ed. Raeder 1933

Scot.   Michael Scotus
         Brug.   Brugensis 99/112
         Caius Gonville & Caius 109
         Got.   Gotoburgensis 8
         Chis.   Vat. Chisianus E viii 251
         Rud.   Rudberg 1911 transcription

Guil.   Guilelmus de Moerbeka: *De hist. an.* ed. P. Beullens and
       F. Bossier, Leiden 1999– (abbrev. B.-B.)
       Tz Toletanus 47.10
       cett. *uide Praef. supra* p. xv, n.10
       Rud. Rudberg 1911 transcription

Gaza   Theodorus Gaza: *Hist. an.* [*uide* Introd. p. 1]
Fel.   Joh. Bernardus Felicianus: *HA* x Lugduni 1560
Scal.   Jul. Caes. Scaliger: *HA* x Lugduni 1584; *HA* I–x Tolosae
       1619

Balme	D. M. Balme ed. (Camb. Class. Texts and Comms.) 2002
Barnes	Rev. Oxford Transl., *HA* x trs. Jonathan Barnes, Princeton 1984
Bk.	I. Bekker, Prussian Acad. ed. Berlin 1831
Camot.	J. B. Camotius ed. Venice 1553
Dt.	L. Dittmeyer ed. (Teubner) Leipzig 1907
Junt.	Juntine ed. Florence 1527
Louis	P. Louis ed. (Budé) Paris 1964
Pk.	N. S. Piccolos ed. Paris 1863
Rud.	G. Rudberg comm. *HA* x Uppsala 1911
Sn.	J. G. Schneider ed. Leipzig 1811
Sylb.	F. Sylburg ed. Venice 1587
edd.	editores nonnulli siue omnes

[*alia nomina—uide Praef.* p. ix]

OUTLINE OF PLAN OF *HA* X

De non generando

CHAPTER I

I Introduction to topic
The first chapter opens with the three possible reasons an adult, sexually active couple may be unable to reproduce:
  (a) the man and woman are both capable of reproduction but incompatible with one another
  (b) the man is infertile
  (c) the woman is infertile
The author will focus on the woman and says that the first thing that needs to be considered in her case is the state of the uterus.

II Definition of health which will suggest problem lies elsewhere than in the womb.
Healthy functioning requires that a part:
  (a) is not in pain after function
  (b) is not incapacitated after function
  (c) is not fatigued after function
Author uses the eye as an exemplum.

III Challenge to this definition and author's response
Some say that sometimes the functioning of an organ proceeds well and painlessly even if the organ itself is disordered in some of its parts or has a growth upon it.
This is not true. The functioning will be adversely affected in some way; analogy of the eye.

IV Importance of the position of the womb for conception
  (a) it should not be out of place

(b) it should move forward down the vagina at appropriate times in order to be able to draw in seed and conceive

(c) it should return to original position afterwards to prevent becoming desensitized and therefore failing to open

Summary: If any of these things are not so, uterus needs treatment.

V Non-healthy condition of uterus revealed by menstruation in a stable body

If the body itself is healthy and the menses are appearing regularly, a woman's infertility is not caused by the state of uterus, but if the body itself is healthy and the menses are irregular in some way, infertility is caused by the state of uterus. Signs of an unhealthy uterus are:

(a) too frequent, infrequent, or erratic menstruation

    (i) too little fluid shows uterus is not opening up to body correctly as a result of its insensitivity—results in infrequent menstruation

    (ii) too much fluid shows it is inflamed—results in frequent menstruation

(b) excessively putrefied menses follow pains in womb (in healthy women whites are putrefied)

Summary: Excessively putrefied or qualitatively disordered menses indicate womb needs treatment. Irregular timing of periods shows that the condition of the womb is variable, and this is an impediment to conception, but one that is self-correcting.

VI Healthy condition of uterus revealed by menstruation in a changeable body

If body itself is becoming wetter or drier, amount and regularity of menses should change:

(a) if body is healthy and changeable, no need of therapy

(b) in case of a diseased body

    (i)   too little menstruation indicates residue is being
        expended elsewhere in body
    (ii) too much menstruation indicates body is purging
        itself in this direction

Summary: When menses fluctuate in accordance with increase
and decrease of fluid in the body, uterus is healthy and it is the
body that needs treatment in order for woman to be able to
conceive.

VII Nature of "whites" in a healthy womb
    (a) at beginning of menses they are milk-white and odorless
    (b) turn red during menstruation per se
    (c) at cessation of menses whites have heavy, acrid, but not
        putrefied smell.

Summary: If menses occur as described in the latter part of
this chapter and a woman cannot conceive, the problem does
not lie in her uterus.

CHAPTER 2

Once the *ergon* of the womb has been examined, the author
turns to the position of the womb. This is indicated by the
alignment of the cervix.

I Necessity of a correctly aligned uterus to draw in seed
    (a) woman emits in front of uterus. This is shown by moist-
        ness in area after orgasm at the end of an erotic dream
    (b) this is same place as that into which the man emits, not
        into the uterus. This is shown by the same place becom-
        ing moist after intercourse
    (c) through the cervix, uterus draws seed into itself by
        pneuma, as nostrils draw in *pneuma*
    (d) women can become pregnant from any sexual position if
        womb is aligned correctly. A woman could not become
        pregnant in any position if she emitted directly into womb

(e) if the uterus is misaligned, it cannot take up the seed because it is not deposited in front of the cervix, the "nostrils" of the womb

Summary: If this is a congenital condition or has become chronic through disease, it cannot be cured, but may be resolved naturally.

II Necessity of appropriate opening of womb, which is affected by its position

 (a) at beginning of menstruation cervix should be soft and not clearly dilated
 (b) whites come at beginning when cervix is not dilated
 (c) fleshy-colored menses show womb has expanded without pain
 (d) cervix should be dilated and dry after menstruation, but not hard
 (e) should remain in this state 1½–2 days.
 (f) at beginning, uterus should not be expanded, but *stoma* should be soft to show uterus is relaxing in concert with body itself.
 (g) first material emitted is whites from mouth of uterus
 (h) uterus expands when body sends forth more
 (i) stoma remaining open after menstruation shows uterus is empty, dry, and thirsty with no residues round the passage

Summary: This behavior shows uterus is in a state to be able to attract seed and to close once it has done so.

CHAPTER 3

If the functioning of both the womb and the cervix appears to be in good order, doctor should consider the general environment of the womb. Anomalies of structure and moistness may not prevent menstruation, but will prevent a woman becoming pregnant.

I Signs that a womb has the necessary attractive power in its cotyledons

Woman should dream she is having intercourse and emit as if she really were having intercourse. At least sometimes she should be dry after such dreams, but later the moisture should be released from the womb. This shows that the cotyledons in the womb attract and retain *sperma*.

II Signs of elasticity in the uterus

This would be needed to bring a pregnancy to term if the *sperma* were successfully drawn into the uterus. Uterus should produce and expel gas just like the stomach. If it does not, this shows it cannot expand to nurture fetus. Both sides of womb should do this equally.

III Necessity for lubrication of vagina during intercourse
    (a) like saliva, shows uterus is ready to take in *sperma*
    (b) like sweat, shows uterus is working hard
    (c) like tears, enables uterus to adjust to environment
    (d) too much can prevent uterus taking up *sperma* from man and woman

IV The significance of a woman's bodily strength after night emission
    (a) to be weaker without being ill, and to be dry at first but later to become moist, shows body is emitting *sperma*
    (b) to be stronger with a dry womb shows body has drawn *sperma* to itself

V Wind-pregnancy
    (a) excessively dry womb draws in mixed male and female *sperma* but dries it up
    (b) in particularly dry wombs this is immediately expelled
    (c) sometimes retained and produces symptoms of pregnancy

(d) remains this way till it falls out

(e) not noticed because it is so small

CHAPTER 4

I Pathological conditions of the uterus which can cause infertility

    (a) spasm

        (i) distention through inflammation

        (ii) pressure of material during childbirth

    (b) growths

    (c) congenital closure of cervix

II Causes of infertility other than conditions of the womb

    (a) man could be infertile

        (i) unspecified "other" signs to show when this is the case

        (ii) if he has children with other women, shows it is not the case

    (b) problem lies in their pairing

        (i) *sperma* must be emitted by both partners simultaneously

        (ii) men tend to emit first

        (iii) woman should be more aroused to begin with than man

CHAPTER 5

Signs which a couple may think indicate infertility but in fact do not. The mechanics of a woman's emission of *sperma* when sexually excited.

I Women and men can be healthier after emission of *sperma*

    (a) if there is a surplus of material to be evacuated

    (b) if the material is not usable in the body anyway

    (c) *sperma* soon regenerates itself

(d) woman who thinks she has not emitted *sperma* because of these circumstances does not think she can become pregnant

II Do not need to become completely dry after intercourse to conceive
  (a) both man and woman can emit more than can be drawn into womb and more than enough for conception
  (b) this explains multiple births; *sperma* is separated into portions of appropriate quantity by falling into separate spaces
  (c) *sperma* must therefore come uniformly from the body as a whole; *sperma* for different body parts cannot be discrete
  (d) *pneuma* draws in the *sperma* from the area before the womb

III Configuration of passage that deposits woman's *sperma* before her womb
  (a) women have the equivalent of a penis, a *kaulos*, inside their bodies
  (b) emit *pneuma* through a *poros* leading from the *kaulos* to the outside air when sexually excited
  (c) *kaulos* empties in front of womb through an opening narrower than the vagina itself
  (d) the configuration of the openings of the nose (inner opening through which air travels to the pharynx is narrow, outer opening through which mucus flows is wide) is reversed in the *kaulos* (inner opening through which *sperma* flows to the vagina is wide, outer opening which expels only *pneuma* is narrow)

Dialectica de De non generando

Topos

Formulation of *Non Gen.*'s premise: a woman emits *sperma* like a man.

Empirical *phainomenon Non Gen.* cited in support of the premise: men and women experience the same affections after orgasm.

Consequence of the belief that the fluid the woman emits parallels male semen: male and female orgasmic ejaculates play the same role in generation.

Phainomenon adduced as evidence for premise: woman's ejaculate is the cause of something else. (This is uterine mole, but it is not expressed in the *topos* itself.)

Refutation of premise: this other condition is a disease or death.

Instruction for *topos*: examine this argument that female *sperma* is the cause of a diseased or fatal affection on the basis of the premise that it is also a source of generation.

Basis for *topos*: show that the theory does not cohere with the basic law of cause and effect.

CHAPTER 6

I Female animals seem to emit something when sexually excited
  (a) hens pursue males and produce wind-eggs
  (b) grasshoppers reproduce without male input
  (c) fact that wind-eggs can become fertile shows they are like the grasshopper's contribution to reproduction, though they need male input
  (d) women emit in dreams and become moist and feel enervated afterwards

II Why do quadrupeds not reproduce parthenogenetically or produce wind-eggs?
  (a) birds produce wind-eggs, other animals produce nothing
  (b) birds have no external depository outside their wombs; *sperma* from male birds flows directly onto the ground if female birds' wombs are not open
  (c) so birds must emit directly into their wombs
  (d) quadrupeds do have a place which acts as an external depository outside their wombs
  (e) female *sperma* does not enter womb from there because it gets mixed up with other fluids

(f) in case of other animals, both partners needed for any sort of generation

CHAPTER 7

Objects to the position of *Non Gen.* that women ejaculate *sperma* at orgasm because they do not develop "wind pregnancies." Dismisses the condition of the uterine mole as a candidate support for this position.

I If women can draw *sperma* into themselves after a night emission, why do other animals not also do so and produce wind-eggs?
  (a) mole is a sort of pregnancy but woman does not give birth or reduce in size
  (b) only released from condition by supervention of a more serious condition

II Does a hot and dry womb cause mole from the unmixed *sperma* of one partner? Why does it stay in the womb so long?
  (a) birds regularly evacuate their wind-eggs because they create so many of them the womb fills up and the body becomes expulsive
  (b) viviparous animals give birth because growing fetus needs a change of nourishment
  (c) neither of these conditions holds for the mole

III Or does mole come about through fluid or through being in a middle state between heat and cold?
  (a) if womb were really cold, it would discharge fluid
  (b) if it were really hot, it would concoct it within a limited time
  (c) because it is not alive it does not move and cause labor
  (d) hardness of mole suggests imperfect concoction, so heat not the cause

IV Doctors too often diagnose mole, which is a rare condition
  (a) dropsical symptoms with retention of menses more often
      come about through flowing of moist residues to wom-
      an's abdomen
  (b) only a mole if womb has increased in size
  (c) womb will be hot and dry to the touch
  (d) cervix will be in the state it is during pregnancy

HISTORIA ANIMALIVM X

ΥΠΕΡ ΤΟΥ ΜΗ ΓΕΝΝΑΝ

CHAPTER 1

[633b12] [προϊούσης δὲ τῆς ἡλικίας] Ἀνδρὶ καὶ γυναικὶ τοῦ μὴ γεννᾶν ἀλλήλοις συνόντας τὸ αἴτιον ὁτὲ μὲν ἐν ἀμφοῖν ἐστιν ὁτὲ δ' ἐν θατέρῳ μόνον. πρῶτον μὲν οὖν ἐπὶ τοῦ θήλεος δεῖ [15] θεωρεῖν τὰ περὶ τὰς ὑστέρας ὅπως ἔχει, ἵν' εἰ μὲν ἐν ταύταις τὸ αἴτιον αὗται τυγχάνωσι θεραπείας, εἰ δὲ μὴ ἐν ταύταις περὶ ἕτερόν τι τῶν αἰτίων ποιῶνται τὴν ἐπιμέλειαν.

ἔστι δ' ὥσπερ καὶ περὶ ἄλλο μέρος φανερὸν εἰ ὑγιαίνει ὅταν τὸ ἔργον τὸ αὐτοῦ ἱκανῶς ἀποτελῇ καὶ ἄλυπόν τε ᾖ [20] καὶ μετὰ τὰς ἐργασίας ἄκοπον, οἷον ὀφθαλμὸς ὅταν λήμην τε μηδεμίαν ποιῇ καὶ ὁρᾷ καὶ μετὰ τὴν ὅρασιν μὴ ταράττηται μηδ' ἀδυνατῇ ὁρᾶν πάλιν. οὕτω καὶ ἡ ὑστέρα ἡ πόνον τε μὴ παρέχουσα, καὶ ὃ ἐκείνης ἐστὶ τοῦθ' ἱκανῶς ἀπεργαζομένη, καὶ μετὰ τὰ ἔργα μὴ ἀδύνατος ἀλλ' [25] ἄκοπος.

λέγεται δὲ καὶ μὴ καλῶς ἔχουσαν τὴν ὑστέραν, ὅμως πρὸς τὸ ἔργον τὸ ἑαυτῆς ἔχειν καλῶς καὶ ἀλύπως ἄν. <ἀλλὰ> μὴν ταύτης χεῖρον τὸ ἔργον ἐστὶν οὕτως ἐχούσης ὥσπερ ὄμμα κωλύεται ὁρᾶν ἀκριβῶς μὴ ἔχοντος τοῦ ὀφθαλμοῦ καλῶς πάντα τὰ μόρια, ἢ εἰ <ἔστι> φυμάτιον.

ὁμοίως δὲ καὶ [30] ὑστέρα, εἰ εὖ ἔχοι τοῦ ἐπικαίρου τόπου, οὐθὲν ἂν πρὸς τοῦτο [634a1] βλάπτοι. δεῖ δὴ τὴν ἔχουσαν καλῶς ὑστέραν πρῶτον μὲν τῷ τόπῳ μὴ ἐν ἄλλῳ καὶ ἄλλῳ εἶναι ἀλλ' ὁμοίως τῇ θέσει· πλὴν γίγνεσθαι τὸ πορρώτερον ἄνευ πάθους καὶ λύπης, καὶ μηδὲν ἀναισθητοτέρας εἶναι θιγγανομένας. τοῦτο δὲ κρίνειν [5] οὐ χαλεπόν. ὅτι δὲ δεῖ τοιαύτας εἶναι ἐκ τῶνδε

633b12 μὴ om. Dᵃ: *non* Scot. Guil.   **26** ἄν. ἀλλὰ μὴν D-J.: ἂν μὴ Dᵃ.   **27** οὕτως ἐχούσης D-J.: αὐτῆς ἔχειν Dᵃ.   **28** κωλύεται D-J.: κωλύει αὐτὸ Dᵃ.   **29** εἰ φυμάτιον Reeve: *si pustula* Guil. (Tz.): εἰ...ὄν om. Guil. (cett.): εἰ φῦμά τι ὄν Dᵃ ἔστι add. D-J.

HISTORIA ANIMALIUM X

ON FAILURE TO REPRODUCE

CHAPTER 1

[633b12] [But as the time of life proceeds] If a man and a woman fail to reproduce after having intercourse with one another, the cause is sometimes attributable to incompatibility in the pairing, sometimes to only one or the other partner. So first, in the case of the female, it is necessary [15] to observe how things stand with the uterus, what state it is in, so that if the cause is located here it can be treated, but if it is not here let them direct their attention to one of the other two causes.

And just as it is clear with any other part whether it is healthy when it fulfills its own function satisfactorily and is free from both pain [20] and fatigue after its tasks, for example, an eye when it both produces no rheum and sees, and after seeing is neither disordered nor incapable of seeing again, so also the womb is healthy which does not cause suffering and satisfactorily carries out its proper function, and after its functions is neither incapacitated nor [25] fatigued.

But it is said that even if the womb is not in a good state, nevertheless with regard to its function it may be in a good and painless state. But surely, its function is worse when it is in this state, just as an eye is prevented from seeing accurately if it is not in a good state with respect to all its parts or if there is a growth present.

Likewise [30] a womb, if it is properly situated, would cause no [634a1] harm to its function. Indeed, the womb which is in a good state should not first be in one place and then in another but should remain in the same position; except for moving to a farther position down the vagina without symptoms and pain and losing no sensitivity if it is being touched. This is [5] not

φανερόν. εἴτε γὰρ μὴ πλησίον προσίασιν, οὐκ ἔσονται ἀνασπα-
στικαί· πόρρω γὰρ αὐταῖς ἔσται ὁ τόπος ὅθεν δεῖ ἀναλαβεῖν.
εἰ δὲ [μὴ] πλησίον μένουσι καὶ μὴ οἶαι ἐπανιέναι πορρωτέρω,
κωφότεραι ἔσονται <τῷ> διαθιγγάνεσθαι [δ'] ἀεί, ὥστε μὴ ταχὺ
[10] ἀνοίγεσθαι· δεῖ <δὲ> τοῦτο σφόδρα ποιεῖν καὶ εὐηκόους
εἶναι. ταῦτά τε οὖν χρὴ ὑπάρχειν, ὅσαις τε μὴ ὑπάρχει αὗται
θεραπείας δέονται τινος.
   καὶ τὰ καταμήνια γίνεσθαι καλῶς, τοῦτο δ' ἐστὶ δι' ἴσων
χρόνων καὶ μὴ πεπλανημένως, ὑγιαίνοντος τοῦ σώματος.
σημαίνει γὰρ οὕτω γινόμενα καλῶς ἔχειν <τὰς ὑστέρας
πρὸς τὸ> [15] ἀνοίγεσθαι καὶ δέχεσθαι τὴν ἐκ τοῦ σώματος
ὑγρότητα ὅταν τὸ σῶμα διδῷ. ὅταν δὲ πλεονάκις ἢ ἐλαττονάκις
ἢ πεπλανημένως ἀφιῶσι, τοῦ ἄλλου σώματος μὴ συναιτίου
ὄντος ἀλλ' ὑγιαίνοντος, ἀνάγκη τοῦτο συμβαίνειν δι' αὐτάς. καὶ
<γὰρ ἢ> διὰ κωφότητα οὐκ ἀνοίγονται ἐν τοῖς καιροῖς, ὥστ'
[20] ὀλίγα δέχονται, ἢ μᾶλλον ἐπισπῶνται τὸ ὑγρὸν διά τινα
φλεγμασίαν αὐτῶν, ὥστε θεραπείας σημαίνουσι δεόμεναι ὥσπερ
καὶ ὀφθαλμοὶ καὶ κύστις καὶ κοιλία καὶ τἆλλα· πάντες γὰρ οἱ
τόποι φλεγμαίνοντες ἕλκουσιν ὑγρότητα τοιαύτην ἢ πέφυκεν
ἐκκρίνεσθαι εἰς ἕκαστον τόπον, ἀλλ' οὐ [25] τοιαύτη ἢ τοσαύτη.
ὁμοίως δὲ καὶ ἡ ὑστέρα πλείω ἀποδιδοῦσα σημαίνει φλεγματικόν
τι πάθος, ἐὰν ὅμοια μὲν πλείω δ' ἀποδιδῷ.
   ἐὰν δ' ἀνόμοια καὶ σεσημμένα μᾶλλον <ἢ> οἷα ταῖς ὑγιαινούσαις
προέρχεται, τότε μὲν ἤδη πάθος καὶ ἐπίδηλον γίνεται· ἀνάγκη
γὰρ καὶ πόνους τινὰς [30] ἐπισημαίνειν ἐχούσης ὡς οὐ δεῖ. ταῖς
δ' ὑγιαινούσαις τὰ λευκὰ καὶ σεσημμένα προέρχεται, ταῖς μὲν καὶ
ἀρχομένων ταῖς δὲ πλείσταις ληγόντων τῶν καταμηνίων. ὅσαις
μὲν οὖν σεσημμένα μᾶλλον γίνεται ἢ ταῖς ὑγιαινούσαις ἢ ἄτακτα,
[πλείω ἢ ἐλάττω,] μᾶλλον δέονται θεραπείας ὡς ἐμποδιζόντων

634a6 ἀνασπαστικαί Sn.: ἅμα σπαστικαί Dᵃ.   **8** μὴ secl. Sn: *et si fuerit
propinqua* Scot.: *si non prope* Guil. (cett.)   **9** τῷ add. Pk.: δ' secl. Pk.: *surdiores
erunt tangi autem semper utique* Guil.   **10** δὲ add. Sn.   **14** τὰς ὑστέρας add.
Dt. πρὸς τὸ add. Sn.: *ad* Guil.   **19** γὰρ ἢ add. Pk ἐν Sn.: δ' ἐν Dᵃ: *autem in*
Guil.   **27** ἀνόμοια Camot.: ὅμοια Dᵃ: *similia* Guil.   **28** μᾶλλον ἢ Sn.:
magis quam Guil.: μᾶλλον Dᵃ τότε Sn.: *tunc* Guil.: τοῦτο Dᵃ.   **34** πλείω ἢ
ἐλάττω secl. D-J.

difficult to discern. That the uterus should be like this is clear
from the following. If it does not move close, it will not draw
up the seed, for the place from which it must take up the seed
will be far away from it. But if it remains close and is not such
as to go back further away again, it will be less responsive as a
result of being constantly touched so that it does not [10] open
readily. It must do this forcefully and promptly. These things
must be so; those uteri for which they do not obtain need some
treatment.

As regards normal menstruation: this is at regular intervals
and not erratically when the body is healthy. For when the menses come in this way they show that the uterus is in the right state
[15] to open and receive the moisture from the body whenever
the body supplies it. But whenever it discharges too frequently
or too infrequently or erratically, and the rest of the body is not
a contributory cause but is healthy, the uterus itself must be the
cause. For either on account of its unresponsiveness it does not
open at the right times so that it [20] receives a small amount
of fluid, or it draws in too much fluid because of some inflammation within it, so that it shows that it is in need of treatment
just as eyes, bladder, intestines, and the rest do. For all inflamed
parts draw the kind of moisture which is naturally secreted into
each part, but not [25] of the same quality and amount as when
healthy. In the same way too, when the womb passes on more
fluid than normal it indicates some inflammatory condition, at
least when it passes on similar but excessive fluid.

But if the fluid is dissimilar and more putrefied than that
which is emitted by healthy women, at this time it is already
a condition and is becoming evident. For some suffering must
[30] be indicating that the womb is not as it should be. In
healthy women the whites come out in a putrefied state, for
some at the beginning of menstruation, but for most when they
are tapering off. Those, then, in whom menses occur more
putrefied than they do for healthy women, or in a disordered
state, certainly need treatment since they are impediments
[35] to reproduction. But, for those in whom it is only the time

ARISTOTLE

[35] πρὸς τὴν τέκνωσιν. ὅσαις δὲ τοῖς χρόνοις μόνον ἀνωμάλοις καὶ μὴ δι' ἴσου, ἧττον μὲν διακωλυτικὸν τὸ πάθος, διασημαίνει μέντοι τῆς ὑστέρας τὴν ἕξιν κινουμένην καὶ οὐκ ἀεὶ ὁμοίως μένουσαν. ἔστι δὲ τοῦτο τὸ πάθος οἷον μὲν βλάψαι τὰς εὐφυεῖς πρὸς τὴν σύλλη-ψιν, οὐ μέντοι νόσος ἀλλὰ [40] τοιοῦτόν τι πάθος οἷον καθίστα-σθαι καὶ ἄνευ θεραπείας, ἂν [634b1] μή τι προσεξαμαρτάνῃ αὕτη.

ἐὰν δὲ μεταβάλλωσι τῇ τάξει ἢ τῷ πλήθει, τοῦ ἄλλου σώματος μὴ ὁμοίως ἔχοντος ἀλλ' ὁτὲ μὲν ὑγροτέρου ὁτὲ δὲ ξηροτέρου, οὐθὲν αἴτιαι αἱ ὑστέραι, ἀλλὰ δεῖ καὶ ἀκολουθεῖν αὐτὰς τῇ τοῦ σώματος [5] ἕξει, δεχομένας καὶ ἀφιείσας κατὰ λόγον. ἐὰν μὲν οὖν ὑγιαίνοντος τοῦ σώμα-τος μεταβάλλοντος δὲ τοῦτο ποιῶσιν, οὐθὲν αὐταὶ δέονται θεραπείας· ἐὰν δὲ νοσοῦντος, ἢ ἐλάττω ἀποδιδῶσι διὰ τὸ ἄλλοθί που ἀναλίσκε-σθαι τὸ περίττωμα ἢ κάμνει τὸ σῶμα, ἢ πλείω ἀφιῶσι διὰ τὸ δεῦρο [10] ἐξερεύγεσθαι τὸ σῶμα, οὐδὲ τοῦτο σημαίνει αὐτάς γε τὰς ὑστέρας δεῖ-σθαι θεραπείας ἀλλὰ τὸ σῶμα. ὡς ὅσαις συμμεταβάλλει ταῖς ἕξεσι τοῦ σώματος τὰ γυναικεῖα, δηλοῖ ὅτι οὐθὲν αἴτιον ἐν ταῖς ὑστέραις ἐστὶν ὅτι ὑγιαίνουσαι διατελοῦσιν. αὐταὶ δ' αὑτῶν ὁτὲ μὲν ἀρρωστότεραι ὁτὲ δὲ ἰσχύουσι [15] μᾶλλον, καὶ ὁτὲ μὲν ὑγρότεραι ὁτὲ δὲ ξηρότεραι. καὶ φοιτᾷ αὐταῖς ὅταν μὲν πλεῖον τὸ σῶμα αὑτοῦ πλείω, ὅταν δ' ἔλαττον ἐλάττω, καὶ ἐὰν μὲν ὑγρὸν ὑδαρέστερα, ἐὰν δὲ ξηρὸν ἐναιμότερα.

καὶ ἄρχονται μὲν ἐκ λευκῶν γαλακτοειδῶν, ἀνόσμων μενου-σῶν· τὰ δὲ φοινικᾶ μέν, ἀπολήγοντα [20] δὲ λευκότερα ἐσχάτης καταλήξεως. ὀσμὴν δ' ἔχει τὰ λευκὰ ταῦτα οὐ σηπεδόνος ἀλλὰ δριμυτέραν καὶ βαρυτέραν, οὐδὲ πύου. καὶ ἄνευ μὲν τήξεως, μετὰ μέντοι θερμασίας, ὅταν οὗτος ᾖ ὁ τρόπος τῶν σημείων.

ὅσαις μὲν οὖν οὕτω συμβαίνει, ταύταις ἔχουσιν ὡς δεῖ τὰ περὶ τὰς ὑστέρας [25] πρὸς τὴν τέκνωσιν.

634a35 τέκνωσιν Junt.: νέωσιν D^a: *pfuth* Guil.   **634b9** ἢ Pk.: ἢ D^a: *aut* Guil. ἢ Dt.: ἐὰν δὲ D^a: *si autem* Guil.   **22** οὐδὲ D-J.: οὔτε D^a.

128

periods which are anomalous and irregular, the condition is less of a complete impediment, although it clearly indicates that the state of the womb is variable and does not always remain the same. This sort of condition harms healthy women in their power to conceive, yet it is not a disease but [40] the kind of condition that sorts itself out even without treatment, as long as she does [634b1] not do anything to exacerbate it.

But if the menses change in regularity or amount and the rest of the body is not in a stable state but is sometimes wetter and sometimes drier, the uterus is not to blame since it has to follow along with the [5] state of the body, receiving and discharging in proportion. If it does this when the body is healthy but changing, the uterus has no need of therapy. But if during an illness, the uterus either passes along less residue because it is being used up elsewhere where the body is suffering, or it discharges more because the body is [10] evacuating itself through this orifice. This too is not a sign that the uterus needs treatment but the body. So for those women in whom the menses change along with the states of the body they show that there is no blame to be accorded the uterus because it fulfills its functions in a healthy fashion. These women are sometimes weaker, sometimes [15] stronger, sometimes wetter, sometimes drier than normal. And the menses come more fully for them when the body is fuller than normal, and less when it is less so. And if the body is moist the menses are more watery, and if dry more bloody.

And menses begin with the milk-like whites, which remain odorless; then they turn red but [20] taper off whiter in color at the very end of the cessation of menstruation. These whites have an odor not of putrefaction, rather a more acrid and heavier smell, but at least not of pus. And they occur without decay, although with heating, whenever the signs occur in this manner.

For those women for whom things turn out this way matters regarding the uterus are as they should be [25] as regards childbearing.

CHAPTER 2

καὶ πρῶτον ταῦτα σκεπτέον εἰ καλῶς ἔχει, μετὰ δὲ ταῦτα πῶς ἔχει τὸ στόμα τῶν ὑστερῶν. δεῖ γὰρ εἰς ὀρθὸν ἔχειν· εἰ δὲ μή, οὐχ ἕλξουσιν εἰς αὑτὰς τὸ σπέρμα. εἰς τὸ πρόσθεν γὰρ αὐτῶν καὶ ἡ γυνὴ προΐεται, ὡς δῆλον [30] ὅταν ἐξονειρώττωσιν αὗται τελέως· τότε γὰρ οὗτος ὁ τόπος θεραπείας δεῖται αὐταῖς ὑγρανθεὶς ὥσπερ εἰ ἀνδρὶ συνεγίνετο, ὡς προϊεμένων ἐνταῦθα καὶ τὸ παρὰ τοῦ ἀνδρός, εἰς τὸν αὐτὸν τόπον καὶ οὐχὶ εἰς τὰς ὑστέρας εἴσω. ἀλλ᾽ ὅταν ἐνταῦθα προϊῶνται, ἐντεῦθεν σπῶσι τῷ πνεύματι, οἷον αἱ [35] ῥῖνες, καὶ αἱ ὑστέραι τὸ σπέρμα. διὸ καὶ παντὶ σχήματι συνοῦσαι κυΐσκονται, ὅτι εἰς τὸ πρόσθεν πάντως <καλῶς> ἐχούσης γίγνεται καὶ αὐταῖς καὶ τοῖς ἀνδράσιν ἡ πρόεσις τοῦ σπέρματος· εἰ δ᾽ εἰς αὑτήν, οὐκ ἂν πάντως συγγενόμεναι συνελάμβανον. ἐὰν δὲ μὴ εἰς ὀρθὸν βλέπωσιν αἱ ὑστέραι ἀλλ᾽ [40] ἢ πρὸς τὰ ἰσχία ἢ πρὸς τὴν ὀσφὺν ἢ πρὸς τὸ ὑπογάστριον, [635a1] ἀδύνατον συλλαβεῖν διὰ τὴν προειρημένην αἰτίαν, ὅτι ἀνελέσθαι οὐκ ἂν δύναιντο τὸ σπέρμα. ἐὰν μὲν οὖν ἰσχυρῶς τῇ φύσει οὕτως ἔχωσιν ἢ ὑπὸ νόσου, ἀνίατον τὸ πάθος· ἐὰν δ᾽ ᾖ ῥῆγμα ἢ φύσει ἢ ὑπὸ τῆς νόσου διὰ φλεγμασίαν [5] συσπασάσης, ἐπὶ θάτερα αὐτῇ τὸ πάθος.

ταῖς δὲ μελλούσαις ἐγκύοις ἔσεσθαι δεῖ, καθάπερ εἴρηται, τὸ στόμα εἰς ὀρθὸν εἶναι, καὶ πρὸς τούτοις ἀνοίγεσθαι καλῶς. λέγω δὲ τὸ καλῶς τοιοῦτον ὅπως ὅταν ἄρχηται τὰ γυναικεῖα, θιγγανόμενον ἔσται τὸ στόμα μαλακώτερον ἢ πρότερον, καὶ μὴ [10] διεστομωμένον φανερῶς. ἀλλ᾽ [εἰ] οὕτως ἔχοντος, τὰ πρῶτα σημεῖα τὰ λευκὰ φοιτάτω. ὅταν δὲ σαρκινώτερα ᾖ τὴν χρόαν τὰ σημεῖα, φανερῶς ἔσται ἀνεστομωμένη ἄνευ ἀλγήματος, κἂν θιγγάνηται [κἂν μὴ θιγγάνῃ], καὶ μήτε κωφότητα μήτε στόμα ἀλλοιότερον αὐτὸ αὑτοῦ. ληξάντων δὲ τῶν γυναικείων

634b27 στόμα Fᵃ Xᶜ: σῶμα Dᵃ: *corpus* Guil.   **36** πάντως Barnes: παντελῶς Dᵃ: *paratius* Guil. καλῶς add. D-J.   **635a10** εἰ secl. Sn; *sed sic habente* Guil. cett.   **13** κἂν θιγγάνηται Sn.: κἂν θιγγάνῃ Dᵃ Lᶜ: κἂν θιγγάνῃ κἂν μὴ θιγγάνῃ codd. nonnulli: *et si tangatur et si non tangatur* Guil.: κἂν θιγγάνηται κἂν μὴ θιγγάνηται Dt.

CHAPTER 2

First of all we need to consider whether the menses are in a good state, and after that the state of the cervix of the uterus. For it must be straight; if it is not, the uterus will not draw the *sperma* into itself. Because it is in fact into the place in front of the uterus that a woman emits, as is clear [30] whenever they have erotic dreams which reach completion. For then this place needs seeing to by them since it becomes moist, just as if she had engaged in intercourse with a man, since they both emit at this place, the *sperma* from the man also, into the same place and not into the interior of the uterus. Whenever they emit here, the uterus draws in the *sperma* from this place by means of *pneuma*, just like the [35] nose. For this reason, women become pregnant when they have intercourse in any position, because the emission of the *sperma* both by them and by men in every position is in front of the cervix, if the womb is properly positioned. If the female emission were into the womb, women would not conceive in any position. But if the uterus is not looking straight but [40] either towards the hips or towards the tailbone or towards the underbelly [635a1], it cannot conceive on account of the reason already mentioned, because it cannot take up the *sperma*. If the uterus is firmly established in this state either by nature or by disease, the condition is incurable. But if there is a rupture either naturally or as a result of a disease which contracts the womb through inflammation, [5] the condition tends the opposite way for the woman.

In those who are intending to become pregnant it will be necessary, as we said, that the cervix be straight and in addition that it should open properly. And by properly, I mean in such a way that whenever the menses begin the cervix will be softer to the touch than it was before, and not [10] clearly dilated. Though again, when it is in this state, the first signs should be the whites. Whenever the signs are more fleshy in color, clearly the womb will have expanded, without pain even if touched, and it will have neither unresponsiveness nor any alteration of

[15] διεστομωμένον ἔστω σφόδρα καὶ ξηρόν, ἀλλὰ μὴ σκληρόν, ἡμέραν ὅλην καὶ ἡμίσειαν ἢ καὶ δύο ἡμέρας· <ὅπερ ἐστὶ στόματος ὑγιεινῶς ἔχοντος.> ταῦτα γὰρ σημαίνει οὕτω γιγνόμενα ὅτι καλῶς ἔχουσιν αἱ ὑστέραι καὶ ποιοῦσι τὸ αὐτῶν ἔργον, τῷ μὲν μὴ εὐθὺς ἀνεστομῶσθαι ἀλλὰ μαλακὸν τὸ στόμα γίγνεσθαι, ὅτι ἅμα τῷ ἄλλῳ [20] σώματι λυομένῳ λύονται, καὶ οὐκ ἐμποδίζουσι, καὶ ἀφιᾶσι πρῶτον τὰ ἀπ' αὐτοῦ τοῦ στόματος, ὅταν δὲ πλείω τὸ σῶμα προῆται, ἀναστομοῦνται. [ὅπερ ἐστὶ στόματος ὑγιεινῶς ἔχοντος.] παυσαμένων δὲ τῶν σημείων, τοῦ μὴ εὐθὺς συμπίπτειν σημαίνουσιν ὅτι, ἂν ἀπορήσῃ, κεναὶ καὶ ξηραὶ γίνονται καὶ [25] διψηραὶ καὶ οὐκ ἔχουσι λείψανα περὶ τὴν δίοδον. προσσπαστικαὶ οὖν οὖσαι σημαίνουσι καλῶς ἔχειν πρὸς τὸ συλλαβεῖν πλησιάσαντος ὅταν οὕτως ἔχωσιν ἄνευ ἄλγους καὶ [μετὰ] ἀναισθησίας. τό τε μὴ ἀλλοιότερον ἔχειν τὸ στόμα ἀγαθόν· καὶ γὰρ τοῦτο σημαίνει ὅτι οὐδέν ἐστιν ὃ κωλύει μὴ [30] συμμύειν αὐτὰς ὅταν δέῃ.

CHAPTER 3

περὶ μὲν οὖν τὸ στόμα τῶν ὑστερῶν ἐκ τούτων ἡ σκέψις ἐστὶν εἰ ἔχει ὡς δεῖ ἢ μή. περὶ αὐτὴν δὲ τὴν ὑστέραν δεῖ συμβαίνειν τοιαῦτα μετὰ τὴν κάθαρσιν, πρῶτον μὲν ἐν τοῖς ὕπνοις ὡς συγγινομένην τῷ ἀνδρὶ καὶ προϊέναι, ὡς ἂν εἰ [35] παρεπλησίαζε, ῥαδίως· ἂν τοῦτο φαίνηται πλεονάκις πάσχουσα, ἄμεινον. καὶ ἀνισταμένην ὁτὲ μὲν δεῖσθαι θεραπείας οἵας ὅταν πλησιάσῃ ἀνδρί, ὁτὲ δὲ ξηρὰν εἶναι. τὴν δὲ ξηρότητα ταύτην μὴ συνεχῆ, ἀλλ' ὕστερον μετὰ τὴν ἔγερσιν ἐξυγραίνεσθαι ὁτὲ μὲν θᾶττον ὁτὲ δ' ὀψιαίτερον καὶ ὅσον [40] εἰς ἥμισυ τῆς ἡμέρας βραχείας προελθούσης. ἡ δ' ὑγρότης [635b1] ἔστω τοιαύτη οἵα ὅταν πλησιάσῃ τῷ ἀνδρί. πάντα γὰρ ταῦτα σημαίνει δεκτικὴν τὴν ὑστέραν εἶναι τοῦ

635a16 ὅπερ ἐστὶ στόματος ὑγιεινῶς ἔχοντος transp. from 1–22 D-J. **22** προῆται Sn.: προΐενται D^a: *emittunt* Guil. (Tz.): *amittat* Guil. (cett.) ἀναστομοῦνται Sylb.: ἀναστομοῦντα D^a: *aperientia* Guil. **28** μετὰ secl. Sn: *cum insensibilitate* Guil. στόμα F^a pr.: os Guil.: σῶμα D^a. **34** προϊέναι D-J.: προϊεμένην D^a: *eicientem* Scot.: *emittentem* Guil. **37** ξηρὰν εἶναι Dt.: ξηρασίας D^a: *debet est sicca* Scot.: *indigere…siccam* Guil.

132

the cervix from its normal state. When the menses have ceased [15], the cervix should be particularly dilated and dry, but not hard, for a whole day and a half or even two days, the very mark of a cervix in a healthy state. For when these things occur in this way they indicate that the uterus is in a good state and performing its proper function by not expanding immediately but becoming soft at the cervix because it is [20] relaxing at the same time as the rest of the body is relaxing and, offering no impediment, it first emits the stuff from the cervix itself and only expands when the body sends forth more. And when the signs have ceased, by not immediately contracting, the uterus shows, if it is looking straight, that it has become empty and dry and [25] thirsty and has no residues around the passage. Therefore, being able to attract it shows that it is well disposed towards conception if she has intercourse, whenever it is in this state without pain and insensitivity. And the cervix having no alteration is a good thing. For this shows that there is nothing which prevents the uterus [30] closing together when it needs to.

CHAPTER 3

Concerning the cervix of the uterus, the investigation over whether it is as it should be or not proceeds from these things. Concerning the womb itself it is necessary that the following things take place after menstruation. Firstly that in her sleep, as if she is having intercourse with her husband, she should actually emit, just as if [35] she were reaching orgasm, readily. If she obviously experiences this frequently, all the better. And on rising sometimes she must require attention just as when she does have intercourse with her husband, and sometimes she should be dry. This dryness should not last, but later after waking up she should become moist, sometimes sooner and sometimes later, even by as much as [40] half a day, if the day in question is short. And the moisture [635b1] should be such as when she has intercourse with her husband, for all these things

ARISTOTLE

διδομένου, καὶ προσπαστικὰς τὰς κοτυληδόνας καὶ καθεκτικὰς
ὧν λαμβάνουσι καὶ ἀκούσας ἀφιείσας.

ἔτι φύσας ἐγγίνεσθαι ἄνευ [5] πάθους, ὥσπερ ἡ κοιλία, καὶ
ἀφιέναι, καὶ μεγάλας γινομένας καὶ ἐλάττους αὐτῶν, ἄνευ νόσου·
καὶ γὰρ ταῦτ᾽ ἀποδηλοῖ αὐτὰς ὅτι οὐδὲν στερεώτεραι τοῦ
δέοντός εἰσιν, οὔτε κωφαὶ οὔτε φύσει οὔτε νόσῳ, ἀλλὰ δύνανται,
ᾧ ἂν δέξωνται, αὐξανομένῳ παρέχειν χώραν. ἔχουσι δὲ καὶ
διάτασιν. ὅταν [10] δὲ τοῦτο μὴ γίγνηται, ἢ πυκνότεραί εἰσιν
ἢ ἀναισθητότεραι ἢ φύσει ἢ νόσῳ. διὸ καὶ οὐ δύνανται τρέφειν
ἀλλὰ καὶ διαφθείρουσι τὰ ἔμβρυα, ἐὰν μὲν σφόδρα τοιαῦται ὦσιν
ἔτι μικρὰ ὄντα, ἐὰν δ᾽ ἧττον μείζω· ἐὰν δὲ πάνυ ἠρέμα, φαυλότερα
ἐκτρέφουσι τὰ ἔκγονα καὶ οἷον ἐν ἀγγείῳ φαύλῳ [15] τραφέντα.

ἔτι δὲ θιγγανομένης τὰ ἐπὶ δεξιὰ καὶ τὰ ἐπ᾽ ἀριστερὰ ὁμαλὰ
αὐτῆς εἶναι, καὶ τἆλλα τούτοις ὁμοίως. καὶ ἐν τῇ πρὸς τὸν ἄνδρα
συνουσίᾳ μεταξὺ ὑγραίνεσθαι, μὴ πολλάκις δὲ μηδὲ σφόδρα.
ἔστι δὲ τοῦτο τὸ πάθος οἷον ἵδρωμα τοῦ τόπου, ὥσπερ καὶ τῷ
στόματι σιάλου πολλαχοῦ [20] μὲν καὶ πρὸς τὴν φορὰν τῶν
σιτίων, καὶ ὅταν λαλῶμεν καὶ ἐργαζώμεθα αὐτοὶ πλέον· καὶ
τοῖς ὄμμασι δακρύομεν πρὸς τὰ λαμπρότερα ὁρῶντες, καὶ ὑπὸ
ψύχους καὶ θερμότητος ἰσχυροτέρας, ἧς κρατεῖ τὰ μόρια ταῦτα
ὅταν τύχῃ ὑγροτέρως ἔχοντα. οὕτω καὶ αἱ ὑστέραι ὑγραίνονται ἐργαζόμεναι, [25] ὅταν τύχωσιν ὑγροτέρας διαθέσεως.
πάσχουσι δὲ τοῦτο τὸ πάθος καὶ αἱ μάλιστα καλῶς πεφυκυῖαι.
διὸ θεραπείας ἀεὶ δέονται αἱ γυναῖκες ἢ πλείονος ἢ ἐλάττονος,
ὥσπερ καὶ τὸ στόμα πτύσεως. ἀλλ᾽ ἐνίαις τοσαύτη ὑγρασία
γίνεται ὥστε μὴ δύνασθαι καθαρὸν τὸ τοῦ ἀνδρὸς <καὶ τῆς
γυναικὸς> ἀνασπάσαι [30] διὰ τὴν σύμμιξιν τῆς γιγνομένης ἀπὸ
τῆς γυναικὸς ὑγρότητος.

635b8 ᾧ Sn.: ὡς Dᵃ: *secundum quantitatem* Scot.   **14** ἐκτρέφουσι τὰ ἔκγονα
Sn.: ἐκτρέφουσι δὲ τὰ ἔκγονα Dᵃ.   **29** καὶ τῆς γυναικὸς add. D-J.

signal that the womb is receptive of what is being given. The cotyledons should have attractive power and be retentive of what they take in and unwilling to give it up.

Further, the uterus should produce wind without [5] symptoms, just like the stomach, and expel it, both inflating and deflating from it without disease. For, with respect to the uterus these things reveal that it is in no way firmer than it ought to be, nor is it unresponsive either by nature or by disease, but it is capable, for whatever it has received, of providing room for the thing as it grows. And it also has the ability to stretch. Whenever [10] this does not happen, it is either too dense or too insensitive either naturally or as a result of disease. For this reason too it is incapable of nurturing and even destroys embryos. If the uterus is badly affected in this way, it will destroy the embryos while they are still small, but if it is less affected, when they are bigger. If it is only mildly affected, it produces inferior babies, and such as are [15] nourished in a poor vessel.

Furthermore, the right and left sides of the womb should be even to the touch, and the other parts of it likewise. And during intercourse with her husband she should become moist, but not constantly and not excessively. This condition is like a local secretion, just as in the mouth there is often a local secretion of saliva [20] both at the expectation of food, and whenever we are chattering and working hard ourselves. And in our eyes we produce tears when we look at rather bright things and as a result of more powerful cold and heat, over which these parts get the mastery when they achieve a moister disposition. So too does the uterus produce moisture when it is exerting itself, [25] whenever it happens to be in a somewhat moist disposition. A uterus that is in a particularly good state experiences this condition. For this reason women always need either more or less attention, just as the mouth does from spittle. But some women produce so much moisture that they are unable to draw up the *sperma* of the man and the woman unalloyed [30] on account of the intermingling of the secretion which comes from the woman.

πρὸς δὲ τούτοις τοῖς πάθεσι καὶ τοσόνδε δεῖ κατανοεῖν, τί συμβαίνει, ὅταν δόξῃ ἐν τῷ ὕπνῳ πλησιάσαι τῷ ἀνδρί· πῶς ἔχουσα ἐξανίσταται, οἷον εἰ ἀσθενεστέρα, καὶ εἰ ἀεί, ἢ ὁτὲ μὲν ὁτὲ δ᾽ οὔ, ἢ ἐνίοτε καὶ ἰσχυροτέρα· εἰ [35] δὲ μὴ ξηροτέρα τὸ πρῶτον, εἶτα ἐφυγραίνεται. δεῖ γὰρ ταῦτα συμβαίνειν τῇ γονίμῳ γυναικί. τὸ μὲν γὰρ ἐκλύεσθαι σημαίνει προετικὸν εἶναι τὸ σῶμα σπέρματος ἀεί, τήν τε ποιοῦσαν ποιεῖ <ἀσθενῆ>· καὶ σωματωδῶν δ᾽ οὐσῶν ἀσθενεστέρα. τὸ δ᾽ ἀνόσως τοῦτο πάσχειν σημεῖον ὅτι κατὰ φύσιν καὶ ὃν δεῖ [40] τρόπον ἡ ἄφοδος τούτου γίνεται· εἰ γὰρ μή, νοσώδης ἦν [636a1] ἀρρωστία. τὸ δέ ποτε καὶ ἰσχύειν μᾶλλον, καὶ ξηρὰν εἶναι τὴν ὑστέραν, [εἶτ᾽ ἐφυγραίνεσθαι,] σημεῖον ὅτι πᾶν τὸ σῶμα λαμβάνει καὶ ἀφανίζει, καὶ οὐ μόνον ἡ ὑστέρα, καὶ τὸ σῶμα ἰσχύει. πνεύματί τε γὰρ ἕλκει ἡ ὑστέρα τὸ προσελθὸν [5] ἔξωθεν αὐτῇ, ὥσπερ πρότερον εἴρηται. οὐ γὰρ εἰς αὐτὴν προΐεται, ἀλλ᾽ οὗ καὶ ὁ ἀνήρ. ὅσα δὲ πνεύματι, πάντα ἰσχύϊ ἐργάζεται. ὥστε δῆλον ὅτι καὶ τὸ σῶμα προσσπαστικὸν τὸ τῆς τοιαύτης.

εἰσὶ δέ τινες αἳ πάσχουσί τι τοιοῦτον ὃ καλοῦσιν ἐξανεμοῦσθαι· [10] δεῖ δὴ καὶ τοῦτο μὴ πάσχειν. ἔστι δὲ τὸ τοιοῦτον πάθος. ὅταν συγγένωνται τῷ ἀνδρί, οὔτε προϊέμεναι δῆλαι τὸ σπέρμα οὔτε κυΐσκονται, διὸ καὶ καλεῖται ἐξανεμοῦσθαι. αἴτιον δὲ τοῦ πάθους ἡ ὑστέρα, ὅταν ᾖ λίαν ξηρά. ἑλκύσασα γὰρ πρὸς αὑτὴν τὸ ὑγρὸν <οὐκ> ἀφίησιν ἔξω· τὸ δὲ κατασκελετεύεται, [15] καὶ μικρόν τι γινόμενον ἐξ αὐτῆς ἀπέπεσέ τε καὶ ἔλαθε διὰ μικρότητα ἐξιόν. καὶ ὅταν μὲν τοῦτο σφόδρα πάθῃ ἡ ὑστέρα καὶ γένηται ὑπέρξηρος, ταχύ τε ἀπέβαλε καὶ ταχὺ δῆλον γίνεται ὅτι οὐ κύει· ἐὰν δὲ μὴ σφόδρα ταχέως ταῦτα ποιῇ, ἐν

635b32 τί Dt.: εἰ Dᵃ.　　**34** ἢ' Louis: μὴ Dᵃ: *aut* Scot.: *non* Guil.　　**38** ἀσθενῆ add. D-J.　**636a2** εἶτ᾽ ἐφυγραίνεσθαι secl. D-J.　　**7** προσσπαστικὸν Dt.: προσπαστικὸν Dᵃ.　　**14** οὐκ add. Dt.　　**15** αὑτῆς Dt.: αὐτοῦ Dᵃ.

In addition to these conditions one should also learn this much, what happens after she thinks she has had intercourse with her husband in her sleep: what state she is in when she wakes up, such as whether she is weaker, and if so whether invariably, or sometimes and sometimes not, or even on occasion stronger, and whether [35] she is not dryer at first and then becomes moist. For these things must happen to a fertile woman. For releasing ejaculate invariably signals that the body is emitting *sperma* and causes the one producing it to become weak. And, moreover, if the ejaculates are more substantive she will be still weaker. To experience this without illness is a sign that the discharge of this material occurs naturally and in the appropriate [40] manner. If this were not the case, the [636a1] weakness would be accompanied by other signs of disease. The fact that on occasion a woman is even stronger, and the womb is dry, is a sign that the whole body and not just the womb seizes on her *sperma* and causes it to disappear, and that the body grows strong from it. For with *pneuma* the womb draws in what has come towards [5] it from outside, just as was said earlier. For the woman's *sperma* is not emitted into the womb but where the man emits too. All things that perform their functions by *pneuma* do so by strength. So it is clear that the body of this sort of woman has an attractive power as well as the womb.

There are some women who suffer the sort of thing which they call wind-pregnancy. [10] And they should not suffer this. The condition has the following nature. Whenever they have had intercourse with their husband, neither are they seen to expel the *sperma*, nor do they become pregnant, and for this reason it is called a wind-pregnancy. The cause of the condition is the womb whenever it is too dry. For having drawn the moisture into itself it does not let it go outside, but the moisture dries up, [15] and becoming a small thing it falls from the womb and when it leaves it is not noticed on account of its smallness. And whenever the womb suffers this particularly and becomes excessively dry, it quickly gets rid of it and it quickly becomes clear that it has not conceived. But if it does not do

τῷ μεταξὺ χρόνῳ δοκεῖ κύειν ὃ ἂν ἔχῃ [20] αὐτὴ πρὸς αὑτήν, ἕως ἂν ἀποβάλῃ. καὶ ὅμοια συμβαίνει ταχὺ ταύταις πάθη οἷα ταῖς ὀρθῶς κυούσαις, καὶ ἐὰν γίγνηται πολὺς χρόνος, αἴρεται ἡ ὑστέρα ὥστε φανερῶς δοκεῖ κύειν, ἕως ἂν ἀποπέσῃ· τότε δ' ὁμοία ἐγένετο οἷα πρὸ τοῦ ἦν. ἀναφέρουσι δὲ τοῦτο τὸ πάθος εἰς τὸ δαιμόνιον. ὅ ἐστι [25] θεραπευτὸν ἐὰν μὴ φύσει τοιαύτη ᾖ σφόδρα πάσχουσα τὸ πάσχον. σημεῖον δὲ τοῦ [μὴ] τοιαύτας εἶναι ἐὰν φαίνωνται μὴ προϊέμεναι, ὅταν λάβωσι παρὰ τοῦ ἀνδρός, καὶ μὴ συλλάβωσιν.

CHAPTER 4

κωλύονται δὲ καὶ ἐὰν σπάσμα ἔχωσιν αἱ ὑστέραι. γίνονται δὲ σπάσματα ἐν ταῖς ὑστέραις ἢ φλεγμασίᾳ [30] διατεινομένης τῆς ὑστέρας, ἢ ἐν τῷ τόκῳ πληρώματος πολλοῦ ἐξαπίνης ἐπιπεσόντος καὶ μὴ ἀνοιγομένου τοῦ στόματος· τότε ὑπὸ τῆς διατάσεως γίνεται σπάσμα. σημεῖον δὲ τοῦ μὴ ἔχειν σπάσμα ἐὰν μὴ φαίνηται εἰς φλεγμασίαν ἀφικνουμένη ἐν τοῖς αὑτῆς ἔργοις ἡ ὑστέρα· ἔχουσα [35] γὰρ σπάσμα φλεγμαίνοι ἂν τότε.

ἔτι δὲ ἐὰν φῦμα ἐπὶ τοῦ στόματος ᾖ <ἢ> πολλὰ ἑλκωθὲν τὸ στόμα, ἐμποδίζει πρὸς τὰς συλλήψεις. σημεῖον δὲ καὶ τοῦ ταῦτα μὴ ἔχειν ἐὰν φαίνηται ἀνοιγομένη καλῶς ἡ ὑστέρα καὶ συμμύ-ουσα ὅταν γένηται αὐταῖς τὰ γυναικεῖα καὶ αἱ πρὸς τὸν ἄνδρα χρήσεις.

[636b1] ἔτι ἔστιν αἷς πως τὸ στόμα συμφύεται, ταῖς μὲν ἐκ γενετῆς ταῖς δὲ διὰ νόσον. γίνεται δὲ τοῦτο καὶ ἰατὸν καὶ ἀνί-ατον. οὐ χαλεπὸν δὲ τοῦτο γνῶναι ἐὰν ᾖ· οὐ γὰρ οἷόν τε οὔτε λαμβάνειν οὐδὲν ὧν δεῖ οὔτε προΐεσθαι. ἐὰν οὖν φαίνηται [5] καὶ δεχομένη παρὰ τοῦ ἀνδρὸς καὶ ἀφιεῖσα, δῆλον ὅτι οὐκ ἂν ἐνσχεθείη τῷ πάθει.

636a26 μὴ secl. Rud.   **34** αὑτῆς Sylb.: αὐτοῖς D^a: *suum* Scot.: *in propriis* Guil.   **35** τότε D-J.: ποτε D^a: *aliquando* Guil.   **36** ἢ add. D-J. ἑλκωθὲν τὸ στόμα D-J.: ἑλκωθέντος D^a: *a magno tempore* Scot.: *multa trahente* Guil.   **636b6** οὐκ ἂν ἐνσχεθείη Dt.: κἂν ἔλεγχος εἴη D^a: *et utique elenchus sit* Guil.

this particularly quickly, in the meantime it seems to be pregnant [20] until it expels whatever it is holding to itself. And such women quickly experience similar symptoms to those women who have genuinely conceived, and if much time elapses the womb is raised up so that it seems clearly to have conceived until it falls out of it. Then it becomes like it was before. They attribute this condition to the supernatural, a thing which is [25] treatable unless the woman is by nature such as to be extremely prone to suffer the suffering. It is a sign that they are like this if they appear not to expel the *sperma* whenever they receive it from the man and do not become pregnant.

CHAPTER 4

The uterus is also impeded if it has spasm. Spasms arise in the uterus either when [30] the womb is distended by inflammation or when in childbirth a large amount of material suddenly presses downward and the cervix does not open. Spasm occurs at that time from distention. If it is not seen to become inflamed while fulfilling its functions, it is a sign that it is not in spasm. For if it had [35] spasm it would at that time be inflamed.

Moreover, if there is a growth on the cervix or it is severely ulcerated, it gets in the way of conception. It is a sign that this is not the case if the womb evidently opens and closes properly whenever women are menstruating or having intercourse with their husband.

[636b1] Furthermore, it is the case for some of them that the cervix grows together somehow, in some women congenitally, in others because of disease. This comes about in both a curable and incurable form. It is not difficult to recognize this if it is present. For it is able neither to take up nor to emit any of the things it ought to. So if she clearly [5] both receives from the man and discharges menses, it is clear that she is not in the grip of the condition.

ὅσαις δὲ τούτων μηδὲν ἐμπόδιον ᾖ ἀλλ᾽ ἔχουσιν ὃν τρόπον
δεῖν εἴρηται ἔχειν, ἂν μὴ ὁ ἀνὴρ αἴτιος ᾖ τῆς ἀτεκνίας ἢ ἀμφότεροι
μὲν δύνωνται τεκνοῦσθαι πρὸς ἀλλήλους δὲ μὴ ὦσι σύμμετροι
τῷ ἅμα προΐεσθαι [10] ἀλλὰ πολὺ διαφωνῶσιν, ἔσονται τέκνα
τούτοις. τῷ μὲν οὖν εἰδέναι <εἰ> τὰ τοῦ ἀνδρὸς αἴτια ἔστι μὲν
καὶ ἄλλα σημεῖα λαβεῖν, ἃ δὲ ῥᾴω μάλιστα <ἂν> φαίνοιτο, πρὸς
ἄλλας πλησιάζων καὶ γεννῶν.
τοῦ δὲ πρὸς ἀλλήλους μὴ συνδρόμως ἔχειν, πάντων τῶν εἰρη-
μένων ὑπαρξάντων, οὐ γεννῶσιν. δηλοῖ [15] γὰρ ὅτι τοῦτο
αἴτιον μόνον. εἴπερ γὰρ καὶ ἡ γυνὴ συμβάλλεται εἰς τὸ σπέρμα
καὶ τὴν γένεσιν, δῆλον ὅτι δεῖ ἰσοδρομῆσαι παρ᾽ ἀμφοῖν. ἐὰν οὖν
ὁ μὲν ταχὺ ἐκποιήσῃ ἡ δὲ μόλις (τὰ γὰρ πολλὰ αἱ γυναῖκες βραδύτεραι), τοῦτο κωλύει· διὸ καὶ συζευγνύμενοι <οὐ> γεννῶσι
μετ᾽ ἀλλήλων [20] [οὐ] γεννῶντες δὲ ὅταν ἐντύχωσιν ἰσοδρομοῦσι πρὸς τὴν συνουσίαν. εἰ γὰρ ἡ μὲν ὀργῶσα καὶ παρεσκευασμένη εἴη καὶ ἐννοίας ἔχουσα ἐπιτηδείας, ὁ δὲ προλελυπημένος
καὶ κατεψυγμένος, ἀνάγκη τότε ἰσοδρομῆσαι αὐτοὺς ἀλλήλοις.

CHAPTER 5

ἔτι δ᾽ ἐνίοτε γυναιξὶ καὶ ἐξονειρωξάσαις καὶ ἀνδράσιν
ἀφροδισιάσασι [25] συμβαίνει εὐρωστοτέροις εἶναι, μὴ ἰσχύϊ ἀλλ᾽
ὑγιείᾳ· γίνεται δὲ τοῦτο ὅταν πολὺ τὸ σπέρμα ᾖ ἠθροισμένον
ἐπὶ τὸν τόπον ὅθεν προΐενται. ἐὰν οὖν τότε ἀπέλθῃ, οὐδὲν
ἀσθενέστεραι γίνονται· οὐ γὰρ ἀεὶ ἐκλύονται ἀπελθόντων, ὅταν
ἱκανὰ ᾖ τὰ λειπόμενα, οὐδ᾽ ἂν εἰ ἐκεῖνα ἄχρηστα ᾖ· [30] ἅμα καὶ
ῥᾷον, οἷον πλησμονῆς ἀπαλλαγέντα· διὸ οὐκ ἰσχύϊ εὐρωστότεραι
ἀλλὰ κουφότητι γίνονται. ἀλλ᾽ ὅταν ἀπὸ τοσούτων ἀπίῃ ὧν
τὸ σῶμα δεῖται, τότε ἀσθενεστέρας ποιεῖ. παύεται δὲ ταχὺ ἂν

636b7 δεῖν Sn.: δὴ Dᵃ: *oportet* Guil. **10** ἔσονται Scot.: οὐκ ἔσονται Dᵃ:
non Guil. τῷ D-J.: τῶ Dᵃ: *ad* Guil. μὲν οὖν Gᵃ Sᶜ Lᶜ: μὲν Dᵃ: *et* Scot.: *autem*
Guil. **11** εἰ add. Pk.: *utrum* Scot.: *si* Guil. **12** ἂν add. Sn. **13** ἀλλήλους Sn.:
ἄλλους Dᵃ: *ad inuicem* Guil. **14** οὐ codd.: μὴ Dᵃ Rᶜ Vᶜ. **19** οὐ transp.
Scal. **24** ἔτι Sylb.: ὅτι Dᵃ: *quod* Guil. **32** ἀπίῃ Scal.: ἐπίῃ Dᵃ.

But in the case of women for whom none of these impediments is present but who are in the state we have said they
ought to be, if it is not the case that the man is a cause of infertility, or that both are capable of engendering children but are
not matched with each other in the time of their emissions [10]
but are very discordant, they will have children. And while it is
indeed possible to take other signs in ascertaining if the causes
lie on the husband's side, it would certainly be apparent more
easily if he has intercourse and conceives with other women.

From not keeping pace with one another, although all the
other things we have talked about are in place, they do not
conceive. For it is clear [15] that this is the sole cause. For if the
woman contributes to the *sperma* and to reproduction it is clear
that it is necessary for both of them to keep pace with each
other. If therefore the man finishes off quickly while the woman
has scarcely started (for in most things women are slower), this
is an impediment. This is the reason why when yoked together
they do not produce children with each other [20] although
they do generate whenever they have intercourse with those
who run at the same pace with regard to copulation. For if the
woman is excited and prepared and has appropriate thoughts,
but the man is preoccupied and chilled, then they must keep
pace with one another.

CHAPTER 5

And again it sometimes happens both to women who have had
emissions during sleep and to men after intercourse [25] that
they are more robust, not in strength but in health. This happens whenever there is a lot of *sperma* collected together at the
place from which they emit it. If it is expelled then, women
become in no way weaker. For they are not always enervated
when *sperma* is released as long as there is sufficient left behind,
nor would they be if the emitted material is unusable. [30] And
at the same time there is an easing for them, as when things are
released from fullness. For this reason they become more robust

ἄλλως τις ὑγιάνῃ τὸ σῶμα καὶ ἐν ἡλικίᾳ ἢ ταχὺ σπερμοποιεῖ· τῶν γὰρ αὐξανομένων τοῦτ᾽ [35] ἐστὶ ταχὺ καὶ τῶν αὐξητῶν. καὶ λανθάνουσι τότε μάλιστα κυΐσκόμεναι. οὐ γὰρ οἴονται συνειληφέναι ἐὰν μὴ αἴσθωνται <προϊέμεναι> (προϊέμεναι δὲ τυγχάνουσιν), ὑπολαμβάνουσαι ὡς δεῖ ἐπ᾽ ἀμφοῖν συμπεσεῖν ἅμα, καὶ ἀπὸ τῆς γυναικὸς καὶ ἀπὸ τοῦ ἀνδρός.

μάλιστα δὲ λανθάνει ὅσαι οἴονται ἀδύνατον εἶναι [637a1] συλλαβεῖν ἐὰν μὴ ξηρανθῶσι καὶ ἐπιδήλως ἀφανισθῇ τὸ δοθέν. συμβαίνει δ᾽ ἐνίοτε πλέον προΐεσθαι καὶ αὐτὴν καὶ τὸν ἄνδρα οὗ ἂν δύνηται ἀφανίσαι καὶ τοῦ ἱκανοῦ. ὅταν οὖν σπάσῃ μὲν ἱκανόν, λειφθῇ δὲ πολύ, τότε λανθάνουσι κυΐσκόμεναι. [5] ὅτι δὲ τοιοῦτον ἐνδέχεται γίνεσθαι καὶ οὐκ ἐξ ἅπαντος γίνεται τὸ πάθος, δηλοῖ ὅσα τῶν ζῴων ἀπὸ μιᾶς ὀχείας πολλὰ τίκτει, καὶ ἡ τῶν διδύμων γένεσις, ὅταν ἀπὸ μιᾶς γένηται. δῆλον γὰρ ὅτι ἐξ οὐχ ἅπαντος ἐγένετο, ἀλλὰ μέρος τι αὐτοῦ ἔλαβέ τις τόπος, τὸ δὲ περιελείπετο πολλαπλάσιον.

[10] ἔτι εἰ πολλὰ ἀπὸ μιᾶς ὀχείας γίνεται, ὅπερ φαίνεται ἐπὶ τῶν ὑῶν καὶ τῶν διδύμων ἐνίοτε γιγνόμενον, δῆλον ὅτι [οὐκ] ἀπὸ παντὸς ἔρχεται τὸ σπέρμα τοῦ σώματος, ἀλλ᾽ ἐφ᾽ ἑκάστου εἴδους ἐμερίζετο. ἀπὸ παντὸς μὲν γὰρ ἐνδέχεται ἀποχωρισθῆναι καὶ τὸ πᾶν εἰς πολλά. ὥστε ἅμα καὶ κατὰ [15] μέρος ἀδύνατον.

ἔτι ἡ γυνὴ προΐεται εἰς τὸ πρόσθεν τοῦ στόματος τῶν ὑστερῶν, οὗ καὶ ὁ ἀνήρ, ὅταν πλησιάσῃ. ἐντεῦθεν γὰρ σπᾷ τῷ πνεύματι, ὥσπερ τοῖς στόμασιν ἢ τοῖς μυκτῆρσιν. πάντα

636b37 προϊέμεναι add. Rud.   **39** ἀδύνατον εἶναι Dᵃ: εἶναι ἀδύνατον Orib.   **637a1** ξηρανθῶσι Dᵃ hic: ἀναξηρανθῇ Dᵃ infra: ἐπιξηρανθῇ Orib.   **2** πλέον προΐεσθαι Dᵃ hic: προέσθαι πλέον Dᵃ infra Orib.   **3** δύνηται Dᵃ infra: δύναιντο Dᵃ hic: δύναιτο Orib.   **4** λειφθῇ Orib.: ληφθῇ Dᵃ hic et infra: remanebit Scot. hic, remanet Scot. infra: relinquatur utrobique Guil.   **7** τίκτει Dᵃ hic et infra: τίκτεται Orib. ἡ om. Orib.   **8** ἐξ οὐχ ἅπαντος Gᵃ Q Fᵃ Xᶜ Lᶜ: ἐξ ἅπαντος Dᵃ hic: οὐκ ἐξ ἅπαντος Dᵃ infra Orib.: non ex toti Guil. hic, ex omni Guil.   **9** μέρος τι αὐτοῦ Dᵃ hic: μέρος τοῦ αὐτοῦ Dᵃ infra Orib.: partem aliquam ipsius Guil. hic, partem ipsius v.l. partem eius Guil. infra περιελείπετο Orib.: περιέλιπε τὸ Dᵃ infra: περιέλιπε Dᵃ hic.   **12** οὐκ secl. D-J.

not by strength but by lightness. But whenever the emission comes out of the amount of stuff that the body needs, then it makes them weaker. But this soon ceases as long as the woman is otherwise healthy in body and at the time of life which produces *sperma* rapidly. For this is one of the things that are capable of [35] rapid increase and of causing increase. And it escapes women's notice in these circumstances particularly that they have become pregnant. For they do not think they have conceived if they do not notice that they are emitting but they are in fact emitting, since they understand that it is necessary for both of their emissions to fall together at the same time, both from the woman and from the man.

Those women who think it is impossible [637a1] to become pregnant unless they are left completely dry after intercourse and what has been supplied has quite clearly disappeared are prone not to notice when they conceive. Often it happens that both she and her husband emit more than she can completely use up and more than enough for conception. Whenever she has drawn up enough but a lot has been left behind, then they are unaware that they have become pregnant. [5] The fact that such a thing can occur and that the condition does not come about from all of the *sperma* is shown by those animals which produce many offspring from one coupling, and by the production of twins, whenever that occurs from one coupling. For it is clear that each fetus came about from not all the *sperma* but a particular place took up some part of it and the multiple of this amount was left behind. [10] Moreover, if many young come from one coupling, which is clear in the case of pigs and sometimes in the case of twins in humans, it is clear that the *sperma* comes from the whole body but is parceled out in respect of each individual. For of course it is possible for an individual to be separated off from all the *sperma* and for all the *sperma* to separate into many individuals. So that it is impossible at the same time for *sperma* to be separated off from the body [15] part by part.

Further, the woman emits to the place in front of the cervix of the uterus, where the man too emits, whenever she reaches

γὰρ ὅσα μὴ ὀργάνοις προσάγεται, ἢ εἴσφυσιν ἔχει ἄνωθεν <ἢ> κοῖλα ὄντα πνεύματι ἕλκονται ὡς ἐκ τούτου τοῦ [20] τόπου. διὸ ἐπιμελοῦνται ὅπως γένηται ξηρὸς οὗτος ὥσπερ πρὶν τοῦτο συμβαίνειν. πέφυκε δ' οὕτως ἡ ὁδὸς δι' ἧς ἔρχεται ταῖς γυναιξίν. ἔχουσι καυλόν, ὥσπερ καὶ οἱ ἄνδρες τὸ αἰδοῖον, ἀλλ' ἐν τῷ σώματι. ἀποπνέουσι διὰ τούτου μικρῷ τε πόρῳ ἀνωτέρω <ἢ> ᾗ οὐροῦσιν αἱ γυναῖκες. διὸ καὶ ὅταν ὀργῶσιν [25] ἀφροδισιασθῆναι, οὗτος ὁ τόπος οὐκ ἔχει ὁμοίως καὶ πρὶν ὀργᾶν. ἀπὸ δὴ τούτου τοῦ καυλοῦ γίνεται ἔκπτωσις, καὶ τὸ ἔμπροσθεν τῆς ὑστέρας πολλῷ μεῖζον ἢ καθ' ἣν εἰς ἐκεῖνον τὸν τόπον ἐκπίπτει. ὅμοιον δ' ἐστὶ τοῦτο κατὰ τοῦτο ταῖς ῥισίν· καὶ γὰρ αἱ ῥῖνες ἔχουσιν εἴσω εἰς τὸν φάρυγγα πόρον τινὰ [30] καὶ εἰς τὸν ἔξω ἀέρα· οὕτω κἀκεῖνος καὶ ἔξω ἔχει πόρον μικρόν τε πάνυ καὶ στενόν, ὅσον πνεύματι ἔξοδον, τὸν δ' εἰς τὸ πρόσθεν τῆς ὑστέρας εὐρύχωρον εὔρουν, ὥσπερ αἱ ῥῖνες τὸν εἰς τὸν ἀέρα μείζω τοῦ εἰς τὸ στόμα καὶ φάρυγγα. ὁμοίως δὲ καὶ αἱ γυναῖκες μείζω τὸν εἰς τὸ ἔμπροσθεν τῶν ὑστερῶν [35] πόρον ἔχουσι καὶ εὐρυχωρότερον τοῦ ἔξω.

ΔΙΑΛΕΚΤΙΚΗ ΥΠΕΡ *ΥΠΕΡ ΤΟΥ ΜΗ ΓΕΝΝΑΝ*

Τόπος

Ὅ τι συμβάλλεται εἰς τοῦτο ποιεῖ <τὸ αἴτιον> τῶν αὐτῶν παθημάτων ὅτι καὶ ἡ γυνὴ γόνιμον προΐεται. τὰ δ' αὐτὰ αἴτια ταῦτα συμβαίνει. καὶ γὰρ οἷς ἢ νόσου ἢ θανάτου δοκεῖ ἑτέρου

637a19 ἢ add. D-J. ἕλκονται Pk.: *trahunt* Guil.: ἕλκων ἢ Dᵃ ὡς add. Dt.   **23** τούτου D-J.: τοῦτο Dᵃ.   **24** ἢ add. Scal.   **35** τοῦ Scal.: τὸ Dᵃ: *quam extrinsecum* Scot.: *eo qui extra* Guil.   **36** τὸ αἴτιον add. D-J.

climax. And from there the womb draws it in by *pneuma*, just as in the case of the mouth and nostrils. For all things that draw things to themselves without tools have either a natural funnel above or, being hollow, they draw it in by *pneuma*, as from this [20] place. And so they are concerned that this place become dry, just as it was before the emission of *sperma* occurred. The route through which *sperma* travels in women is of the following nature. They have a *kaulos* just as men have a penis, but within the body. They breathe out through this, and at a small opening above the place where women urinate. And for this reason, whenever they are [25] sexually excited, this place is not in the same state as it was before the excitement. From this *kaulos* there comes an emission, and the area in front of the womb is much greater than the passage through which the emission falls into that place. And in this respect the configuration of the *kaulos* is similar to the nose. For the nose too has a passage inside to the pharynx [30] and to the outside air. Similarly the *kaulos* also has a small and very narrow passageway outside, large enough to be an outlet for the *pneuma* while that towards the front of the womb is capacious and wide, just as the nose has the one towards the air larger than that towards the mouth and pharynx. Similarly, women have the passage to the place in front of the uterus larger [35] and more spacious than the one to the outside.

DIALECTIC ON *ON FAILURE TO REPRODUCE*

Topos

Whatever is contributed to this (i.e., the mixture of fluids in the area before the uterus), the author makes the cause of the same experiences (in women as in men, i.e., excitement and lassitude) because <he believes that> the woman too is emitting a generative fluid. And it follows that these things (i.e., male and female ejaculate) are the same causes (i.e., in reproduction itself). And in fact, those to whom it (i.e., the female ejaculate) also seems to

τὸ αἴτιον εἶναι, <οὐ> θεωροῦσι τὸ [637b1] τελευταῖον ἐπὶ τὰς ἀρχάς, ὃ δεῖ ὁρᾶν. τοῖς μὲν γὰρ ταὐτὰ αἴτια τὰ πάντα, τοῖς δὲ οὐδέν, τῶν δὲ τὰ μὲν τὰ δ᾽ οὔ. ἀποδίδωσιν οὖν κατὰ λόγον καὶ τὰ ἀποβαίνοντα· καὶ τοῖς μὲν διὰ πάντων συμβαίνει διελθεῖν τῶν αὐτῶν παθημάτων, [5] τοῖς δὲ διὰ πολλῶν οἷς πολλά· τοῖς δὲ δι᾽ ὀλίγων· τοῖς δὲ δι᾽ οὐθενὸς ὅσοις μηδέν.

CHAPTER 6

φανερὰ δὲ τὰ ζῷά ἐστιν ὅταν ὀχευθῆναι δέηται. διώκει γὰρ τὰ ἄρρενα, οἷον αἱ ἀλεκτορίδες διώκουσι καὶ ὑφιζάνουσιν αὐταὶ ἐὰν μὴ ὀργᾷ ὁ ἄρρην. τοῦτο δὲ ποιεῖ καὶ ἄλλα ζῷα. εἰ δὴ ταῦτα πάθη πᾶσι τοῖς ζῴοις [10] φαίνεται ὄντα περὶ τὴν συνουσίαν, δῆλον ὅτι καὶ ταῦτα αἴτια συμβαίνοντα. ἀλλὰ μὴν ἥ γε ὄρνις οὐ μόνον τοῦ λαβεῖν ἐπιθυμίαν ἔχει, ἀλλὰ καὶ τοῦ προέσθαι. σημεῖον δὲ τούτου· ἐὰν γὰρ μὴ παρῇ ἄρρην, πίπτει ὑπ᾽ ἄλλην καὶ ἔγκυος γίγνεται καὶ τίκτει ὑπηνέμια, [ὡς] ἐπιθυμοῦσα καὶ τοῦ [15] ἀφεῖναι τότε, ὡς ἀφεῖσα ὅταν καὶ τῷ ἄρρενι συνῇ. ποιεῖ δὲ τοῦτο καὶ τἆλλα, ἐπειδὴ καὶ τῶν ἀδουσῶν ἀκρίδων ἤδη τις ἐπειράθη τρέφουσα, ἔτι ἁπαλὰς λαβοῦσα· καὶ ἐγένοντο αὐξηθεῖσαι αὐτόματοι ἔγκυοι. ἐκ δὴ τούτων δῆλον ὅτι συμβάλλεται εἰς τὸ σπέρμα πᾶν τὸ θῆλυ, εἴ γε καὶ ἐφ᾽ [20] ἑνὸς γένους φαίνεται τοῦτο γιγνόμενον. οὐδὲν γὰρ διαφέρει τὸ ᾠὸν τὸ ὑπηνέμιον τούτου, ἀλλ᾽ ἢ τῷ μὴ γεννᾶν ζῷον. τοῦτο δ᾽ ὅτι οὐ παρ᾽ ἀμφοῖν ἦλθεν. διὸ οὐδὲ τὰ ἀπὸ τοῦ ἄρρενος ἅπαντα γόνιμα φαίνεται, ἀλλ᾽ ἔνια ἄγονα ὅταν μὴ ἐξ ἀμφοῖν ὡς δεῖ συναρμοσθῇ. ἔτι γυναῖκες ἐξονειρώττουσι, καὶ [25] ταύταις γίνεται, ὡς ὅταν συγγένωνται ἀνδρί, ταὐτὰ παθήματα μετὰ τὸν ὀνειρωγμόν, διάλυσις καὶ ἀδυναμία. δῆλον τοίνυν, εἰ ἐν τῷ ἐξονειρωγμῷ φαίνονται προϊέμεναι <ὡς> καὶ

637a38 οὐ add. Barnes.   **637b2** πάντα D-J.: πρῶτα Dᵃ.   **10** ταὐτὰ Dt.: τὰ Dᵃ.   **13** ἄλλην Dt.: αὐτὴν Dᵃ.   **14** ὡς secl. D-J.   **15** ὡς D-J.: καὶ Dᵃ.   **21** ᾠὸν Dt.: ζῷον' Dᵃ: ouum Scot. ἀλλ᾽ ἢ Sn.: ἀλλὰ Dᵃ: nisi Scot. Guil.   **22** οὐ Dt.: καὶ Dᵃ.   **24** ἔτι Scal.: et accidit Scot.: ἐπεὶ Dᵃ: quoniam Guil.   **27** ὡς add. Scal.

be the cause of something else, either disease or death, are not examining their [637b1] conclusion with a view to their initial premises, which they ought to keep in view. Because for some experiences all the causes are the same, in others none, and of others some causes are the same and others are not. And so they produce outcomes in proportion. In some <conditions> they (i.e., sufferers of any condition) go through all the same experiences, [5] in those which have many causes the same they go through many of the same experiences, in others they go through few, and in those conditions which have no causes the same they go through none of the same experiences.

CHAPTER 6

Female animals make it clear when they need mating; they pursue the male, for example hens pursue and get under the cock themselves if he is not excited. Other animals also do this. So, if the same conditions are [10] apparent in all animals in respect to intercourse, it is clear that the same causes are indeed occurring. But surely, the female bird at least not only has a desire for taking something on but also for emitting something. A sign of this: if a male is not present, she falls under another female and becomes pregnant and lays wind-eggs since she desires to discharge [15] at that time too, as she discharges whenever she does in fact couple with a male. Other animals do this too, since there was once some woman who, catching some singing grasshoppers while they were still tender, raised them to see what would happen. When they had grown, they became pregnant by themselves. From these things it becomes clear that every female contributes to the *sperma* even if this is seen to come about in [20] just one type of animal. For there is no difference between the wind-egg and the grasshopper pregnancy except that the wind-egg does not produce a living animal. And this is because it does not come from both parents. And so it is also apparent that not all the emission from the male is generative, but some is unproductive, whenever the emission from

ARISTOTLE

τότε συμβάλλονται, ὅτι μετὰ τοὺς ἐξονειρωγμοὺς ὁ αὐτὸς τόπος
ἀφυγραίνεται καὶ θεραπείας δέονται τῆς αὐτῆς αὐταὶ [30] ὑφ'
αὑτῶν ὥσπερ ὅταν συγγένωνται ἀνδρί. ὥστε φανερὸν ὅτι παρ'
ἀμφοῖν γίνεται πρόεσις σπέρματος εἰ μέλλει γόνιμον ἔσεσθαι.
προΐενται δ' οὐκ εἰς αὐτὰς τὰς ὑστέρας ἀλλ' ἔξω, οὗ καὶ ὁ
ἀνήρ· εἶτ' ἐκεῖθεν ἕλκει εἰς αὐτάς. ὡς τὰ μὲν γεννᾷ ἀφ' αὑτῶν τὰ
θήλεα οἷον ὄρνις (τὰ [δ'] ὑπηνέμια), τὰ δ' [35] οὐθὲν οἷον ἵπποι
καὶ πρόβατα; ἢ ὅτι ἡ μὲν ὄρνις εἰς τὴν ὑστέραν προΐεται, καὶ οὐκ
ἔστιν ἔξω τόπος εἰς ὃν ἀφίησιν οὐδὲ ὁ ἄρρην· διὸ ἐὰν μὴ τύχῃ
ὀχεύων, εἰς τὴν γῆν ἐκχεῖ· τοῖς δὲ τετράποσιν ἔστιν ἔξω τόπος
ἄλλος εἰς ὃν καὶ τὸ θῆλυ [638a1] προΐεται καὶ τὸ ἄρρεν· ὅπερ τοῖς
μὲν ἄλλοις μετὰ τῶν ἄλλων ὑγρῶν συγχεῖται καὶ οὐ συνίσταται
ἐν τῇ ὑστέρᾳ διὰ τὸ μὴ εἰσιέναι, ταῖς δ' ὄρνισι λαβοῦσα ἡ ὑστέρα
συμπέττει καὶ σῶμά τι ὅμοιον τὰ ἄλλα πλὴν οὐ ζῷον· διότι δεῖ
ἐξ [5] ἀμφοῖν τὸ ζῷον εἶναι.

CHAPTER 7

ἔστι δ' ἐνστῆναι, εἰ ἀληθῆ λέγουσι φάσκουσαι, ὅταν ἐξονειρώτ-
τωσι, ξηραὶ ἀνίστασθαι. δῆλον γὰρ ὅτι ἕλκει ἡ ὑστέρα ἄνωθεν·
ὥστε διὰ τί οὐ γεννᾷ αὐτὰ καθ' αὑτὰ τὰ θήλεα, ἐπείπερ καὶ
μιχθὲν ἕλκει τὸ τοῦ ἄρρενος; διὰ τί οὐχὶ καὶ ἀμιγὲς τὸ αὐτῶν
ἕλκει, ὅπερ εἰς τὸ ἔξω διατείνει;

637b32 αὐτὰς τὰς ὑστέρας D-J.: αὐτὰς αἱ ὑστέραι Dᵃ: uterque…in se Scot.: in
se ipsas matrices Guil.　33 αὐτάς D-J.: αὐτάς Dᵃ: attrahit ipsum femina ad se Scot.:
trahunt in se ipsas Guil. ὡς Scal.: ὧν Dᵃ: quarum Guil.　34 δ' secl. Dt.: ouum
uenti Scot.: hec autem ypenemia Guil.　638a4 διότι Dt.: διὸ Dᵃ: propter quod
Guil.　6 ὅταν Sn.: ὅ τι ἂν Dᵃ: quod si Guil.　9 ἀμιγὲς Pk.: αἱ αἶγες Dᵃ:
capre Guil.: om. Scot. αὐτῶν D-J.: αὐτῆς Dᵃ: proprium Guil.

both does not harmonize as is necessary. Furthermore, women have emissions in dreams and [25] for them there occur the same experiences after the dream emissions as when they have sex with a man, relaxation and loss of power. And so it is clear, if in the dream they clearly emit, that they also contribute <to the fetus> at that time (i.e., when they become pregnant after having intercourse with a man), because after the dream emissions the same place becomes moist and they require the same treatment [30] from themselves as when they have had sex with a man. And so it is clear that the emission of *sperma* happens on both sides if it is to be fertile.

And women do not emit into the uterus itself but outside, where the man also emits, and then from there she draws it into her uterus. How is it that some females reproduce by themselves, such as a bird (wind-eggs), but others produce nothing, such as horses and sheep? Now, is this because the female bird emits into the [35] womb and there is not any external place into which even the male discharges? For this reason, if he does not manage to mate, it flows onto the ground. But in quadrupeds there is another place outside into which both [638a1] the male and the female emit. In the other female animals this emission is mixed up with the other fluids and does not take shape in the womb because it does not go into it, while in female birds the womb receives it and even concocts a sort of body similar in other respects except it is not a living animal. Because [5] the living thing must come out of both.

CHAPTER 7

It is possible to object, if women are telling the truth when they say that whenever they have a wet dream they wake up dry. For it is clear that the womb draws their emission in upwards. So why do females not impregnate themselves since they do draw in the emission once the emission from the male has been mixed in? Why do they not also draw up their own emission unmixed when it reaches the place outside?

[10] αἷς γίνεται τοῦτο τὸ πάθος κυούσαις ἔτη πολλά. τίκτουσι
γὰρ ὃ καλοῦσι μύλην, οἷον συνέβη τινὶ γυναικί. συγγενομένης τῷ
ἀνδρὶ καὶ δοξάσης συλλαβεῖν ὅ τ᾽ ὄγκος ηὐξάνετο τῆς ὑστέρας
καὶ τἆλλα ἐγίγνετο τὸ πρῶτον κατὰ λόγον. ἐπεὶ δ᾽ ὁ χρόνος ἦν
τοῦ τόκου, οὔτε ἔτικτεν οὔτε ὁ ὄγκος [15] ἐλάττων ἐγίγνετο,
ἀλλ᾽ ἔτη τρία ἢ τέτταρα οὕτω διετέλεσεν, ἕως δυσεντερίας
γενομένης καὶ κινδυνευσάσης αὐτῆς ἔτεκε σάρκα εὐμεγέθη, ἣν
καλοῦσι μύλην. ἐνίαις δὲ καὶ συγκαταγηράσκει τὸ πάθος καὶ
συναποθνήσκει.

πότερον δὲ διὰ θερμότητα γίνεται τὸ πάθος τοῦτο, ὅταν τύχῃ
ἡ ὑστέρα θερμὴ καὶ [20] ξηρὰ οὖσα καὶ διὰ ταῦτα σπαστικὴ
πρὸς αὐτήν, καὶ οὕτως ὥστ᾽ ἔστιν ἀνελέσθαι καὶ φυλάξαι πρὸς
αὐτήν; οὕτω γὰρ ἐχούσαις, ἐὰν μὴ μεμιγμένον ἐστὶ τὸ ἀπ᾽ ἀμφοῖν,
ἀλλ᾽ ὥσπερ τὸ ὑπηνέμιον ἐνδέξαιτο ἀπὸ θατέρου, τότε γίνεται ἡ
καλουμένη μύλη, οὔτε ζῷον, διὰ τὸ μὴ παρ᾽ ἀμφοῖν, οὔτ᾽ ἄψυχον,
[25] διὰ τὸ ἔμψυχον ληφθὲν εἶναι, ὥσπερ τὰ ὑπηνέμια. πολὺν
δὲ χρόνον ἐμμένει διά τε τὴν τῆς ὑστέρας διάθεσιν, καὶ διότι ἡ
μὲν ὄρνις πολλὰ εἰς αὐτὴν τίκτουσα, ὑπὸ τούτων οἰγνυμένης
τῆς ὑστέρας, προσάγει καὶ τίκτει· καὶ ὅταν ἅπαξ οἰχθῇ, καὶ τὸ
τελευταῖον ἐξέρχεται. οὐ γάρ ἐστι τὸ εἶργον, [30] ἀλλὰ καὶ τὸ
σῶμα προετικὸν γενόμενον ὅτε ἐπληροῦτο, οὐκέτι τὴν ὑστέραν
ποιεῖ ἀντισπαστικήν. ὅσα δὲ ζωοφορεῖ, διὰ τὸ μεταβάλλειν τὴν
δύναμιν αὐξανομένου καὶ ἄλλοτε ἀλλοίας δεῖσθαι τροφῆς, ἐπιφλεγμαίνουσά τι ἡ ὑστέρα ποιεῖ τακτὸν τὸν τόκον. ἡ δὲ σάρξ,
διὰ τὸ μὴ ζῷον εἶναι, ἀεὶ τῶν ὁμαλῶν. [35] δεῖ γὰρ ὃ βαρύνει

638a11 συγγενομένης...δοξάσης Dᵃ: συγγενομένη...δοξάσῃ Orib.: *commixte...
credenti* Guil. **14** ὅ² om. Orib. **15** ἕως Orib.: ὡς Dᵃ. **16** post
γενομένης add. αὐτῇ Orib. post αὐτῆς add. δηλονότι Orib. **17** ἣν καλοῦσι
μύλην Dᵃ: ἣν καὶ μύλην κατωνόμασας Orib. om. καὶ ante συγκαταγηράσκει
Orib. **18** συναποθνήσκει Dᵃ: ἀποθνήσκει Orib. ante πότερον add. καὶ
γὰρ Orib. δὲ Bk.: δὴ Dᵃ: *igitur* Guil. **19** ante γίνεται add. δηλονότι Orib.
θερμὴ καὶ ξηρὰ Dᵃ: ξηρὰ καὶ θερμὴ Orib. **21** ὥστ᾽ Dᵃ: ὡς Orib. ἔστιν om.
Orib. **22** ἀπ᾽ Dᵃ: ἐξ Orib. **23** τὸ om. Orib. **25** διὰ τὸ ἔμψυχον
om. Orib. **26** διὰ...ἔτι δὲ 638b7 om. Orib. **28** οἰγνυμένης Gohlke:
γινομένης Dᵃ: *facta* Guil. **30** καὶ τὸ Scal.: κατὰ Dᵃ: *secundum* Guil. **33**
τακτὸν τὸν Pk.: ταὐτὸν Dᵃ: om. Guil.

[10] This condition is present in women who have been pregnant for many years. They give birth to what they call a mole, such as happened to one particular woman. For after she had had intercourse with her husband and believed she had conceived, the bulk of the womb increased and everything else occurred at first according to expectations. But when the time of birth arrived she neither gave birth nor did the bulk [15] become any less, but she went on this way for three or four years, until having contracted dysentery and become very sick she gave birth to a lump of flesh of considerable size, which they call a mole. And in some women the condition persists into old age and even death.

A further question then is does this condition arise because of heat, whenever the womb happens to be hot and [20] dry and for this reason is disposed to draw <female seed> into itself and is so hot and dry that it is able to draw it up and keep it within itself? For when the uterus is in this state, if the *sperma* from both parents is not mixed but were to be received from one of the two as in the case of the wind-egg, then the so-called mole is generated, neither an animal—since it is not from both of them—nor is it without soul [25] because it was taken up with some soul in it, just like wind-eggs. And it remains a long time because of the state of the womb, whereas the bird produces many eggs within herself and when the womb is opened by these pushes them forward and lays them. And when once the womb has been opened even the last one comes out, for there is nothing holding it back, [30] rather the body too becoming expulsive when it has been filled up causes the womb to be no longer retentive. On the other hand, in the case of those animals which are viviparous, because of the change in the capacity of the growing fetus and its need for different nourishment at different times, the womb, becoming somewhat inflamed, causes its birth at the right time. But flesh, since it is not an animal, is always one of the uniform things, [35] for what weighs

τὴν ὑστέραν οὐδὲν ποιεῖν <αὐτὴν> φλεγμαίνειν. ὡς ἐνίαις γε
καὶ συναποθνήσκει τὸ πάθος, ἐὰν μὴ δι᾽ εὐτύχημα ἀσθενήματος
συμβῇ, οἷον τῇ ληφθείσῃ ὑπὸ τῆς δυσεντερίας.

[638b1] πότερον δ᾽, ὥσπερ εἴρηται, διὰ θερμότητα γίνεται
τὸ πάθος ἢ μᾶλλον δι᾽ ὑγρότητα [ὅτι καὶ ἔστι τὸ πλήρωμα οἷον
μύει], [ἢ] ὅταν μὴ οὕτως ᾖ ψυχρὰ ἡ ὑστέρα ὥστε ἀφεῖναι, μηδ᾽
οὕτω θερμὴ ὥστε πέψαι; διὸ καὶ χρόνιον τὸ πάθος, ὥσπερ [5]
τὰ ἐν ἑψήσει πολὺν χρόνον διαμένει. τὰ δ᾽ ἑψόμενα πέρας ἔχει καὶ
παχυτῆτα. αἱ δὲ τοιαῦται ὑστέραι ἀκρόταται οὖσαι τὸν χρόνον
ποιοῦσι πολύν. ἔτι διὰ τὸ μὴ ζῷον εἶναι, οὐ κινούμενον οὐ ποιεῖ
τὴν ὠδῖνα· ἡ γὰρ κίνησις τῶν συνδέσμων ὠδίς ἐστιν ἤ, διὰ τὸ
ζῆν, προΐεται τὸ ἔμβρυον. [10] καὶ ἡ σκληρότης δ᾽ ἡ γιγνομένη
τοῦ πράγματος μωλύσεως ἔργον ἐστίν. οὕτω γὰρ γίνεται
σκληρὸν ὥστε πελέκει οὐ δύνανται διακόπτειν. τὰ μὲν οὖν ἑφθὰ
καὶ πάντα τὰ πεπεμμένα μαλακὰ γίνεται, τὰ δ᾽ μεμωλυσμένα
ἄπεπτα καὶ σκληρά.

[15] ὅ τι πολλοὶ ἰατροὶ ἀγνοοῦντες, δι᾽ ὁμοιότητα μύλας εἶναι
τὸ πάθος φάσκουσιν, ἂν μόνον ἴδωσι τάς τε κοιλίας ἐπαιρομένας
ἄνευ ὕδρωπος καὶ τῶν ἐπιμηνίων σχέσιν, ὅταν χρονίζῃ τοῦτο
τὸ πάθος. τὸ δ᾽ οὐκ ἔστιν, [ἀλλ᾽] ὀλιγάκις <γὰρ> γίνονται [αἱ
γιγνόμεναι] μύλαι. ἄλλοτε μὲν σύρρους γίνεται ψυχρῶν [20]
καὶ ὑγρῶν περιττωμάτων καὶ ὑδαρῶν, ἄλλοτε δὲ παχυτέρων,
εἰς τὸν περὶ τὴν κοιλίαν τόπον, ἐὰν τὴν φύσιν τοιαῦται ἢ τὴν

638a35 ποιεῖν Louis: οἴει Dᵃ: om. Scot. Guil. αὐτὴν add. D-J.   **638b3** ἢ
secl. D-J.   **6** παχυτῆτα D-J.: ταχυτῆτα Dᵃ: om. Scot.: uelocitatem Guil. **7**
διὰ Sn.: δὲ Dᵃ: adhuc autem propter Guil.: τῷ γὰρ Orib.   **9** ἢ D-J.: ἦν Dᵃ:
que Guil. προΐεται Orib.: προΐεσθαι Dᵃ: emittit Guil.   **10** μωλύσεως Orib.:
κωλύσεως Dᵃ.   **13** μεμωλυσμένα Orib.: ἀπολελυμένα Dᵃ.   **15** ὅ τι Dᵃ:
om. Orib. πολλοὶ ἰατροὶ Dᵃ: πολλοὶ δ᾽ ἰατροὶ Orib.   **16** φάσκουσιν Orib.:
πάσχουσιν Dᵃ: dicunt Scot.: patiuntur Guil.   **18** χρονίζῃ Dᵃ: χρονίσῃ Orib.
ἀλλ᾽ secl. Orib. γὰρ add. Orib.: non accidit nisi raro Scot.: sed raro fiunt facte
Guil.   **19** αἱ γιγνόμεναι secl. Orib. οὖν add. Orib.: alias quidem Guil.   **20**
post περιττωμάτων add. καὶ λέπτων Orib.: subtiles Guil.   **21** τοιαῦται D-J.:
τοιαῦτα Dᵃ Orib.: talia Guil.   **22** ἢ Orib.: ἦ Dᵃ.

down the womb must in no way cause it to be inflamed. So in some women at any rate the condition persists even to death, unless good fortune comes to them by way of falling ill, as in the case of the woman taken by dysentery.

[638b1] But does the condition come about through heat, as has been said, or rather through a fluid (because it is in fact the fullness which closes <the *stoma*>), whenever the womb is not so cold as to discharge it and not so hot as to concoct it? And for this reason the condition is chronic, just as [5] things which are simmered for a long time remain the same; simmered things have a limit to their thickening. Wombs of this sort, in the extreme state, cause the condition to last for a long time. Again, since the thing is not alive, because it is not moving it does not cause labor. For movement of the ligaments is labor which, because the fetus is alive, expels the embryo. [10] And the hardness that develops in the thing is the effect of under-cooking. For it becomes so hard that they are unable to cut it with an axe. Now, some things that have been simmered and all things that have been concocted become soft, but undercooked things are unconcocted and [15] hard.

Not knowing this, many doctors, as long as they have seen the rising of the bellies without dropsy and the retention of menses—whenever this condition lasts for a long time—, affirm the condition to be moles, because of the similarity. But it is not; for moles develop rarely. Sometimes there is a collocation of cold, moist [20] and watery residues, sometimes of thicker ones, to the area in the abdominal region, if women are such in nature or disposition. These fluids produce neither pain nor heat on account of their coldness. And when they increase, some more than others, they do not draw in any other disease apart from

ἕξιν ὦσιν. ταῦτα γὰρ οὔτε ὀδύνην παρέχει οὔτε θερμότητα διὰ ψυχρότητα. αὔξησιν δὲ λαβόντα τὰ μὲν μείζω τὰ δ᾽ ἐλάττω, οὐδεμίαν ἄλλην ἐπισπῶνται νόσον παρ᾽ ἑαυτά, [25] ἀλλ᾽ ὥσπερ πήρωμά τι ἡσυχάζει. ἡ δ᾽ ἀπόλειψις τῶν καταμηνίων γίνεται διὰ τὸ δεῦρο καταναλίσκεσθαι τὰ περιττώματα, ὥσπερ καὶ ὅταν θηλάζωνται· καὶ γὰρ ταύταις ἢ οὐ γίνεται ἢ ὀλίγα. ἔστι δ᾽ ὅτε καὶ εἰς τὸν μεταξὺ τόπον τῆς ὑστέρας καὶ τῆς κοιλίας συρρέον ἐκ τῆς σαρκὸς [30] δοκεῖ μύλη εἶναι, οὐκ οὖσα.

ἔστι δ᾽ οὐ χαλεπὸν γνῶναι, ἂν μύλη <ἢ> θιγγανομένης [ἢ] τῆς ὑστέρας. ἐὰν γὰρ ἦ εὐσταλὴς καὶ μὴ ἔχουσα αὔξησιν, δῆλον ὅτι οὐκ ἐν ἐκείνῃ τὸ πάθος. ἐὰν δὲ τοιαύτη ἦ οἷα ὅταν παιδίον <ἔχῃ>, ἔχει μύλην· θερμή τε [καὶ ψυχρὰ] καὶ ξηρὰ ἔσται διὰ τὸ εἴσω τετράφθαι τὰ ὑγρά, καὶ [35] τὸ στόμα τοιαύτη οἷα ὅταν κύωσιν. ἐὰν δέ τι ἄλλο ἦ ὁ ὄγκος, ἔσται ψυχρὰ θιγγανομένη καὶ οὐ ξηρά, καὶ ἀεὶ τὸ στόμα ὅμοιον.

638b22 ὀδύνην Orib.: ὀδυνηρὰν D^a: *dolorem parturitionis* Guil.   **23** θερμότητα D^a: *caliditatem* Guil.: θερμαίνεται Orib.   **25** πήρωμά τι D^a: *orbatum aliquid* Scot.: πληρώματα Orib. ἀπόλειψις D^a: ἀπολύσις Orib.   **27–8** καὶ γὰρ τ. ἢ οὐ γ. ἢ ὀλίγα om. Orib.   **31** ante μύλη add. ἡ Orib. ἢ transp. Orib. θιγγανομένης D-J.: θιγγάνουσα D^a Orib.: *apud tactum matricis* Scot.: *tacta matrice* Guil.   **33** οἷα ὅταν D-J.: οἷον ὅτε D^a ἔχη add. Orib. ἔχει secl. Orib.: *uelut quando puerum habet* Guil. καὶ ψυχρὰ secl. Orib.: *durus apostematus et frigidi tactus* Scot.: *calida frigida sicca* Guil.   **34** ἔσται D^a: ἐστι Orib.   **35** τοιαύτη οἷα ὅταν κύωσιν om. Orib. οἷα Rud.: οἷον D^a τι ἄλλο D^a: τις ἄλλος Orib.: *aliquid aliud* Guil.   **36** ἔσται D^a: ψυχρὰ ἔσται Orib.

themselves, but lie dormant [25] just like an inert fetus. The cessation of the menses occurs because the residues are used up here just as when they are nursing. For in these women, menses either do not come at all or are very scanty. And sometimes a collocation of fluids from the flesh into the place between the womb and the belly [30] seems to be a mole when it is not.

It is not difficult to recognize if there is a mole if the womb is palpated. For if it is compact and has not increased in size, it is clear the condition is not in that place. But if it is like it is when it has a child, it has a mole. It will be both hot and dry on account of the fluids turning inwards and it will be [35] such in respect of the cervix as when they are pregnant. But if the mass is something else the womb will be cold to the touch and not dry, and the cervix will be as it always is.

COMMENTARY

The italic headings preceded by upper case Roman numerals reflect the major divisions of the chapters as indicated in the Outline of Plan of *HA* X, pp. 114–123.

CHAPTER 1

I *The author introduces the topics he will deal with in explaining failure to reproduce.*

633b12 [προϊούσης δὲ τῆς ἡλικίας]: For arguments that these four words are not the original introit to *Non Gen.* see Introduction pp. 2–8, 109–10. If we have lost the original beginning of *Non Gen.* and these words came at a later stage in the treatise, they could indicate either that the author had been explaining why children could not reproduce (in which case τῆς ἡλικίας would mean "age," with the definite article indicating the generic noun) or why the capability to reproduce was not coincident with the onset of puberty (since ἡλικία can also mean a particular time of life, and in this case the definite article would be specific). If the latter, this would be a view shared by Aristotle. At *HA* V.14, 544b14, he says that in most animals the first appearance of *sperma* does not immediately herald the ability to reproduce, and at 25–7 he puts the age at which *sperma* first appears in humans at age 14 and the capacity to reproduce at 21. In *HA* IX(VII).I, 581a14, he states that in humans the male (τὸ ἄρρεν) first produces *sperma* around 14 and at 31–581b1 that in females (θήλεσιν) menses are first produced at around the same time. However, later in the chapter, at 582a16–29, he argues that until the age of 21 τὰ σπέρματα are at first infertile and then weak so that the offspring of young males and females (οἱ νέοι and αἱ νέαι) are small and imperfect, and although young females conceive quickly they have trouble with childbearing. The terms ἄνδρες and γυναῖκες are used to refer to males and females once past the age of 21, at which time women "have reached a favorable state for childbearing while the men continue to improve in this regard." In contrast, the Hippocratics generally agree with the cultural norm that it was best for a girl to become sexually active and pregnant as soon as possible after menarche, sometimes even to pre-empt it, *Virg.* (VIII.468.21–3); cf. King 1983, 109–27; Dean-Jones 1994, 47–55. However, they do not indicate how often they expected very young sexually active girls to become pregnant, so they too may not have been overly perturbed at a young woman's not becoming pregnant until several years after the onset of puberty. The menstrual cycles of adolescent girls are usually anovulatory for the first two years after menarche (Sato 2002). Ages are not usually given in the Hippocratic Corpus, but the youngest mother mentioned is 17, *Epid.* III, case 12 (first set) (III.62.14–66.11).

13 συνόντας: Acc. as subject of γεννᾶν rather than dat. in agreement with ἀνδρὶ καὶ γυναικί; see Smyth 1062. The corrector of Gᵃ and its apographa have συνιόντας, which may have been influenced by *convenientes* in Guil.

ἀμφοῖν: Literally "in both," but it is more probable that the circumstance the author means to indicate by this word is that in which neither of the partners is infertile *per se*, but they are incompatible with one another; see 636b8–10 and 13–23. It is sufficient cause of the failure to produce children if one partner is infertile. It would be a case of extreme bad luck—and it would take some time to prove—if both were, and would involve positing no distinct cause of infertility that would call for a different therapeutic approach (although obviously both partners would need to be successfully treated for there to be any chance of a happy outcome). However, the case where both partners are fertile and simply unable to produce children with each other requires a different type of intervention, explained at 636b10–23; see notes ad loc.

14 πρῶτον μὲν οὖν: "Sometimes μὲν οὖν (like *igitur*) shows that a subject announced in general terms is now to be treated in detail," Smyth 2900c. In focusing on various conditions of the womb in Chapters 1–4 the author assumes the woman herself is healthy. This narrower focus on the causes of infertility compared with the gynecological treatises of the Hippocratic Corpus may be why Aristotle chose *Non Gen.* as his *endoxon*; see Introduction pp. 78–81. *Non Gen.* acknowledges that there are conditions of the body which could affect the functioning of the womb at 634b7–14, but discussing such conditions in detail is not part of the topic of the treatise. The author's primary concern with the condition of the womb is not balanced by any equivalent discussion of the male in the treatise; see Introduction pp. 36–9.

15 θεωρεῖν: Ancient practitioners could, and did, palpate the womb, see note to 635a8, but the verb θεωρεῖν is typically used in the Hippocratic Corpus to signify observation of external signs rather than any direct examination of a body part, e.g., *Epid.* II.1.6 (VI.76.16), *Acut.* 20 (II.268.5), *Sept.* 9 (VII.448.29), *Coac.* 483 (V.692.21). By contrast, the basic sense of the verb in Aristotle is "consider," often in a fairly theoretical manner, and it is frequently directly associated with Aristotelian *theôria*, intellectual contemplation; although for Aristotle too it can have the more general sense of "observe," particularly in biological contexts (see, e.g., *HA* VIII(IX).6, 612b5; 7, 612b18; 37, 620b10; 40, 624b9; 44, 629a6).

ὅπως ἔχει: An example of the author's predilection for prolepsis; see Introduction p. 107.

16 τυγχάνωσι θεραπείας: Here and at 634a11, 21, 34, 40, b7, and 11 θεραπεία clearly means medical intervention, but at 634b31, 635a36, b26, and 637b29 it means simply that a woman should attend to drying off her moisture after she has emitted. For the lack of discussion of therapy in *Non Gen.*, see Introduction pp. 78–81.

17 ἕτερόν τι τῶν αἰτίων: That is, either the man or mutual incompatibility.

ποιῶνται. For the argument that the subjects of this verb are the man and woman who are trying to conceive, see Introduction p. 77.

II *Having delimited the issue with which he will be dealing, conditions of the uterus, the author proceeds to give a definition of what would constitute a healthy uterus.*

633b18 ἔστι δ' ὥσπερ: For the Aristotelian nature of this phrase, see p. 93. The prolepsis of ἔστι in an extended analogy is not common in Greek (i.e., "And just as…so also…" as opposed to "It is just as if…"). The only use of it in the classical period is by Aristotle, who uses it once in *Phys.* and twice in *de An.* The analogy in *Phys.* is a very short one in which both comparans and comparandum are very simply stated: ἔστι δ' ὥσπερ τὸ ἀγγεῖον τόπος μεταφορητός. οὕτω καὶ ὁ τόπος ἀγγεῖον ἀμετακίνητον, "And just as a vessel is a transportable place, so also is place an unmovable vessel" (*Phys.* IV.6, 212a14–16). The two occurrences in *de An.* appear very close together and also introduce very simple analogies in which the comparandum (in both cases the sense of smell) is not postponed by an elaboration of the comparans: ἔστι δ' ὥσπερ χυμὸς ὁ μὲν γλυκὺς ὁ δὲ πικρός, οὕτω καὶ ὀσμαί, "And just as one liquid is sweet and another bitter, so also are smells" (*de An.* II.9, 421a26–27); ἔστι δ' ὥσπερ ἡ ἀκοὴ καὶ ἑκάστη τῶν αἰσθήσεων. ἡ μὲν τοῦ ἀκουστοῦ καὶ ἀνηκούστου, ἡ δὲ τοῦ ὁρατοῦ καὶ ἀοράτου, καὶ ἡ ὄσφρησις τοῦ ὀσφραντοῦ καὶ ἀνοσφράντου, "And just as each of the senses, hearing, for one, is of the audible and the inaudible, and sight, for another, is of the visible and the invisible, smell also is of the odorous and the non-odorous" (*de An.* II.9, 421b3–6). It should be noted that in both the *de An.* passages, after one sentence Aristotle continues the analogy with the words ὁμοίως δὲ καί (*de An.* II 9, 421a30, and 421b8). In *Non Gen.* this locution appears at 633b30 but it is introducing a new point about the correct condition of the womb—its position. It is not a continuation of the simile. The use of these phrases in an extended analogy may argue for Aristotle paraphrasing an original analogy in *Non Gen.*

φανερὸν εἰ ὑγιαίνει: φανερόν followed by an indirect question rather than a statement is unparalleled. The conditional force of the indefinite subordinate clause may have affected this construction. Dt.'s emendation ὅτι may be correct, but Guil. shows *manifestum et si sana est.*

20 ὀφθαλμός: The eye is used as an example of a generic body part in the first part of the sentence and as an analogy for the womb in the last part. The eye is also used as an analogy for the womb at 634a22 (for a pathological state) and 635b21–4 (for a physiological condition). At *GA* IV.1, 766a8–9, in a discussion about the male generative parts and the womb, Aristotle uses the eye as an illustration of the way in which animals receive a function and its corresponding body part simultaneously, but the term he uses for "function" is δύναμις, not ἔργον, and for "body part" ὄργανον, not μέρος.

20–1 ὅταν λήμην τε μηδεμίαν ποιῇ: This clause has no parallel in the criteria of the malfunctioning of a generic body part—pain and fatigue—given in the previous two lines. The phrase used to refer to the correct functioning of a generic body part, τὸ ἔργον τὸ αὑτοῦ ἱκανῶς ἀποτελῇ, is answered in the case of the eye as seeing, ὁρᾷ; in the case of the eye, μὴ ταράττηται parallels ἄλυπον and μηδ᾽ ἀδυνατῇ ὁρᾶν πάλιν parallels ἄκοπον. It may be that the author of *Non Gen.* thought λήμη an appropriate specific example of an ophthalmic disturbance because he is anticipating the analogy with the womb and the womb too can produce a pathological discharge, such as that described at 634a27–30. However, absence of a discharge is not listed as a criterion of the satisfactory functioning of the womb at 22–5, where τὸ ἔργον τὸ αὑτοῦ ἱκανῶς ἀποτελῇ is answered by ὃ ἐκείνης ἐστὶ τοῦθ᾽ ἱκανῶς ἀπεργαζομένη, ἄλυπον by πόνον τε μὴ παρέχουσα, and ἄκοπον by μὴ ἀδύνατος ἀλλ᾽ ἄκοπος. This extra criterion for the health of the eye—that in addition to performing its own function (seeing) without pain or fatigue, it also produce no discharge, because a discharge would hamper an eye in performing its function even if it caused no pain or fatigue—may be included in preparation for the challenge to the claim that a womb could fulfill its ἔργον (menstruation) well even when it is not in a completely healthy condition.

λήμη: λῆμαι περὶ τὰς ὄψιας are listed among signs which are κακὰ καὶ ὀλέθρια at *Prog.* 2 (II.116.7), but at *VM* 19 (I.616.9) λήμη is considered a more benign concocted form of the acrid ῥεύματα which eat into the eyelids and cheekbones. In *Vid. Ac.* 2 (IX.152.16) the author says that the eyesight of children can be healthy despite the presence of λῆμαι (accepting Craik's conjecture), though the text goes on to remark that the λῆμαι have to be dealt with by scraping and cauterizing the eyelid when the child finishes growing (Craik 2006, pp. 38–40). λήμη is one of the words that Rud. describes as rare in Aristotle; see Introduction p. 100. Apart from this passage, the word occurs in the Aristotelian Corpus at *Metr.* IV.2, 379b32, and *Rh.* III.10, 1411a16. However, it is similarly rare in the Hippocratic Corpus. Apart from the *Prog.*, *VM* and *Vis.* passages, it appears 11 times in *Prorrh.*

22 ὑστέρα: The change from the plural to the singular form of the word is not unusual for the Hippocratic gynecological works (e.g. *Mul.* I.13 (VIII.50.17 and 21, and 52.5), I.24 (VIII.64.8 and 9), II.110 and 127 (VIII.238.6 and 11,

272.15 and 20)). Aristotle can also change from singular to plural within a short passage, e.g., *HA* I.13 and 14, 493a24 and b5 and even more strikingly at *HA* I.17, 497a31 and 33, but more often uses only one or the other throughout a passage; see Introduction pp. 96-7.

23-4 ὃ ἐκείνης ἐστὶ τοῦθ᾽ ἱκανῶς ἀπεργαζομένη: The ἔργον of a womb under discussion here cannot be simply pregnancy and parturition. If the womb were producing children well and painlessly, there would be no question of observing it to look for an explanation for infertility. The author must therefore be discussing an ἔργον the womb performs when not pregnant. Most of Chapter 1 is spent describing what constitutes normal menstruation, and at the very end of the chapter the author says that if everything is as he has described then the womb is in the condition it needs to be for childbearing, τέκνωσις. Therefore, although τέκνωσις may be one function of the womb, it is not the one that has been under discussion. There are two more places in the treatise where the phrase "the ἔργον of the womb" clearly refers to menstruation. At 635a18 the author states that the womb is performing its proper function (ποιοῦσι τὸ αὐτῶν ἔργον) when it has responded appropriately to the body during menstruation. At 636a28-35 the author discusses spasm. He states that one sign that the womb does not have spasm is if it does not become inflamed during its own functions (ἐν τοῖς αὐτῆς ἔργοις) because spasm is caused by inflammation. Distention during childbirth is treated as a different cause of spasm than inflammation "during its own functions."

The Hippocratics thought that menses could be problematic for some otherwise healthy women because they descended through the body all at once at regular intervals if the woman did not become pregnant. The problem was generally dissipated after a woman gave birth because the abundant lochial flow widened the passages in her body; see Dean-Jones 1994, pp. 125-6. At *HA* IX(VII).2, 582b7-9, Aristotle indicates that he believes ordinary menstruation causes distress to the bodies of women, πονοῦσι γὰρ τὰς ἡμέρας ταύτας...τὸ δὲ σῶμα βαρύνεται πάσαις ἕως ἂν ἐξέλθῃ.

III *Aristotle challenges the author's assumption that menstruation could proceed normally if the womb was not healthy.*

633b25-9 λέγεται...φυμάτιον: As the app. crit. in Balme 2002 indicates there are several problems with this sentence which scholars have attempted to correct in a number of ways. Pk. made 4 emendations. Dt. accepted 2 of these and added a further 3 of his own. Most later editors and translators accept some combination of these emendations, plus a reading found in Scot and the earliest ms. of Guil. but not in D^a; see below at 633b27. I believe the problems have arisen because neither the early copyists nor the later translators and editors have given due weight to the introductory λέγεται, which does not commit the author of the sentence to concurring with the statement it reports. The sentence is translated by Tricot, Louis, Balme, and Barnes as if the author of *Non Gen.* would concur with it, though if the author did concur, there would be no need for him to attribute the observation to somebody else. More importantly, the content of the reported statement contradicts what the author has just stated about correct functioning indicating the health of a part. And furthermore, as Scot realized, only very specific types of diseases of the eye would leave its vision unimpaired. I believe these problems can all be explained if we take the sentence to be Aristotle's gloss on the apparent contradiction of the immediately preceding definition of a healthy womb with what *Non Gen.* says in the rest of the treatise, where the physician is directed to look at other possible problems with the womb that could prevent conception, apparently even when menstruation was proceeding normally. This seems to be the case, for example, in the condition that the text deals with immediately after this passage, a womb that fails to move up and down the vagina as it should. As the emendations I have made to the text to support this reading are quite far-reaching, I will spend some time explaining the problems I see with other solutions.

The reported statement up to the term ἀλύπως in l.26 conflicts with the author's immediately preceding claim that performing a function correctly without pain or fatigue guarantees the health of a part. It claims that even if the womb is not healthy (καὶ μὴ καλῶς ἔχουσαν), it is in a good and painless condition (ἔχειν καλῶς καὶ ἀλύπως), as regards its own function (πρὸς τὸ ἔργον τὸ ἑαυτῆς), i.e., menstruation, if it is possible to obtain its function in no worse state from it (ἂν μὴ ταύτης χεῖρον τὸ ἔργον ἐστὶν αὐτῆς ἔχειν in Balme's text following Dᵃ). At the outset there is something very clumsy and tautological about this statement. In the reading of Dᵃ, the analogy following ὥσπερ introduces a counter-example; it describes an eye that, although feeling no pain or fatigue, is not completely healthy and is impaired in its function. It is unclear whether we should distinguish between ὄμμα and ὀφθαλμός here. They cannot always be differentiated as clearly as Tricot asserts: "ὄμμα désigne précisément la partie principale de l'œil ou sa vision même, tandis que le mot ὀφθαλμός indique l'organe entire" (1957, p. 698, n. 1). Sometimes they are clearly synonyms. ὄμμα is generally considered a poetic word, but it is not uncommon in prose where it is frequently used for *variatio*, e.g., Pl. *Phd.* 118a13. Aristotle uses ὀφθαλμός 249 times to 160 occurrences of ὄμμα. The Hippocratics prefer ὀφθαλμός over ὄμμα 291 times to 71. That they can be used without any difference in meaning is shown clearly where they appear close together, e.g., in the Hippocratic Corpus at *de Arte* 11 (VI.20.2–3) the author says of things known only through reason that these are harder to know "than if they had been seen by the eyes; for whatever escapes the sight of the eyes, these things are mastered by the sight of the mind," ἢ εἰ τοῖσιν ὀφθαλμοῖσιν ἑώρατο γινώσκεται· ὅσα γὰρ τὴν τῶν ὀμμάτων ὄψιν ἐκφεύγει, ταῦτα τῇ τῆς γνώμης ὄψει κεκράτηται. At *GA* II.6, 744a20, Aristotle says "on account of the fluid in the eyes, the eyes appear large," διὰ δὲ τὸ ὑγρὸν τὸ ἐν τοῖς ὄμμασιν οἱ ὀφθαλμοὶ μεγάλοι φαίνονται, and at *HA* I.9, 491b32, when describing in what way a mole both has and does not have eyes like other vivipara, he says that if the skin is removed, the mole has "the place for the eyes and the black part (i.e., the iris) of the eyes," τήν τε χώραν τῶν ὀμμάτων καὶ τῶν ὀφθαλμῶν τὰ μέλανα. On occasion both terms can be used for vision itself, or, by synecdoche, for the face. Neither of these uses makes sense in this context. I think it is more likely that they are being used as synonyms here since the eye is functioning as an analogy for the womb as a whole, though I cannot rule out the possibility that ὄμμα refers to something like the pupil, iris and fluid, and ὀφθαλμός to the whole eyeball. In either case, unless the eye is taken to be different from every other part of the body, the fact that disease in the eye leads to impaired function appears to challenge the statement introduced by λέγεται.

The most problematic part of this sentence is the clause ἂν μὴ ταύτης χεῖρον τὸ ἔργον ἐστὶν αὐτῆς ἔχειν. It is generally taken to be the second protasis of the conditional within the indirect statement, but it is very difficult to construe as it stands in Dᵃ. Guil.'s Latin seems to be a word for word translation of the same phrase, *si non huius deterius opus est ipsius habere*, which must, then, have been in Wᶜ. The Latin is even harder to construe than the Greek. I suspect Guil. could not make sense of the Greek and chose simply to record the words as closely as possible.

Balme renders the whole sentence as:

> It is said too that even if the uterus is not in its right condition, nevertheless for the purpose of its own function its condition is right and undistressed if its function can be obtained from it without being impaired in the way that accurate eyesight is prevented if the eye does not have all its parts in the right condition or if some growth is present.

In the previous sentence, the author claimed that one way to tell if the womb, or eye, was healthy was to check that it could fulfill its function painlessly and without fatigue. As translated by Balme, the author here first says this is not the case for the womb (it can perform its function well even if not in a good state itself), and then uses the eye as a counter-example (it cannot function well if it is not in a good state itself) without explaining why it has ceased to be a viable comparandum.

The problem with this sentence is reflected in Scot's translation of the Arabic version, which, as with much of Scot's rendition, is more a paraphrase than a translation:

et possibile est, ut non sit matrix sana, quamuis compleat opus suum sine nocumento quando non fuerit infirmitas in tota matrice; quoniam non est remotum, ut uideat oculus visu bono, quamuis aliqua parcium illius sit laesa, sicut si macula fuerit in aliqua parte ipsius, quoniam hoc non prohibet ipsum uidere bene; tamen hoc non accidit, nisi quando occasio non fuerit in aliqua parte nobili oculi.

(Rud. 1911, pp. 109–10)

And it is possible that if the womb is not healthy, nevertheless it will fulfill its own function without detriment when the weakness is not in the whole womb; since it is not unlikely that an eye may see with good vision even when there is a lesion in some part of it, as if there were a little spot in some part of it, since this does not prevent it from seeing well; however this does not happen except when it <i.e., the lesion> is not in some important part of the eye.

In Scot's version *dicitur* (λέγεται) appears in the previous sentence as part of the definition of a healthy womb. This means that some other verb had to be supplied to govern ἔχειν in l.26, and the modality of possibility, which was imported either by Scot himself or by his Arabic exemplar, does ameliorate somewhat the inconsistency with *Non Gen.*'s claim in the preceding paragraph that fulfilling its function guarantees the health of a part. In referring to conditions which are not "in the whole womb" he may be thinking of the condition of φύματα on the womb discussed at 636a35–b1, which are said to affect the correct opening and closing of the womb for menstruation but not necessarily menstruation itself. Scot or his exemplar dealt with the problem of the apparently inappropriate analogy of the eye by reading οὐδὲν before κωλύει (which is not present in Q as reported by Dt., Balme 2002, p. 19), so that, just as a less than completely healthy womb is said to be able to fulfill its function (to menstruate) well, it is said that nothing hinders an imperfect eye from seeing; but then Scot immediately makes an editorial comment on the unlikelihood of a diseased eye being able to see accurately.

Barnes accepts Scot's οὐδὲν and translates:

It is said that even a womb not in good condition may nevertheless be able to perform its function well and painlessly if it is not impaired in respect of its function (translating Dt.'s text ἂν μὴ ταύτῃ χεῖρον, ὃ ἔργον ἐστὶν αὐτῆς, ἔχῃ), just as nothing prevents an eye from seeing accurately even when not all its parts are in good condition or there is a stye in it.

Like Scot, although his translation denies the possibility of determining the health of a body part through painless and fatigueless function, which the author asserted in the previous paragraph, and although it is a reported opinion, Barnes takes the author to be agreeing that there are conditions under which the function of the womb is unaffected even if the womb itself is not in the right condition. But he too feels compelled to import the modality "may," as if an ἄν accompanied the infinitive ἔχειν. Like Barnes, Tricot 1957, p. 698, "apte à accomplir sa function propre, comme il faut et sans souffrance," and Louis 1969, p. 156, "capable de exercer convenablement et sans souffrance sa function propre," take ἔχειν in its meaning "to be able to" and supply an infinitive to govern the adverbs καλῶς and ἀλύπως rather than the idiom ἔχω + adverb as a periphrasis for εἶναι + adjective, as in the opening participial phrase after λέγεται.

One of the problems with the protasis ἄν μὴ ταύτης χεῖρον τὸ ἔργον ἐστὶν αὐτῆς ἔχειν is the use with ἄν of the present indicative ἐστί, which is present in Dᵃ and all its apographa except Xᶜ and appears in Guil.'s translation as est. This would not be a problem if the treatise was a later work, but Balme accepts it even though he believes it is an early work of Aristotle. Pk. makes ἐστί into the verb of a relative clause within the protasis by emending ταύτης to ταύτῃ, inserting a relative pronoun ὅ after τὸ ἔργον and emending the infinitive ἔχειν to ἔχῃ: "If the function which belongs to it is not worse for this (i.e., the womb)." Dt. refines Pk.'s solution by simply correcting the τό to ὅ, but he shows his dissatisfaction with the solution in his app. crit. when he comments "Sed fort nihil mutandum, at ἐστὶν delendum est." ἐστί is secluded by Rud. (p. 95), though he does think it possible that Aristotle could use the indicative with ἐάν/ἄν, see note to 638a22.

The problem of the apparent counter-example of the eye is addressed by most editors by accepting Scot's οὐδέν, though we have already seen that Scot himself thought there was something dubious in the assertion that nothing stops a diseased eye from seeing well. Rud. prefers a simple οὐ, noting "die Negationen sind in unseren Hss. sehr nachlässig behandelt worden." Dt.'s solution replacing κωλύει with ἰσχύει has not found favor.

I believe it is not the ἐστί that is the problem but the ἄν. To support my contention that λέγεται introduces a gloss by Aristotle I suggest three emendations to the Dᵃ's and Guil.'s reading, two of which can be accounted for by typical copyist errors. To ameliorate the baldness of the contradiction between the reported conditional and the preceding paragraph, which leads to the importation of modality and qualification in earlier translations, I take ἄν with ἔχειν as the conclusion of the apodosis. ἀλλὰ μήν (a favorite form of Aristotle's to introduce a caveat; see Introduction pp. 91–3) originally introduced a challenge to *Non Gen.*'s assumption in the later chapters that an unhealthy womb could, sometimes at least, menstruate normally. ἀλλά was accidentally omitted at an early juncture, at which point a copyist took μήν for μή and ἄν μή as introducing a protasis in which the foregoing overly general statement could be true. αὐτῆς ἔχειν could have been written from ἑαυτῆς (αὐτῆς) ἔχειν in the line above by dittography in place of οὕτως ἐχούσης. Rud. notes that even accepting a negation, αὐτό in the phrase ὄμμα οὐδὲν κωλύει αὐτὸ ὁρᾶν, is peculiar, "Eigentümlich ist auch das αὐτό" (p. 95). It would still be unusual, but more understandable, if we read it as reflexive by the simple expedient of giving it a rough breathing. Better still is to read κωλύεται, though I cannot explain the corruption to κωλύει αὐτό.

The emendations I suggest not only obviate the need for explaining the use of the present indicative with ἄν, they also allow λέγεται to introduce a challenge to the author's definition of health rather than an opinion of someone else with which the author concurs. Furthermore, they explain the apparent contradiction of the reported statement with the definition of health that the author has just given, and restore to the analogy the likelihood of impaired vision resulting from a diseased eye.

There is a further, minor, difficulty at the very end of the sentence. Balme reads ἢ εἰ φῦμά τι ὄν as a conditional participial phrase in the accusative absolute following the genitive absolute μὴ ἔχοντος τοῦ ὀφθαλμοῦ. This reading has not found favor with most edd. because there is no reason to import εἰ when the conditional force of the participle has already been established, and the subject of an acc. absol. is very rarely a substantive. For ὄν Pk. wrote ἐνείη, Dt. inserted τυγχάνει, and Louis wrote ἔνεστιν. Michael Reeve suggested to me that we should read εἰ φυμάτιον (misprinted as πυμάτιον in Balme's app. crit.) following the *si pustula* of the best ms. of Guil.; see also *Mul.* II.133 (VIII.282.10). This seems to me an elegant solution, though the ellipsis of the existential ἔστι is unusual and should be supplied.

IV *The importance of the womb being in its correct position.*

633b29 ὁμοίως δὲ καὶ ὑστέρα: There is no question here of a womb which has something wrong with its situation continuing to perform its functions. ὁμοίως is referring back not to an unhealthy yet functioning womb but to the definition of a healthy womb in 633b18–25, a further indication that the passage at 25–9 is a gloss inserted by Aristotle and not part of the author's original argument.

30–634a2 τοῦ ἐπικαίρου τόπου...ἀλλ᾽ ὁμοίως τῇ θέσει: Plato states that the womb can move around and even issue from a woman's body (*Ti.* 91c), and the Hippocratics believe that the womb can relocate to other organs in the body (head, heart, liver, diaphragm—the phenomenon of the "Wandering Womb," e.g. *Mul.* II.123 and 124 (VIII.266.11–268.8), *Nat. Mul.* 44 (VII.388.4–19)), which Aristotle denies (*GA* I.13, 720a11–13); see Manuli 1983, Hanson 1991, pp. 81–7, Dean-Jones 1994, pp. 69–77, King 1998, p. 36 and pp. 222–4. This phenomenon is to be distinguished from both the supposed normal physiological descent and retraction of the cervix up and down the vaginal canal (which *Non Gen.* assumes is necessary) and the misalignments of the womb discussed at 634b39–635a5 (a problem frequently addressed in the Hippocratic Corpus; see notes to 634b27–8).

While Chapter 2 discusses misalignments of the cervix, *Non Gen.* nowhere discusses far-flung peregrinations of the womb, and it may be the possibility of misalignment that the author is referring to here. However, *Non Gen.*'s implication that an unhealthy womb <u>could</u> move to different τόποι seems more radical than a simple tipping backwards or forwards and possibly aligns the author with the Hippocratic camp on this issue; see Introduction pp. 82–3.

The author introduces this topic at this point because after discussing the ἔργον of the womb in Chapter 1 he will turn to the position of the womb in Chapter 2.

30: For βλάπτοι with πρός, cf. *EN* VII.13, 1153a20.

634a3 πορρώτερον: πορρώτερον signifies the initial movement of the womb <u>away</u> from its usual position to a point where it is more likely to be touched, a position close to the vaginal opening. The term is relational, so it is not surprising that the same movement is described at 633b6 as coming close, πλησίον προσίασιν, or that πορρωτέρω is used in the same line to mean the movement away from the vaginal opening back <u>towards</u> its original position. Balme (1991, pp. 479–81) thinks πορρώτερον and πορρωτέρω have to signify the same position here.

Nat. Puer. 30 (VII.534.5–6) says that many women become pregnant after menstruation, when the womb gapes open and moves down the vagina, αἱ μῆτραι ἔχανον καὶ κατὰ τὸ αἰδοῖον ἐστράφησαν, and *Mul.* I.13 (VIII.52.7) that conception would be hampered if the womb was too close, presumably to the opening of the vagina, so it needed to be drawn back to its proper place, but no Hippocratic treatise emphasizes the regular movement up and down the vagina as facilitating conception. Aristotle did believe that the womb could descend to facilitate conception (*HA* IX(VII).2, 582b24, *GA* II.4, 739a31, IV.5, 774a12). In all three Aristotelian passages the verb used to describe the womb's movement down the vaginal canal is καταβαίνω, which is not used by *Non Gen.* πορρώτερον occurs 41 times in Aristotle and never in the Hippocratic Corpus. πορρωτέρω occurs 24 times in Aristotle and 4 times in the Corpus including twice in the gynecology, at *Mul.* I.34 (VIII.80.8) and *Oct.* 13 (VII.460.5). πάθους. See Introduction pp. 97–8.

4 ἀναισθητοτέρας, θιγγανομένας: Note the abrupt change from the singular to the plural in reference to the womb.

The author is describing the normative action of the womb, so I do not think he imagines either the woman herself or a doctor constantly touching the cervix. It is more likely that the touching agent is the penis, which will come up against the cervix if it moves down the vagina as it should. The cervix needs to be sensitive to open up to discharge menses and receive *sperma*.

4–5 τοῦτο δὲ κρίνειν οὐ χαλεπόν: The verb κρίνειν implies some expertise in discernment; *Aph.* I.1 (IV.458.2) states ἡ δὲ κρίσις χαλεπή. The person ascertaining if the womb is in the correct position is the doctor. It is true that the individual making the judgment about whether or not the womb had drawn in all the *sperma* would probably be the woman, unless we are to imagine the doctor examining the woman immediately after intercourse, which seems unlikely but is perhaps not impossible. However, *sperma* remaining in the woman's vagina is not a sign unique to the condition of the womb failing to move down the vagina far enough. It can also occur on account of the misalignment of the womb (Chapter 2), the closure of the cervix (Chapters 2 and 4), the lack of drawing power of the cotyledons (Chapter 3), or an excessive emission of *sperma* (Chapter 5). Because the position of the cervix in the vaginal canal can be directly observed, the doctor will find it easy to judge if this is the cause of the *sperma* left in the vagina.

ἐκ τῶνδε φανερόν: See Introduction p. 93.

7 ἀνασπαστικαί: At *GA* II.4, 739b5, Aristotle says that the womb draws in (εἴσω σπᾷ) the male semen (γονή) when it is in a suitable condition and hot because of the evacuation of the menses. At 739b11–16 he likens the womb's attractive power to that of cupping instruments and denies that it can be attributed "as some assert to the parts involved in copulation," ὡς δέ τινες λέγουσι, τοῖς ὀργανικοῖς πρὸς τὴν συνουσίαν μορίοις, a comment probably directed at the description of the female pudenda at 637a15–34; see notes ad loc.

On balance, Sn.'s conjecture seems more probable than Dᵃ's reading, especially given προσσπαστικαί at 635a25, b3, and 636a7; see Rud. pp. 27–8 and 32. However, there is something to be said for the reading retained by Balme, which is translated by Guil. as *simul tractiue*. Balme's suggestion that the author means simultaneous with coition is not attractive because it would imply the womb was drawing in throughout coition, which is not the implication elsewhere in the treatise. It is more likely to mean simultaneity with the emission, though this would not give the emissions of the man and the woman much time to mingle outside the womb, which the author of *Non Gen.* believes is necessary; see 634b29–39, 635b37, 636a4–6, 637a15–17. Perhaps ἅμα σπαστικαί resulted from a misreading by Aristotle. The adjective σπαστικός is used in *Non Gen.* at 638a20 and at *PA* IV.6, 683a22. It also occurs in the Ps.-Aristotelian *Prob.* at V.9, 881b15. At *GA* II.4, 739b8 Aristotle says because the wombs of birds and viviparous fishes are close to their diaphragms (and therefore farther from the vaginal opening) they have to draw in the male's *sperma* after it has been emitted (expressed by the aorist participle ἀφεθέν) since they are unable to draw it in ἐκεῖ. This seems to be a rare temporal meaning of ἐκεῖ, akin to ἅμα (LSJ ad loc. III).

7 ὁ τόπος ὅθεν δεῖ ἀναλαβεῖν: The object of ἀναλαβεῖν is not specified, but it is worthy of note that no differentiation between male and female *sperma* is made at this point. If the woman's *sperma* was emitted b̲y̲ the womb, its place of deposition would never be far away from its opening.

8 εἰ δὲ πλησίον μένουσι: Although μή is present in Dᵃ, it is absent in Scot and the best mss. of Guil. and rightly secluded by Sn., Dt., Rud., and Tricot. Louis prints εἰ δὲ μή, εἰ to get the necessary sense. It has just been stated that one of the possible affections that could afflict a womb on descending down the vagina is a loss of sensitivity (ἀναισθητοτέρας), which is due to its constantly being touched by the penis. If we retain the μή the text then says that it is n̲o̲t̲ remaining in the descended position which will cause it to be too insensitive (κωφότερα). The further description of such a womb as being of the sort that does not go back up again (καὶ μὴ οἶαι ἐπανιέναι πορρωτέρω) also points to the fact that the author is here discussing a womb that remains in the descended position. A womb which returns to its higher position in the vagina will not become desensitized.

9 κωφότεραι: κωφός is usually used in reference to lack of the ability to hear or speak, but Homer uses it to refer to generally senseless things such as weapons, sea, and earth, *Il.* XI.390, XIV.16, XXIV.54, and Theophrastus uses it to refer to generally dull senses, *Sens.* 19. Its use here anticipates the use of εὐηκόους in l.10 to mean responsive. In Dᵃ the sentence following κωφότεραι ἔσονται is difficult to construe because it lacks a finite verb; see Rud. p. 37. Scot translates, *efficitur quasi sine sensu, quoniam semper id, quod apropinquat ei, tangit eam,* "it will become, as it were, without sensation, since that which comes near it will always touch it." I have adopted the suggested emendation of Pk. The particle is similarly out of place at 634a19, 635b14, and 637a34. διαθιγγάνεσθαι is a *hapax*; see Rud. p. 27. The touching in question is that of the penis during intercourse. The womb should not descend during periods when it is not ready to conceive.

10 ἀνοίγεσθαι· δεῖ δὲ τοῦτο: This refers not only to the opening of the womb to receive *sperma* but also to the opening of the womb's inner mouths to allow the menstrual fluid to descend into the womb from the body; see notes to 634a15 and 19–20, and 635a12–13, 19–20, and 21–2.

The inferior mss. of Guil. add *autem* and Sn. inserts δέ. Asyndeton is not common in Aristotle, nor in the more literary treatises of the Hippocratic Corpus, though, as is to be expected, it is more common in the less polished, more clinically inclined treatises.

12 θεραπείας: See Introduction pp. 78–81.

V *The author proceeds to discuss the specifics of the* ἔργον *that will be performed* καλῶς *if the womb is healthy. Pain and fatigue do not need to be explained further; what is involved in a womb's functioning* καλῶς *does. Three major conditions indicate there may be something wrong with the womb: infrequent menstruation, overly frequent menstruation, and putrefied menses. The last of these is the most serious. The other conditions can be self-correcting.*

634a12 δι' ἴσων χρόνων: This is a sign of clinical experience which Aristotle did not take to heart. The Hippocratics knew women had divergent menstrual timetables, which was generally not a problem as long as each woman menstruated at roughly monthly intervals, e.g. *Prorrh.* II.24 (IX.54.14–15), *Mul.* I.4, II.128, 133 (VIII.26.5, 274.17, 298.3–4), *Nat. Mul.* 59 (VII.398.7). Too abundant menstruation results in fever and anorexia, *Mul.* I.5 (VIII.28.9–30.5). Aristotle, on the other hand, believed all women menstruated with the waning moon, though not necessarily every month (*GA* IV.2, 767a2–6; *HA* IX(VII).2, 582a34–b3). See Dean-Jones 1994, pp. 94–101.

πεπλανημένως: This is the only passage in which the word occurs in Aristotle. It is used 10 times in *Epid.* I and III, once in *Coac.*, and πεπλανημένον occurs at *Prog.* 24 (II.182.4).

13–14 ὑγιαίνοντος τοῦ σώματος: The author begins by describing what can be learned from menstruation when the woman herself is healthy. The phrase is closely echoed at 17–18 and b6. Because menstrual blood originates in the body as a whole, problems with the menstrual flow are not always due to the womb itself. The author deals with this later (634b3–18). If the body seems healthy, however, the womb itself is the cause of the aberrant flow. The author is not concerned with extreme cases of menstrual dysfunction which result in complete suppression, pain, fever, abscesses, etc., conditions which are dealt with at length in the Hippocratic gynecology. In these cases it is fairly obvious that the prevailing disease needs to be attended to before the woman has a chance of conceiving. Our author is explaining how to eliminate the womb as a cause of sterility in an otherwise apparently healthy woman. In contrast the Hippocratics are not particularly concerned to discuss normal menstruation, though there are some general remarks on normal menstruation in *Mul.* I.6 (VIII.30.6–22).

14 τὰς ὑστέρας πρὸς τό: Sn.'s conjecture of πρὸς τό from Guil.'s *ad aperiri* seems likely; see Rud. 1911, p. 96. Dt.'s insertion of τὰς ὑστέρας is less necessary given that the subject of ἀνοίγεσθαι and δέχεσθαι can be readily assumed, but it helps the flow of the argument since the subject of the sentence to this point are the menses; see also 635a17.

15 ἀνοίγεσθαι: This could refer to the expansion of the uterus, or to the opening of the "horns" or inner mouths of the womb. The Hippocratics believed that the womb had inner mouths (probably the beginnings of the fallopian tubes) through which it drew the blood to itself from the body at menstruation (see Dean-Jones 1994, p. 66). The Hippocratics had to believe that these inner mouths were open during the month to facilitate female *sperma* reaching the womb either from the head or from the rest of the body. In this theory menstrual blood was retained in the flesh of the body until the flesh became too saturated. *Non Gen.* does not believe the female *sperma* entered the womb through the internal mouths (see Introduction pp. 26–31 and notes on 637a15–35), so the author may have thought of the inner mouths of the womb as closing over during the month and opening to admit the blood when necessary, providing an empty womb to receive the initial mingled male and female *sperma*. However, this would be the only reference to the opening of the inner mouths, whereas the expansion of the womb to admit blood is discussed in Chapter 2.

τὴν ἐκ τοῦ σώματος ὑγρότητα: This refers to the menstrual fluid which has been building up in the body over the month. Scot's paraphrase shows that he takes the ὑγρότης to be *sperma*, but this only works in the context of the rest of the passage if *sperma* is thought to be synonymous with menses. καταμήνια have been announced as the subject and are clearly the fluid which is discussed in the rest of the section as being scanty, excessive, or putrefied. The condition of those women whose only problem lies in the periodicity of their menses is compared favorably with those in whom there is also a problem in the quantity or putrefaction of the fluid. The comparison would make little sense if the fluid in question were something other than the fluid produced at menstruation. *Non Gen.* does not believe a woman's *sperma* is καταμήνια, nor does he believe *sperma* follows the same route into the womb as καταμήνια.

ὅταν τὸ σῶμα διδῷ: Hippocratic authors never talk about an incremental collecting of menses in the womb of a non-pregnant woman but of a sudden descent of fluid from the body to the womb which leads to its immediate discharge, unless the cervix is closed by some pathology, e.g., *Nat. Puer.* 15 (VII.492.21–494.2); see Dean-Jones 1994, p. 62. This is the view of our author; the beginning of menstruation is marked by the body giving the fluid to the womb, not the womb discharging the fluid, though this is what would ensue in the normal course of things. For those authors who believed, like the author of *Non Gen.*, that female *sperma* was a different fluid from menses, menstrual fluid had to be held at bay through most of the month to give time for the male and female *sperma* to mingle and set in the womb. By contrast, Aristotle argues that conception is only possible if the right amount of menstrual fluid is present in the womb, ἰκμὰς ὑπάρχῃ σύμμετρος (*GA* I.19, 727b11–12), ἐντὸς ἱκανῆς οὔσης (*GA* II.4, 739a28). The menstrual blood is carried to the uterus by λεπταὶ φλέβες running from the great blood vessel and the aorta (*GA* II.4, 738a11). Some part of this blood passes into the womb throughout the month. *GA* III.1, 750b34–751a3, suggests sometimes it is drawn there by the heat that is generated during intercourse, though at *GA* II.4, 737b27–34, Aristotle states that the seminal residues are carried to their proper places without any force, and at 739b10–11 says it is the collection and discharge of menses which kindles the heat (ἐμπυρεύει θερμότητα) in the womb. The heat in the womb concocts the blood to the point where it is able to act as a generative residue, but some of the residue of nutrition remains in the fine blood vessels, and when these vessels become full and cannot hold any more blood they overflow and menstruation takes place, usually with the waning moon (HA IX(VII).2, 582a34–b3, GA II.4, 738a 10–21). Though there may be a time of the month when the body releases the majority of accumulated blood, unlike the author of Non Gen., Aristotle believes the body is "supplying" the womb with blood throughout the month.

16–17 πλεονάκις, ἐλαττονάκις, πεπλανημένως: Although Greek doctors realized that women's menstrual periods could vary widely, they did believe there were limits to what was a healthy period. In the case of each individual woman, regularity was the most important aspect of menstruation, but too frequent or too infrequent menstruation was not conducive to childbearing no matter how regular the intervals; see Dean-Jones 1994, pp. 94–101.

τοῦ ἄλλου σώματος μὴ συναιτίου ὄντος ἀλλ᾽ ὑγιαίνοντος: Certain disturbances in normal menstruation could be attributed to the body both in health and disease. In these situations the womb itself is not the cause of sterility. This situation is dealt with at 634b1–18.

συναιτίου: This word appears 15 times in Aristotle and only 3 times in the Hippocratic Corpus.

19 κωφότητα: See note on l.9. The terminology of failure to open due to unresponsiveness echoes that of the discussion in the immediately previous section about the failure of the cervix to open and draw in the *sperma*, but despite that, this is not the fluid or the part of the womb in question here. See following notes. For the correlation in sensitivity at both ends of the womb, see notes on 635a5–22.

ἐν τοῖς καιροῖς: The "right time" for opening is when the body tries to release ("supply," διδῷ, l.16) its menstrual fluid into the womb.

20 ὀλίγα δέχονται: This explains why some women menstruate ἐλαττονάκις. The amount of menses a body produces if it is healthy and not changing (see note to 634b6) will remain constant. If the womb, intermediary between the body's production and the evacuation of menses, does not open properly (probably expand) when this amount is ready, it will only accept a small portion. If it is inflamed, it will draw fluid beyond what the body is ready to give up. The former situation results in infrequent, the latter in overly frequent menstruation because the womb releases menstrual fluid when and only when it reaches a certain volume. Note that when it is not inflamed the womb is said to "receive," δέχομαι, the fluid rather than to "draw," σπάω, the action it exerts on the *sperma* to draw it in through the cervix. δέχομαι is the verb used of the reception of menses in the uterus at 634b5.

μᾶλλον ἐπισπῶνται: This is what explains menses that occur πλεονάκις. The author lists the causes of the conditions introduced in l.16 in chiastic order. The use of μᾶλλον rather than πλέον in agreement with ὑγρόν shows that the author is thinking of excess rather than simply a larger amount of fluid than the small amount just referred to. The author uses the term ἐπισπῶνται here because he is describing an inflamed womb that draws a pathological amount of fluid to itself, more than the body is "supplying." This drawing is shortly to be contrasted with a more normal secretion.

φλεγμασίαν: Inflammation and phlegm.

21 θεραπείας σημαίνουσι δεόμεναι: Spengel (see Rud. p. 38) considers this a lexical violation. Generally σημαίνω uses the participle with an object rather than the subject, e.g. 634a37. Rud. says he has found no parallel to this expression but that it is easy to understand that σημαίνουσι is equivalent to φανεραί εἰσι.

22 ὀφθαλμοί, κύστις, κοιλία: All these organs have different points of ingress and egress for fluid. If these parts are to work as an explanation of what is happening in a womb which produces too much or too little fluid in menstruation, we have to assume the fluid is something that is normally received from inside the body, not drawn in through the orifice which discharges the fluid. If the fluid under discussion were to be equated with female *sperma* (which it is not), this would still mean that the unresponsiveness and failure to open referred to in l.19 is different from the action the terms were used for in the previous section, where the womb's degree of responsiveness depended on its moving closer to or further away from the place from which it was to draw the fluid.

When eyes, bladder, and intestines are healthy, fluid from the body flows naturally to them, πέφυκεν ἐκκρίνεσθαι, and out of them at the appropriate times. Inflammation causes them to draw, ἕλκουσιν, more fluid than necessary from the body. Aristotle (*GA* II.4, 737b31–2) agrees that within the body, fluids flow naturally to their appropriate receptacles and do not need to be drawn as if by cupping vessels (though at one point Aristotle says that a womb heated by intercourse will draw the menses to itself, τὸ πλησιάζειν τοῖς ἄρρεσι κατασπᾷ τὴν τῶν γυναικείων ἀπόκρισιν (*GA* III.1, 751a1)). This is in contrast to *VM* 22 (I.626.22–628.4), which says the bladder, head, and womb draw fluid like cupping vessels.

23 φλεγμαίνοντες: A very common word in medical writing. It occurs in some form 83 times in the Hippocratic Corpus, 3 times outside of *HA* X in Aristotle.

25 τοιαύτη ἢ τοσαύτη: We would expect the accusative as the words are properly the object of ἕλκουσιν, but they have been attracted into the nominative by the intervening relative; see Rud. p. 35. The apparent oxymoron in τοιαύτην...οὐ τοιαύτη is easily understood. Just as the eyes do not draw urine to themselves when inflamed, so the womb does not draw tears. The sort of fluid it draws is still menstrual, but it can be diluted or corrupted.

ἀποδιδοῦσα: The full meaning of this word is "to pay back" or "to render what is due." It emphasizes the process the author has in mind. The womb takes in at one end and gives out at the other. This is made plain at 634b5, δεχομένας καὶ ἀφιείσας κατὰ λόγον.

26 φλεγματικόν: This word occurs nowhere else in either Aristotle or the Hippocratics, but 5 times in Diocles.

27 ἀνόμοια: An emendation adopted by several eds. and evident in Guil. which seems to be necessary. The author has previously discussed menstrual fluid which is similar to that of normal menstruation but abnormal in quantity. Now he contrasts menses which are of a different quality from normal menstruation. καί specifies what this abnormality is.

σεσημμένα μᾶλλον: The fact that the menses of healthy women are "putrefied" to some degree is touched on again in l.33, though there the term may just refer to the "whites." Aristotle constantly refers to menses as concocted blood, albeit less concocted than male semen. At *GA* IV.8, 777a11, he says that concoction and putrefaction are opposites (σαπρότης γὰρ καὶ πέψις ἐναντίον), so he is unlikely to have described normal menses as even a little putrefied; see commentary on ll.30–1 for his view on "whites." Healthy menstrual fluid can range from black to brown to dark red, light red, orange, and pink, and be more or less liquid, more or less clotted (www.healthline.com/health/womens-health/period-blood). Since pus is white and the author also describes the "whites" as putrefied (see below note on ll.30–1), it is likely he is referring to conditions which could cause pus to appear in the menses or to a type of amenorrhea in which menses are replaced by a heavy whitish-brown discharge streaked with blood. Though menstrual fluid is frequently described as bilious or phlegmatic in the Hippocratics, it is not often described as putrefied, and then usually only when it has been suppressed in the womb for some time, e.g., *Mul.* I.2 and 3 (VIII.20.6, 24.5 and 10); *Nat.Puer.* 15 (VII.496.3–5). However, they do frequently refer to a ῥόος λευκός, which they describe as looking like the urine of an ass, as a serious condition in women, e.g., *Nat. Mul.* 15 (VII.332.14–21); *Mul.* II.116–19 (VIII. 250.19–260.22), and at *HA* III.19, 521a27, Aristotle says that when menses become diseased they are referred to as a ῥόος. *Nat. Mul.* 10 (VII.324.22–326.5) and *Mul.* I.11 and 57 (VIII.44.10–17 and 114.8–15) discuss τὰ ἐπιμήνια λευκά as a serious condition requiring treatment. The authors attribute the condition to bile or phlegm and say it involves such symptoms as painful urination, fever, swelling, vomiting, etc. There is no terminology of putrefaction, however, with these conditions. The *gonê*, probably of just the man, is said to putrefy at *Mul.* I.10, (VIII.42.3). *Mul.* I.14–16 (VIII.52.17–54.13) describe remedies for when the semen from the male is retained but putrefies and a recipe for foul-smelling menses. See Dean-Jones 1994, p. 124.

28–9 τότε μὲν ἤδη πάθος καὶ ἐπίδηλον γίνεται: Sn. suggests τότε for τοῦτο on the basis of Guil.'s *tunc*, though Rud. thinks this is just a palaeographic error (p. 81). However, the emendation makes better sense of the argument. Women will already be suffering when the putrefied menses become visible. The case is more serious than simple inflammation. *Mul.* I.8 (VIII.34.6–38.5) details different degrees of the condition of bilious menses. Symptoms include very black menses, insufficient menses, fever, loss of appetite, stomach ache, pains in hips, and dizziness. If the menses are suppressed, among other exacerbations the patient becomes distressed, suffers from insomnia, and belches frequently. This ailment can be cured by a moderate evacuation of bilious matter in vomit, feces, or a ῥόος, but if the discharge becomes too prolonged the womb itself becomes inflamed and the menses become purulent. This seems to be similar to the condition which is being referred to here, where the preceding paragraph focused on an inflamed womb and the following paragraph begins by describing cases in which the womb is not the cause of the ailment. *Non Gen.* (or Aristotle) is not concerned with detailing the pathological conditions preceding putrefied menses. It would be patently obvious why a woman in the grip of a serious illness would not be able to conceive, so it is dismissed in one sentence.

30–1 τὰ λευκά: "Whites," leukorrhea, are a uterine discharge that can precede or follow menses, or occur at any time between menstrual discharges. They are not in and of themselves a pathological symptom. Aristotle believes the whites are unconcocted (μὴ πεπεμμένου) menstrual fluid and pays them no undue attention if they are moderate in amount (*GA* II.4, 738a25–33). Given the strong contrast he draws between concoction and putrefaction (see note on 634a27), if he had wanted to indicate that he believed whites were putrefied menses he would have used a much stronger term than simply the negation of πεπεμμένος to describe them. The Hippocratics do not discuss physiological whites, though a comment at *Mul.* I.24 (VIII.64.5–6) that a woman in whom the *sperma* is flowing away continuously does not welcome intercourse may be a reference to pathological leukorrhea.

34 [πλείω ἢ ἐλάττω]: Since this phrase is in the first half of an antithesis contrasted with women who menstruate at irregular intervals, the author would seem to be drawing a contrast between women who produce more or less menstrual fluid and those who menstruate more or less often; but the previous section collapsed these conditions—the former causing the latter—and contrasted them with menses which were ἀνόμοια. The term ἄτακτα refers to menses that are distinguished from normal menses in some aspect other than quantity. πλείω ἢ ἐλάττω has been mistakenly added as a gloss by a copyist who has not followed the argument.

35 τέκνωσιν: The conjecture of Junt. and accepted generally for νέωσιν. Guil. shows *perfectum* (*pfuth*, though the word is missing in Tz.). On this basis Rud. suggests τελέωσιν. However, the whole thrust of Chapter 1 is that the womb should be performing its ἔργον of menstruation properly for conception to take place. There are many other problems which could prevent successful completion of the whole process after conception with which the author is not concerned.

36 διακωλυτικόν: Occurs nowhere else in Aristotle or the Hippocratic Corpus, though it is used in Plato, *Pol.* 280d in defining *technai* which provide defences against things that people do not want to happen, such as theft and violence.

37 τῆς ὑστέρας: The prolepsis emphasizes what the author has been discussing so far before he proceeds to discuss the ἕξις of the body beginning in 634b1.

38 πάθος: In contrast to putrefied menses which are a νόσος, though they are also referred to as a πάθος at l.28. πάθος runs the gamut of conditions which depart from the usual state of a thing; see Introduction p. 105.

40 καθίστασθαι καὶ ἄνευ θεραπείας: *de Arte* 5 (VI.6.22–8.22) asserts that anybody who appears to recover from an illness without the services of a doctor has unwittingly used medicine, by chance hitting on the right treatment.

634b1 προσεξαμαρτάνῃ: This word is not found again until Galen, and he uses it only once, *MMG* I, K 11.6.17. The effect of this ominous phrase (what is covered by τι?) is to absolve the author if the health-threatening conditions he describes do not in fact self-correct but get worse. *de Arte* 7 (VI.10.15–12.13) asserts that failed recoveries were more often the fault of patients who could not or did not follow doctors' orders than of incompetent physicians.

VI *Having considered the evidence about the state of the womb shown in the menstrual processes of women who cannot conceive but are otherwise healthy and whose bodies are in a constant state,* Non Gen. *now moves on to consider cases in which the condition of the menses follows the general condition of a woman's body. Some of these women too are healthy, but their bodies are changing (perhaps gaining or losing weight)* *and by responding correctly to the greater wetness or dryness of the body a womb fulfills its* ἔργον *correctly; cf.* Mul. *I.11 (VIII.42.9–48.7). If women are sick, it is to be expected that their menstrual cycle would be disrupted and there would be no point in trying to remove the impediments to conception until the general illness had been dealt with. Indeed, if the womb is functioning in a healthy fashion, it should help the ailing body evacuate excess fluid.*

634b2 μεταβάλλωσι: Plural verb with a neuter plural subject; menses is the implied subject.

5 δεχομένας καὶ ἀφιείσας κατὰ λόγον: A clear and concise statement of the author's view of the dual nature of the womb's ἔργον of menstruation.

6 μεταβάλλοντος: That is changing from a wetter to a dryer ἕξις, or vice versa, through a change in regimen, location, or some other non-pathological change.

8 ἀναλίσκεσθαι: In many cases in the Hippocratic gynecology a woman's problems are caused by menses retained elsewhere in the body, e.g., headaches, *Nat. Mul.* 18 (VII.338.7), gout, *Aph.* VI.29 (IV.570.6), fever, *Mul.* I.4 (VIII.26.10–12), loss of reason, *Virg.* (VIII.468.8–17); see Dean-Jones 1994, pp. 131–5. At 638b26–7 Aristotle uses the term καταλίσκεσθαι for cessation of menses due to their being expended upon a uterine mole.

περίττωμα: Normally considered an Aristotelian term; see Introduction pp. 103–4.

9 ᾗ: D^a's reading ἥ is not untenable, but there is no explanation about why a sick body should be too fatigued to menstruate when we have been told of conditions during which a sick body might menstruate more.

10 ἐξερεύγεσθαι: This is not a common verb among classical authors. It is used once each by Herodotus (I.202.3) and Aristotle (*HA* VII(VIII).20, 603a14) in reference to the discharge of a river. It may be worth noting that in both these instances there is some "pathology" involved, either in the excessive discharge of the river itself or to the testacea which are affected. However, it is used in six different Hippocratic treatises (*Epid.*, *Prorrh.*, *Nat. Hom.*, *Vict.*, *Mul.*, *Oss.*), which marks it as a technical medical term. *Morb.* IV.41 (VII.562.8–10) says there are four ways a patient could purge themselves of diseased humors: mouth, nose, rectum, and urethra. In the gynecological works menstruation is the most important way a woman could purge, and it could be viewed as a prophylactic which led to women falling severely ill less often than men; see Dean-Jones 1994, pp. 136–47.

11 θεραπείας: See Introduction pp. 78–81.

13–14 ὑγιαίνουσαι διατελοῦσιν: See note on 633b23–4. It is also possible that this phrase refers to the women themselves rather than the wombs, as

Balme translates, "The fact that they (women) remain healthy shows that... "
However, the author has just said that sometimes the bodies of women whose
menses are disturbed need treatment while their wombs do not.

14 αὐτῶν: Lit. "than themselves," i.e., than normal.

ἀρρωστότεραι: Rare in Aristotle.

16 φοιτᾷ: The subject is the menses. The same verb is used of the whites
at 635a11. It is used by Aristotle of the menses in *HA* IX(VII).2, 582b4, 3,
583a26, and *GA* I.19, 727b27. It is not so used in the Hippocratic Corpus,
where the most common subject of the verb is ὀδύνη.

At *HA* IX(VII).2, 582b8, Aristotle mentions that menses can come ἀθρόα
or κατ' ὀλίγον, but he attributes this to differences in women, ταῖς μὲν...ταῖς
δὲ..., not differences in bodily states within one woman.

VII *The author proceeds to discuss the nature of "whites" in a healthy
womb.*

634b18 ἄρχονται: Plural verb with neuter plural subject τὰ καταμήνια.

19 γαλακτοειδῶν: This is probably just a reference to the color of the
first fluid evacuated in menstruation, though an actual connection between
menses and milk is made at *Epid.* II.3.17 (V.118.10–11), where milk is called
"sister of the menses," and by Aristotle at *GA* IV.8, 777a8, "Milk is concocted
(πεπεμμένον) not decomposed blood." This comment may have been made
in answer to Empedocles' statement, "On the 10th day of the 8th month <of
pregnancy>, the blood becomes white pus" (DK 31 B68). (The mss. read
"milk," not "blood," in the Empedocles fragment, but the correction seems
obvious.) The Hippocratics generally thought the source of milk was the
menstrual fluid, *Alim.* 37 (IX.110.16–18), *Aph.* V.39 (IV.544.14–15), though *Nat.
Puer.* 21 (VII.512.16) says milk is formed when a pregnant uterus squeezes the
fatty part of material that comes from nourishment through the omentum
and the heat from the uterus causes part of it to become sweeter; see Dean-
Jones 1994, pp. 215–17.

ἀνόσμων: The lack of smell is considered noteworthy because the whites
are putrefied.

20 ἀπολήγονται: Plural verb with a neuter plural subject.

καταλήξεως: This is generally a late word, but it is found in Aeschylus at
Choe. 1075, and in Hecataeus, frag. 145 a 2 bis.

22 οὐδὲ πύου: For D^a's οὔτε. Even though they are putrefied and at the
end of menstruation the whites do have an odor, nevertheless this odor is
not that of pus. Some pus could be odorless. *Coac.* 396 (V.674.11) says that in
some cases of fever the expectoration of odorless, white pus can bring about
remission. By contrast *Aph.* VII.44 (IV.590.3) says that a flow of evil-smelling
(δυσῶδες) pus signifies death.

22–3 ἄνευ μὲν τήξεως, μετὰ μέντοι θερμασίας: In this case, although there is some heat present it is not enough to cause putrefaction. At *Morb.* I.6 (VI.152.7), heating and promoting the maturation of pus is listed as an important form of correct therapy. In discussing "whites" at *GA* II.4, 738a26–33, Aristotle says that in women small amounts of residue are secreted from time to time (n.b. not specifically at the beginning and end of menstruation) if they have not been concocted into blood (μὴ πεπεμμένου δὲ κατὰ μικρὸν ἀεί τι ἀποκρίνεται). These can occur in females even when they are quite small children. This seems to indicate that for Aristotle "whites" have been exposed to <u>less</u> heat than normal menses, not more. Although we have no Hippocratic discussion about non-pathological leukorrhea in the Hippocratic Corpus, *Non Gen.*'s account seems closer to their ideas of putrefaction and heat.

σημεῖον: This term is also used for the very beginning and ending of menstruation at 635a10 and 23. It seems that this part of menstruation was considered especially significant for diagnostic purposes. Aristotle uses the term at *HA* VI.18, 572b33 to refer to estrus, which shows when animals are ready to mate or give birth.

24 ἔχουσιν: With neuter plural subject.

CHAPTER 2

I *Having finished discussing the* ἔργον *of the womb when it is not pregnant, the author proceeds to discuss the position of the womb, introduced at 633b29–634a7 in Chapter 1. He begins by explaining the need for the womb to be correctly aligned to draw in* sperma. *The necessity for the womb to move down the vagina to be close to the emitted* sperma *is not reiterated.*

634b27 τὸ στόμα τῶν ὑστερῶν: D^a and Guil. read σῶμα here, followed by most editors and translators. This was corrected to στόμα in F^a and X^c, followed by Bk., Dt., and Balme. When discussing the alignment necessary for conception, the difference is irrelevant for the author of *Non Gen.* In his model, any failure of the mouth of the womb to be straight is caused by the misalignment of the body of the uterus itself (cf. 634b39–40). If we accept the reading of D^a here, we should then correct στόμα to σῶμα at 635a6. This would be possible because it is clear that in the following passage the author is discussing the opening of the womb to receive menstrual fluid from the body, not just the opening of the cervix to discharge it. However, Chapter 3 begins περὶ μὲν οὖν τὸ στόμα τῶν ὑστερῶν, with no ms. authority for σῶμα, and goes on to talk περὶ αὐτὴν δὲ τὴν ὑστέραν, so it seems best to accept that the topic of Chapter 2 is the στόμα. The term στόμα can refer either to the whole cervix or simply to the os uteri. I have translated the term as cervix throughout the treatise because the author is dealing throughout with a non-pregnant womb, for which the differentiation between the cervix and the os uteri proper is not usually an issue.

27–8 ὀρθόν: The author means the cervix should lie parallel to the walls of the vagina. Deviations from this appear to be visualized as the result of the anteflexion or retroflexion of the womb itself. The Hippocratics recognized these obliquities of the cervix (e.g., *Mul.* I.10 (VIII.40.15–42.1), *Nat. Mul.* 8 (VII.322.11–324.9), *Steril.* 213 (VIII.408.4–8)). See Rud. pp. 11–12 for a more complete list. Sometimes the Hippocratics talk of the cervix twisting or folding back on itself (e.g., *Mul.* I.2 (VIII.14.10), *Nat Mul.* 7 (VII.320.18)). There is no sign of this condition in *Non Gen.*

28–38 σπέρμα: The sentence immediately following makes it clear that here the author is discussing female *sperma* as well as male *sperma* and that it is different from menstrual fluid. The previous chapter and the later sections of this chapter make clear that menstrual fluid enters the womb from the body, not through the cervix. If τὸ σπέρμα here were to refer to menstrual fluid, it would mean it had been discharged by the womb before it had to be drawn back in again. Aristotle declares this would be contrary to nature at *GA* II.4, 739b17–20. Balme (1991, p. 491, n.a) acknowledges this contradiction but does not deal with it further. His assumption that the woman's *sperma* "is conveyed in a fluid which the uterus emits during coition" (Balme 1991, p. 488, my emphasis) is perhaps the main reason he equates menses and female *sperma*. See Introduction pp. 15–36 for a detailed explanation that the female fluid referred to in this passage is *sperma*, not menstrual fluid or vaginal lubricant.

29 εἰς τὸ πρόσθεν γὰρ αὐτῶν: Placing the prepositional phrase at the beginning of the sentence by prolepsis emphasizes the author's point. If orthosis of the στόμα is necessary for the uptake of the woman's *sperma*, this *sperma* cannot be discharged by the στόμα, because then the *sperma* would be discharged in front of the στόμα whatever its orientation in the vagina. As it is, the woman's *sperma* is discharged in front of the uterus (αὐτῶν), and if the cervix is oblique this will not coincide with the στόμα.

καί: This is not conjoining the site of the woman's emission to an assumed knowledge that it is the same site into which a man emits. The site of the male emission will be introduced later (l.32) with a καί dependent on this statement.

ἡ γυνὴ προΐεται: The author is here taking for granted that women emit *sperma*; it is the locus of discharge that is at issue. Nowhere in *Non Gen.* does the author argue that women emit *sperma* as a man does. Tricot, Louis, and Balme all avoid making the woman the subject here: Tricot, "Car c'est à la parte antérieure de la matrice que s'effectue aussi l'émission chez la femme";

Louis, "C'est, en effet, au devant de l'utérus qu'a lieu l'émission même chez les femmes"; Balme, "For the woman's emission too is into the region in front of the uterus."

30 ἐξονειρώττωσιν: Aristotle discusses erotic dreams in women at *GA* II.4, 739a23–6, saying that they are the best evidence for believing a woman contributes to the fetation but that in fact they prove nothing because some young men come to the point of ejaculation but do not and others ejaculate *sperma* which is ἄγονον. It is hard to follow the point Aristotle is making here. He clearly agrees with the author of *Non Gen.* that women have erotic dreams, and presumably that they are sometimes, maybe often, accompanied by the release of some fluid, which Aristotle would no doubt identify with the vaginal lubricant (see Introduction pp. 31–6). Mentioning that some young men reach the point of ejaculation but do not emit is perhaps meant to illustrate that women could climax in an erotic dream without emitting any fluid beyond the vaginal lubricant, which is emitted during the course of the dream. The point about young men emitting ἄγονον σπέρμα, though, is opaque to me. In the *GA* a woman's *sperma* is menses and Aristotle does not associate its emission with sexual stimulation. The verb takes the plural form although ἡ γυνή was used in the singular in the same sentence only three words earlier. The author regularly alternates between singular and plural forms with this generic noun; see Introduction p. 96. This confusion of number is un-Aristotelian.

τελέως: For this author, coming to completion in an erotic dream signifies ejaculation. The fluid emitted at this point is to be differentiated from the vaginal lubricant which appears during (μεταξύ) sexual activity; see 635b15–31, 637a15–34, and Introduction pp. 33–4. Current medical research defines orgasm as the clonic contraction of the pelvic and genital muscles without any necessary ejaculation of fluid, though it is known that women can reach orgasm multiple times in quick succession and in those women who believe they do ejaculate (a possibility about which sex researchers are divided; see Salam et al. 2015), ejaculation signals the final orgasm and what they consider to be their true climax, Lloyd 2005, pp. 21 and 109. Vaginal lubrication is recognized as part of pre-orgasmic excitement, necessary but not sufficient for orgasm, Lloyd 2005, p. 38.

Night emissions are mentioned by Hippocratic authors at *Dis.* II.51 (VII.78.19, in a patient suffering from consumption of the back), *Int.* 43 (VII.274.7, in a patient suffering from typhus), 47 (VII.282.18, in a serious condition arising from phlegm), *Vict.* I.35 (VI.520.18, in people whose souls are too fiery and are called "half-mad," ὑπομαινομένους) and II.54 (VI.558.18-19, nightshade can be used to prevent nocturnal emissions). All these should be thought of as primarily male patients, but women are also said to have emissions in dreams at *Mul.* II.175 (VIII.358.1, a case of hydropsy that is worsening). *Genit.* 1 (VII.470.21–472.4) states:

181

καὶ οἱ ἐξονειρώσσοντες διὰ τάδε ἐξονειρώσσουσιν· ἐπὴν τὸ ὑγρὸν ἐν τῷ σώματι διακεχυμένον ἔῃ καὶ διάθερμον, εἴτε ὑπὸ ταλαιπωρίης, εἴτε καὶ ὑπὸ ἄλλου τινός, ἀφρέει· καὶ ἀποκρινομένου ἀπ' αὐτοῦ ὁρᾶν παρίσταται οἷα ἐν τῇ λαγνείῃ· ἔχει γὰρ τὸ ὑγρὸν τοιοῦτο ὅπερ λαγνεύοντι· ἀλλ' οὔ μοι περὶ ὀνειρωσσόντων καὶ παντὸς τοῦ νοσήματος ἔτι ἐστί, καὶ ὁκόσα ἐργάζεται, καὶ διότι πρὸ μανίης.

Moreover, those who have nocturnal emissions do so for the following reasons. When the moisture in their bodies becomes thoroughly diluted and heated through, whether from hard work or any other cause, it foams up; and as this is being emitted from their bodies the sorts of images present themselves that occur in intercourse, for the moisture is the same sort of material as in intercourse. But I will not concern myself further with those who have erotic dreams and the whole sickness, the sorts of things it causes and why it precedes madness.

Non Gen. clearly does not share this pathological view of nocturnal emissions.

31–2 θεραπείας: The woman simply needs to dry herself. She does not need to provide the area with any elaborate therapy.

αὐταῖς...ὥσπερ εἰ ἀνδρὶ συνεγίνετο: Another rapid change from plural to singular with the generic ἡ γυνή, here under the influence of ἀνδρί. There is no need to emend to the plural form. If the fluid is just like that of intercourse, it will not be bloody, another sign that the author is not referring to menses with the term *sperma* here; see 635a40–635b1 and Introduction pp. 24–6.

32 προϊεμένων ἐνταῦθα καί...εἴσω: This form of the genitive absolute is awkward but not impossible in Greek. Rud. suggests the participle refers to both genders, but he then sees the final words of the sentence as a sign of carelessness on the author's part. But this is the first time the author makes a very important point for his theory so he wants to emphasize it: there is no reason to necessitate that women emit directly into their womb because men do not do so and yet still contribute effectively to conception.

34 ἐνταῦθα προϊῶνται, ἐντεῦθεν σπῶσι: From context, here ἐνταῦθα must mean in front of a correctly oriented womb, i.e., in front of the στόμα. Grammatically, the subject of προϊῶνται could be men, women, both sexes, or the womb. But men and women have been the ejaculatory agents in the preceding sentence, and the contrast between the adverbs and the action designated by the verbs προϊῶνται and σπῶσι is so strong that if the womb was to be taken as the subject of both verbs we would expect an adverb such as πάλιν with σπῶσι to make the meaning clear. Since men have not been the subject of any finite verb form thus far in this section, and women are the subject of κυΐσκονται in the next sentence, women are the most likely subject of προϊῶνται here, either alone or as joint subjects with men. The passage is differentiating strongly between the action of the women themselves, in ejaculating, and the action of the uterus, in drawing in.

τῷ πνεύματι, οἷον αἱ ῥῖνες: Note the proleptic position of οἷον αἱ ῥῖνες here. The process is elucidated a little more at 637a17–20; see notes ad loc. Aristotle believes the male semen is drawn into the womb by heat, as cupping instruments draw fluid to themselves. At *GA* II.4, 739b15–16, he states that this drawing in "does not in any way come about, as some say, through the parts used in intercourse," ὡς δέ τινες λέγουσι, τοῖς ὀργανικοῖς πρὸς τὴν συνουσίαν μορίοις οὐ γίνεται κατ᾽ οὐθένα τρόπον. The author of *Non Gen.* would be among these τινες. *VM* 22 (I.626.20–628.5), in discussing the attractive power of the womb on fluids within the body, describes the shape of those structures in the body best adapted to draw fluid to themselves. The best shape, according to *VM*, is that of a broad tapering hollow which acts like a cupping instrument or that of a pursed mouth with a reed inserted. The author of *VM* does not explain further, but it would seem that he is not simply describing capillary action by the image of the reed inserted into the mouth, but is imagining some inhalation also, which could be interpreted as the force of *pneuma*. *VM* thus accommodates both the Aristotelian image of cupping instruments and *Non Gen.*'s image of the inhalation of the nostrils (referred to as mouth and nostrils in 637a17).

36 τὸ πρόσθεν πάντως καλῶς ἐχούσης: Here τὸ πρόσθεν signifies in front of the στόμα and the adverbial phrase has conditional rather than simply possessive connotations. Barnes suggests reading πάντως (see l.37) and omitting ἐχούσης, "because in every case the emission of both male and female sperma is into the <place in> front of the womb," and Dt. inserts ὁπωσοῦν between παντελῶς and ἐχούσης, "because in every case the emission of both male and female sperma is into the <place in> front of the womb in whatever state it is," but the author has been making the case that this only happens if the womb is straight. This is evidence that the female *sperma* is not emitted by the womb, otherwise the woman's *sperma* would always be emitted in front of the στόμα. Inserting καλῶς maintains the author's argument, allows us to retain ἐχούσης and explains how πάντως became παντελῶς.

ἐχούσης: Modifying αἱ ὑστέραι. The singular is no more abrupt than the αὐτήν at the beginning of the following clause. See Introduction pp. 96–7 for rapid changes between singular and plural to refer to the womb.

38–9 εἰ δ᾽ εἰς αὐτήν...συνελάμβανον: The only reason the emission of a woman's *sperma* directly into her womb would prevent conception is if the male and female emissions have to mingle instantaneously, as this author believes is the case; see notes on 636b13–23. The author's theory of pangenesis is also dependent on the *spermata* mingling outside the womb before a portion is drawn into it; see notes on 636b39–637a15.

39 μὴ εἰς ὀρθὸν βλέπωσιν: The use of βλέπωσιν recalls the use of the eye as an analogy for the womb in the previous chapter. The Hippocratics do not use this verb in its figurative sense, but Aristotle uses it of the teeth at *HA* II.5, 502a1, and of a goat's udder at *HA* III.21, 523a2.

40 πρὸς τὰ ἰσχία...ὀσφὺν...ὑπογάστριον: This tilting of the womb towards the front or back of the vagina is the extent of womb dislocation in *Non Gen*. Hippocratic texts do describe such retroversion and anteversion (see notes to 634b27–8) but also imagine much more far-flung uterine peregrinations; see Introduction pp. 82–3. This malpositioning of the womb is one explanation why a woman might not become dry after a night emission, but it may also be that she emitted too much *sperma* to be entirely drawn in by the *pneuma*; see notes to 635a36–7 and 636b39–637a15.

635a2 τὸ σπέρμα: Here the singular must refer to the mixture of male and female *sperma*. Taking up either the male or female *sperma* alone would not result in conception.

3 τῇ φύσει...ἢ ὑπὸ νόσου, ἀνίατον τὸ πάθος: Aristotle recognizes both congenital and disease-caused deformity of the genitals at *GA* II.7, 746b32–747a1. He states that some of these are curable but some are not: γίνεται δὲ τὰ μὲν ἰατὰ τὰ δ' ἀνίατα.

πάθος is here differentiated from νόσος, but again as an abnormal condition; see Introduction p. 105.

3–5 ἐὰν δ' ᾖ ῥῆγμα...συσπασάσης: The situation the author envisages here is very unclear. Scot has extensive paraphrasing in this chapter and omits the beginning entirely up to 635a7. Guil.'s text is lacunose and omits a translation of ῥῆγμα. Balme translates as if the ῥῆγμα is the condition itself, "but if it is a rupture, either natural or due to disease that causes contraction because of inflammation" (1991, p. 490). So too does Louis, "S'il s'agit d'une rupture soit naturelle, soit consecutif par suite d'une inflammation (1969, p. 160). But this raises the question, "A rupture of what?" The misalignment of the cervix is not a rupture of anything. However, if the significance of ἰσχυρῶς is that the cervix has become firmly established in its misalignment by becoming attached to another organ or the wall of the vagina, and so is ἀνίατον by human physicians, ῥῆγμα could mean the tearing away of a misaligned cervix either through some natural non-pathological event or a supervening disease which contracts the womb back to its correct position. The ῥῆγμα then is not the cause but the cure of an otherwise untreatable condition. Barnes begins as if to distinguish the rupture from the condition itself, "But if there is a rupture..." but leaves the end of the passage untranslated, asserting simply "Text uncertain" (1985, p. 986).

Steril. 213 (VIII.408.12) says that if the mouth of the womb has been completely averted blood can force it to straighten out, but it will bring disease with it. Perhaps we should read ῥῆξις.

II *After the discussion of the correct alignment of the cervix in the first half of the chapter, the author turns to the importance of the correct opening of the cervix, which he mentioned after the discussion of the movement of the womb in section IV of Chapter 1 (634a8–12). This section explains how the ability of the cervix to open correctly can be affected by the womb's movements up and down the vagina even if the cervix is straight.*

635a7 ἀνοίγεσθαι καλῶς: A στόμα that does not open properly results in reduced menstruation, e.g., *Mul.* I.4 (VIII.24.20–28.8).

8 ὅπως ὅταν ἄρχηται τὰ γυναικεῖα: τὰ γυναικεῖα is also used for menses at 634b12 and 635a14; see Introduction p. 100.

θιγγανόμενον: References to the touching of the cervix are usually made in the passive because it could be the doctor, the woman herself, or an intermediary who did the touching. The Hippocratic authors tend to use the verbs ἅπτομαι, ψηλαφάω, or ψαύω for palpation of the uterus, though the verb θιγγάνω is used for touching the woman generally in a case of flux from the womb at *Mul.* II.112 (VIII.240.8) and for palpating the κοιλία in a case of inflammation of the womb at *Mul.* II.170 (VIII.350.16). The woman examines herself at *Mul.* I.59 and II.157 (VIII.118.3 and 332.16), *Steril.* 213 and 230 (VIII.408.17, 410.3, and 438.11), and *Nat. Mul.* 2 (VII.312.18); the doctor examines the woman at *Mul.* I.20, 60 and II.160, 163, 165, 168, 171 and 177 (VIII.58.17, 120.8, 338.5, 342.13, 344.5, 346.20, 352.2, and 360.8) and *Nat. Mul.* 6 (VII.320.1); another woman acts as an intermediary at *Mul.* I.21 (VIII.60.16); and in other places it is unclear who is doing the examination, *Mul.* II.146 (VIII.322.7), *Steril.* 213 (VIII.410.13, 20, 23). Whoever does the initial examination, the use of imperatives, etc., implies that the doctor would usually be expected to administer the therapy directly to a woman's genital parts.

9 μαλακώτερον: Softness and openness of the womb as necessary conditions for conception are a recurring theme throughout the Hippocratic gynecology, e.g., *Mul.* II.115 and 133 (VIII.248.16–18 and 296.6–8), *Nat. Mul.* 39 and 107 (VII.382.15–4.3, 422.6–15). The remedies suggested for a hard and closed στόμα involve not just emollients but frequently the insertion of probes of ever-widening diameters into the στόμα. In this section the author is dealing with a womb that is open in some way. Closure of the womb is dealt with at 636a28–b6.

10 and 15 διεστομωμένον: A *hapax*. The author coins the term to differentiate the dilation of the cervix from the expansion of the womb itself. Both of these actions are referred to with the neutral ἀνοίγνυμι in Chapter 1. At the beginning of menstruation, the opening of the cervix may not be discernible, but this does not mean it was closed completely. A healthy cervix

185

has to stay open to facilitate the entry of the *sperma* at any time of the month, though immediately after menstruation when it is at its widest is the easiest time to conceive.

ἀλλ᾽ οὕτως ἔχοντος: Rud. considers deleting εἰ the simplest solution. Barnes and Louis believe there is a lacuna after εἰ, but there does not seem to be anything missing in the sense. Because the condition described by the genitive absolute is health, a temporal rather than a conditional force of the participle seems more appropriate anyway. The author is describing the beginning of menstruation, but he reminds his readers that when the *stoma* is healthy, before the menses show, the whites will appear. This is the progressive use of ἀλλά which Denniston, p. 21, says "is commoner in Hippocrates than in other writers."

σημεῖα: See note to 634b23.

11 φοιτάτω: See note to 634b16.

σαρκινώτερα: The "fleshier" signs are the menses proper (cf. 634b20, φοινικᾶ), which could not exit if the womb were not open.

12 ἀνεστομωμένη: The change in gender shows that the subject has changed from the cervix to the womb itself without any other indication. The author is now discussing not the emission of the menses from the womb, but the arrival of the menses in the womb, which requires the inner mouths of the womb to open up and the body of the womb to expand too (see 634a15–20). ἀναστομοῦνται is used at *HA* IX(VII).1, 581b19 to refer to the opening of the πόροι of the body which make it εὔρουν. The word is used 3 times in this passage, here and at ll.18 and 22. In each case it is the womb rather than the στόμα that is the subject (see notes ad locc.). ἀναστομόομαι, then, appears to be a technical term for the opening up of the body of the womb. In contrast, διαστομόομαι is used twice in the perfect participle form, at 635a9 and 15, to refer to the στόμα of the cervix. To differentiate these two technical terms from each other and the non-specific ἀνοίγνυμι (which is used generally to cover all the opening up involved, including the womb's inner mouths, the womb itself, and the στόμα of the cervix) I have translated διαστομόομαι as "to dilate" and ἀναστομόομαι as "to expand."

12 ἀλγήματος: The womb is performing its ἔργον without pain, as was specified at 633b23. This word is a very common term for pain in the Hippocratics but is used only 4 times in the Aristotelian Corpus, twice in *Prob.* XXVIII.6, 948b32 and 34 (discussing why we can endure thirst more easily than hunger), and twice in *HA* III.3, 512b18 and 25, where Aristotle is quoting more or less verbatim from *Nat. Hom.* When discussing pain Aristotle prefers to use the term ἀλγηδών, λύπη, or ὀδύνη.

13 θιγγάνηται: Balme translates the mss. reading as "it will be evident that the uterus has opened at the mouth without pain, whether one touches it or not" without noting in his app. crit. that the second arm of the disjunction is

missing in Dᵃ as well as Lᶜ; see Rud., p. 99. It is true that if the woman was menstruating there would be no need for anybody to palpate it to see if it was open, but it is unclear why the author would bother to point this out. Barnes, translates Dt.'s text as "the womb will be noticeably distended without any pain, whether it is touched or not," which is more ambiguous about who or what is doing the touching, but it begs the question "what is doing the touching?" and why pain should suddenly be introduced as a possible concomitant of the opening of the cervix.

The explanation of the expression is that the touching at issue is not an examination to make clear whether or not the womb has expanded. In the previous chapter a womb which failed to retract back up the vagina was said to become more insensitive (κωφότεραι) through constantly being touched (διαθιγγάνεσθαι δὲ ἀεί) by the penis and therefore to open less readily (μὴ ταχὺ ἀνοίγεσθαι) (634a9–10, 19–20). In this passage the author is describing a womb which has opened up at the appropriate time to menstruate and is therefore, as the author states immediately after this reference to touching, not insensitive (μήτε κωφότητα). In these circumstances the touching in question is best understood as that of the penis: even if the cervix does not retract back into the vagina during the rest of the month and is touched by the penis whenever sexual intercourse takes place, if menstruation occurs the womb has not been desensitized and is still fulfilling its ἔργον. The corruption of passive to active voice would be easy to account for since θιγγάνηται is followed immediately by καὶ, so –ται could have fallen out through haplography. Rud. notes that Dᵃ has only the positive arm of the disjunction, albeit in the active voice. Once the verb became active, the copyist producing Gᵃ assumed the touching was of the sort that gave evidence of a softened στόμα, and seeing that in the case of full menstruation what was needed was a statement that such touching was not necessary added the negative arm of the disjunction. This conj. would seem to have been adopted by Sᶜ, Rᶜ, and Vᶜ. Guil.'s translation, *tangatur et si non tangatur* reflects a parallel conjecture made by a copyist of a ms. in which the original passive voice had been retained.

13–14 μήτε στόμα ἀλλοιότερον αὐτὸ αὑτοῦ: Chiasmus. The author opens the paragraph with a reference to the soft, l.9, and dilated, l.10, condition of the cervix, then discusses the expansion of the womb itself during menstruation. When menstruation has finished he remarks that the cervix should be dilated, l.15, and not hard, l.15.

14 ληξάντων δὲ τῶν γυναικείων: The use of the aorist participle suggests that unlike Aristotle the author believed that menstruation had to have ceased completely in order for conception to take place; see Introduction p. 21.

16 ἡμέραν ὅλην καὶ ἡμίσειαν ἢ καὶ δύο ἡμέρας: It was a common belief that the best time for conception was the one or two days after menstruation was finished, e.g., *Vict.* I.27 (VI.500.19–20), *Mul.* I.17 and 24 (VIII.56.15–19 and 62.20–1), *Nat. Puer.* 15 (VII.494.18–20), *HA* IX(VII).2, 582b11–19.

ὅπερ ἐστὶ στόματος ὑγιεινῶς ἔχοντος: These words are out of place in l.22. They signal the end of the στόμα as the main topic of the section. The immediately following ταῦτα γὰρ σημαίνει begins a section on a well-functioning <u>womb</u>.

18 τὸ αὐτῶν ἔργον: This is immediately defined in terms that make it clear that the womb's ἔργον which is under discussion is menstruation. It performs its ἔργον well by responding to the body throughout the process.

18–19 τῷ μὲν μὴ εὐθὺς ἀνεστομῶσθαι ἀλλὰ μαλακὸν τὸ στόμα γίγνεσθαι: The agent that has just been described as doing something is the womb, and the activity of the womb is the subject of the rest of the section, including the causal phrase immediately following, so it is natural to take the womb as the subject of ἀνεστομῶσθαι, especially as it was the subject of this verb the last time it was used in l.12 and ἀναστομόομαι has not been used in connection with the στόμα. The similar construction at l.23 of which the womb is clearly the subject also argues for this interpretation. It must be admitted, however, that this makes the second part of the articular infinitive phrase as preserved in Dᵃ rather difficult to construe. If the subject of γίγνεσθαι is τὸ στόμα, we would have expected the conjunction to be τῷ δέ rather than ἀλλά. Perhaps we should read μαλακαί. Because it was the στόμα which was described as μαλακώτερον (l.9) and μὴ σκληρόν (l.15), it is easy to see how a copyist would take στόμα here to be the subject.

19–20 ἅμα τῷ ἄλλῳ σώματι λυομένῳ λύονται: Cf. 634b4–5. The Hippocratics believed menses were drawn to the womb all at once at one point in the month (*Nat. Puer.* 15, VII.492.21–494.2), Aristotle that they flowed there gradually over the course of the month (see note to 634a15). The author of *Non Gen.* believes that the blood is given up by the body, not drawn to the womb, at one point in the month when the body relaxes. The womb relaxes in preparation for receiving the blood, hence the softening of the cervix, but does not expand before it is necessary.

21 πρῶτον τὰ ἀπ' αὐτοῦ τοῦ στόματος: Dᵃ reads στόματος here. Only Guil. and Fel. translate *corpore*, but this cannot be right given the contrast between στόμα and σῶμα indicated by the use of αὐτοῦ with στόματος and δὲ introducing the σῶμα clause.

The fluid that is emitted first, according to 634b19–21, is the "milk-white whites," differentiated from the whites which occur at the end of menstruation by issuing from an odorless womb and not being putrefied (see note to 634a30–2). It is not clear why the author thinks their origin in the στόμα itself explains their white but unputrefied appearance.

21–2 ὅταν δὲ πλείω τὸ σῶμα προΐηται, ἀναστομοῦνται: Dᵃ's reading, προΐενται ἀναστομοῦντα, is untenable. Some verb has to be supplied for σῶμα. Most of the mss. of Guil. translate προΐενται as singular. Sylb. conjectured προΐεται and this was adopted by Sn., Dt., and Bk. as προΐηται in acknowledgement of ὅταν. Balme accepts this in his translation, but assumes it was omitted through haplography rather than corrupted from the plural, "and on the other hand when the body emits more, the uterus emits it by opening up" (Balme 1991, p. 493). Balme's translation acknowledges that following the subordinate temporal clause we need a finite verb of which the womb is subject, but by supplying this by προΐενται he is forced into taking the neuter accusative plural participle, ἀναστομοῦντα, to be functioning like an articular infinitive. Guil. translates ἀναστομοῦντα as a neuter plural participle, *aperientia*, in reference to what is not immediately clear, as is often the case in Guil.'s translation. The easiest solution is Sylb.'s conjecture, ἀναστομοῦνται, which has been accepted by most editors.

The indefinite temporal clause is balancing the fact that the womb does not immediately open up (τῷ μὲν μὴ εὐθὺς ἀνεστομῶσθαι, l.18) when the body begins to relax. προΐηται is used here of the fluid emitted into the womb from the body, equivalent to διδῷ in 634a16, as ἀναστομοῦνται is equivalent to ἀνοίγεσθαι καὶ δέχεσθαι in 634a15 (see above, notes on 635a12 and 18). Although προΐημι is used mainly for the ejaculation of *sperma* at orgasm, it is also used for the emission of menses at 636b4, for the release of unused *sperma* at 636a11 and 27 and by Aristotle for the expulsion of the embryo at 638b9. See Introduction pp. 102–3.

23 παυσαμένων δὲ τῶν σημείων: See note on 634b23.

τοῦ μὴ εὐθὺς συμπίπτειν: The genitive of the articular infinitive here would seem to indicate the source of, or foundation for, the statement about the womb's condition. Sn. and Dt. both conjecture τῷ, which is accepted by Barnes and Louis and would increase the similarity with l.18. However, there is a similar construction with the genitive of the articular infinitive (and with a genitive absolute appended to the main clause) at 636b13. If the womb collapsed in on itself, it would not be capable of attracting the *sperma* by πνεῦμα. It is not simply a question of the στόμα remaining dilated.

24 ἂν ἀπορήσῃ: If the verb is a form of ἀπορέω this phrase is difficult to make sense of. The verb is aorist subjunctive, but is it third person active or second person middle? In the first case the subject would presumably be the woman herself, in the second the attendant physician, who is sometimes addressed directly in the Hippocratic Corpus. This is how Louis takes it, "si l'on hésitait." But the treatise is full of signs that a physician can use to help him identify the cause of infertility; there is no need to address him personally at this particular juncture. This problem is not solved by Balme's impersonal "in case of doubt." Tricot simply ignores the word. Barnes remarks "Text uncertain." It may make more sense to take the verb as an Ionic form of ἀφοράω. The end of the chapter is recapitulating what has been said so far about the necessary conditions for conception. As well as discussing the dilation of the womb and the healthy flow of menstruation, the author has discussed the alignment of the στόμα and at l.39 had used the metaphor ὀρθὸν βλέπωσιν to characterize this. For the same Ionicism, whether we take Dᵃ's reading or the conjecture, see 637a32.

24–5 κεναί, ξηραί, διψηραί: In Aristotle's theory conception in an empty womb is impossible; there has to be a certain amount of menstrual fluid in the womb for the male semen to set.

25 τὴν δίοδον: Since *Non Gen.* has used στόμα so consistently to refer to the cervix throughout this chapter, it seems strange for the author to introduce a new term for it here. Aristotle uses the term δίοδος at *HA* I.14, 493b5, to refer to the "urethra" outside the womb which serves as a δίοδος for the male sperm, by which he seems to be referring to the vagina (see Introduction pp. 12–13 for Aristotle's failure to differentiate the vagina and urethra). However, the vagina is not at issue here since it is open to examination and gives information about the womb rather than vice versa. Perhaps the term is used to refer to the channel within the cervix as opposed to the exterior opening in the vagina. *Mul.* I.4 (VIII.26.2) uses it to distinguish the passages by which blood flows from the womb into the vagina from the στόμα per se.

25–6 προσσπαστικός: This word occurs only in this treatise, here and at b3 and 636a7. The prefix may emphasize the womb's enhanced attractive power immediately after menstruation.

27 πλησιάσαντος: This must refer to the woman's husband.

28 ἄνευ ἄλγους καὶ ἀναισθησίας: μετά seems to have been added by a copyist who took insensitivity in this context to be the antonym of pain.

ἀλλοιότερον...τὸ στόμα: This is a clear repetition of the phrase at 635a14, which, as here, followed immediately upon a reference to the womb not being insensitive.

30 συμμύειν αὐτὰς ὅταν δέῃ: συμμύειν is the complete closing of the cervix, differentiated from συμπίπτειν of the womb. The phrasing shows this is not something that happens as a matter of course every month after menstruation, which is why conception can take place any time during a woman's cycle, though immediately after menstruation when the cervix is most widely dilated and before the womb contracts is the most propitious.

CHAPTER 3

I *If the woman is menstruating and the cervix is in good order but she does not become pregnant, in the interests of examining* πάντα τὰ μόρια *(633b29) the doctor should next examine the environment of the womb itself and its ability to draw in* sperma. *The first structural element considered is the cotyledons.*

635a32 αὐτὴν δὲ τὴν ὑστέραν: The taking up of *sperma* is an ἔργον of the womb, but here the doctor is not considering either menstruation or the activity of the στόμα, but whether the womb is correctly formed so as to be able to attract.

33 μετὰ τὴν κάθαρσιν: If menstruation itself proceeded normally although the womb is not in perfect condition, this would seem to contradict the author's definition of the health of a part in Chapter 1. But here he is discussing a different ἔργον of the womb in which menstrual blood is not involved, that is the drawing in of *sperma*.

34 προϊέναι: δεῖ can be understood from l.32. A copyist mistakenly corrected the infinitive to the participial form because he treated the adverbial καὶ as a conjunction joining προϊέναι to συγγινομένην. If we leave προϊεμένην as a participial form, it is very difficult not to take the καὶ as conjunctive and have both participles governed by ὡς. But the ὡς should not govern the verb indicating ejaculation because although the woman only <u>seems</u> to be having intercourse she must <u>actually</u> ejaculate. Both Balme and Barnes translate as if the infinitive rather than the participle follows καί. Note that the emission takes place after menstruation has finished; it is not part of menstruation.

35 παρεπλησίαζε: The prefix is unusual with this verb. Here, in what would otherwise be a redundant clause if it meant no more than συγγινομένην or προϊέναι, it seems to be intensifying the action of having intercourse and emitting. ὡς ἂν εἰ further intensifies the phrase.

ῥαδίως: Postponed for emphasis.

φαίνηται: This verb is used here because sometimes when the woman has emitted it will not be obvious to her, i.e., when her body draws in the *sperma* and does not release it later; see notes to 636a1–4. There can be no sense of an appearance that is misleading here.

36 ἄμεινον: This is in stark contrast to the Hippocratic view of night emissions; see note to 634b30.

36–7 ὁτὲ μὲν…ὁτὲ δέ: The author has already mentioned a couple of reasons that <u>none</u> of the woman's emission may have been attracted into her womb: the cervix may have retracted back up the vagina, in which case the emission will remain in her vagina because the womb will be too far away to draw in her *sperma*, or the womb may be misaligned. At 636b39–637a15 he explains that a healthy womb does not have to draw in <u>all</u> the emission for conception to take place, so here, the fact that the woman is sometimes moist after a nocturnal emission does not mean that the womb is not performing its ἔργον of drawing in the *sperma*.

36–40 καὶ ἀνισταμένην...βραχείας προελθούσης: Rud. p. 36 comments on the long intervening sentence between the first infinitive dependent on δεῖ in l.32 (συμβαίνειν, l.33) and the other accusative and infinitive constructions dependent on it beginning in l.36. If we read προιέναι instead of προιεμένην in l.34, the postponement of the continued construction is not that long.

36 δεῖσθαι θεραπείας: See note to 634b31.

37 ξηράν: ξηρασία means a state of desiccation. Dᵃ's genitive would make the term dependent on δεῖσθαι, in parallel with θεραπείας. This is obviously not what is meant, but it is easy to see how the ὅτε...ὅτε construction could lead to this.

37–9 τὴν δὲ ξηρότητα ταύτην μὴ συνεχῆ: The author does not explain why a woman does not hold onto her own *sperma* if it is not mingled with a man's. This is the main objection that Aristotle lodges against the author's theory in the *Dialectic*. The longest the womb retains a woman's unmingled *sperma* (unless the woman's body draws it into itself; see 636a2) is half of a short day.

38 ἔγερσιν: This is a rare word in the Hippocratics, used only in *Coac.* 82 (V.602.1) and *Epid.* III.3.17, case 11 (III.134.9). In the Aristotelian Corpus it appears twice in the Pseudo-Aristotelian *Prob.* (X.31, 894a26 and XI.17, 900b36) and once in *EN* III.8, 1116b30, where it is used metaphorically of the stirring of the θυμός. On the other hand, Aristotle uses the word ἐγρήγορσις 35 times for waking up. This term appears 3 times in the Hippocratics, *Hum.* 2 and 9 (V.478.8 and 488.15) and *Vict.* I.10 (VI.486.10)

40–635b1 ἡ δ᾽ ὑγρότης ἔστω τοιαύτη οἵα ὅταν πλησιάσῃ τῷ ἀνδρί: The woman's unmingled *sperma* looks like the fluid that results from the mingling of both male and female *sperma*, further evidence that the woman's *sperma* is like the man's and is not menstrual fluid; cf. 634b31–2.

2 δεκτικὴν τὴν ὑστέραν εἶναι τοῦ διδομένου: This phrasing further argues against the woman's *sperma* originating in the womb.

3 τὰς κοτυληδόνας: See Rud. pp. 22–3, van der Eijk 2001, vol. II, pp. 38–41. A cotyledon is a cup-shaped hollow, such as the suckers on an octopus' tentacles (Hom. *Od.* 5.433, *HA* IV.1, 524a2, *PA* IV.9, 685b3). What sort of structure they are meant to represent inside the womb is something of a mystery. Hippocratic authors refer to them at *Aph.* V.45 (IV.548.2–3), *Nat. Mul.* 17 (VII.336.14), *Mul.* I.58 (VIII.116.5), and *Steril.* 230 (VIII.444.20). As in *Non Gen.* they seem to play a role in keeping the fetus attached to the uterus, perhaps for nourishment, but nothing is said about their role in attracting the *sperma* into the womb to begin with. Galen records that Diocles and Praxagoras believed them to be the protruding ends of the blood vessels which entered the uterus (frag. 22, van der Eijk 2001, vol. I, p. 32), and Soranus records that Diocles (frag. 23d, van der

Eijk 2001 vol. I, p. 34) believed that Nature had created cotyledons within the womb to prepare the fetus for suckling at the nipple. At *GA* II.7, 746a19–20, Aristotle criticizes this belief without using the term κοτυληδών. He refers to the thing fetuses suck on as "a fleshy thing," σαρκίδιόν τι. In reference to the womb, Aristotle uses the term cotyledon to signify the numerous small pits in the uterine wall of some animals (those that have teeth in only their lower jaw and those, such as the hare, mouse, and bat, that have a cluster of blood vessels running through the womb) to which the umbilicus is attached and through which the fetus receives nourishment, *GA* II.7, 745b22–746a28, *HA* III.1, 511a30, IX(VII).8, 586a32–586b15. At *GA* IV.4, 771b27–30, Aristotle denies the attractive force of cotyledons, "The claim that these places in the womb draw the *sperma* and on this account multiple offspring are generated, because of the multiplicity of the places and the cotyledons not being a single structure, is nonsense," τὸ μὲν οὖν ἕλκειν φάναι τοὺς τόπους τῆς ὑστέρας τὸ σπέρμα, καὶ διὰ τοῦτο πλείω γίνεσθαι, διὰ τὸ τῶν τόπων πλῆθος καὶ τὰς κοτυληδόνας οὐχ ἓν οὔσας, οὐθέν ἐστιν. *Non Gen.* does not refer to the cotyledons in its explanation of multiple births (see 636b39–637a15), but it is the only extant text that allots a role in attracting the *sperma* into the womb to these structures.

καθεκτικάς. Only here and *Top.* IV.5, 125b18, and the Pseudo-Aristotelian *Prob.* XXXIII.15, 963a21. No explanation is given as to why the cotyledons would be less retentive of the woman's *sperma* when it is drawn in unmixed with the male's.

II *The author next turns to discussing the elasticity of the womb. If the womb can attract the* sperma, *it will need to be able to expand to bring a pregnancy to term.*

635b4 φύσας: *Steril.* 238 and 239 (VIII.452.5–454.2) say a woman who has had several spontaneous abortions around the second month of pregnancy has a womb that fails to expand with the growing embryo and detail how a doctor should engender wind in a woman's womb if it does not occur naturally. *Mul.* I.57 (VIII. 114.8–116.4), II.177, and 211 (VIII.358.19–360.17 and 406.11–15) record cases of pathological wind in the uterus.

ἐγγίνεσθαι: Note the return to the accusative and infinitive after δεῖ in 635a32. Grammatically φύσας is the subject here, but the subject of the other infinitives and participles in the sentence is the womb.

5 καὶ μεγάλας γινομένας καὶ ἐλάττους αὐτῶν: The uterus does not produce gas like the intestines. It is unclear to what the author is referring here, unless there is some confusion with intestinal gas.

7 αὐτάς: Prolepsis.

8 φύσει…νόσῳ: Cf. 11 and 635a3 and 4.

ᾧ: There is little difference in meaning if one retains the mss. ὡς, but all the φῦσαι do is show that the womb is expandable and so will provide room as the fetus grows. The differences in the amount of *sperma* the womb draws in at conception would not result in immediately greater or lesser expansion, so the manner of the womb's reception of the *sperma* is not appropriate here.

11–12 διαφθείρουσι τὰ ἔμβρυα: See *Genit.* 9–10 (VII.482.3–484.13), which compares the way the size of a womb can constrain growth to the way cucumber frames can dictate the size of cucumbers.

12–13 σφόδρα...μικρά...ἧττον μείζω: If the womb will not expand at all, the embryo cannot grow very large; if it expands a bit further, the embryo will grow somewhat larger before it is stifled.

14 ἀγγείῳ: The term is used of both rigid and pliable receptacles; see LSJ. It is true that cucumber frames are rigid, but elsewhere the image of the womb is much more like that of the expandable wineskin (ἀσκός, *Mul.* I.61 and II.170, (VIII.124.15–21 and 350.16–17)) than the jug or jar which Hanson conceives it as (1990, p. 317, followed by King 1989, p. 23).

III *The author explains the necessity for the vagina to be moist during intercourse, prior to the emission of* sperma *by either the man or the woman. The moisture serves the same sorts of functions as saliva, sweat, and tears.*

635b15–16 ἔτι δέ: Introducing a new topic, though the sentence fits better with the earlier section. Smoothness of the womb does not seem to fit in the discussion either of the elasticity of the womb or of vaginal lubrication. However, if we take ὁμαλά to mean "equal" rather than "smooth," it would fit well with the previous paragraph; both right and left sides of the womb, and upper and lower parts, should be of the same size and elasticity in case it has to nourish twins (see below, 637a9).

τὰ ἐπὶ δεξιά...ἀριστερά: Empedocles believed the left and right sides of the womb played a role in determining the sex of the fetus, but it is not clear whether he thought there were distinct right and left pockets inside the womb. *Superf.* I (VIII.476.3) refers to the "horns," κέρατα, of the uterus, which may mean distinct pockets or be a reference to the fallopian tubes. Oribasius (*Med. Coll.* 24.31.24 (*CMG* VI.2, 1, vol. III, p. 44.27–32 Raeder)) says Herophilus described the offshoots from the sides of the uterus, ἐπὶ τῶν πλαγίων ἀποφύσεις, as semi-circular, which would accord well with the fallopian tubes, and adds that Diocles called these structures "horns," κεραῖαι, because of their shape. However, this was with the benefit of both animal and human dissection, and it is not clear that the Hippocratics did either. Aristotle (*GA* I.3, 716b32–3) believed the womb not only had right and left sides but two distinct chambers, because they parallel the man's two testicles: "The uterus for all females is double, just as all males have two testicles," αἱ δ' ὑστέραι πᾶσι μέν εἰσι διμερεῖς, καθάπερ καί οἱ ὄρχεις τοῖς ἄρρεσι δύο πᾶσιν. He did not call the two parts horns, though Leroi 2014, pp. 185–7, argues that his view of the womb was based on that of the sheep's womb, which is "mostly made of two large uterine horns which humans lack." See King 1998, pp. 33–5, for a discussion of ancient womb anatomy.

17 μεταξύ: That is, <u>before</u> emission of *sperma* at orgasm, 634b30 (τελέως). See Introduction pp. 31–6. This is recognized as a necessary precursor to orgasm in women among contemporary sexologists, Lloyd 2005, p. 38.

18 μὴ πολλάκις δὲ μηδὲ σφόδρα: μὴ πολλάκις signifies that during intercourse the woman does not have to produce this fluid over and over again, though it does not necessarily limit it to one emission. Because this fluid aids in conception, μὴ πολλάκις cannot mean that she should only emit this fluid during a few occasions of intercourse. μηδὲ σφόδρα signifies that however many emissions of the local fluid there are during one act of intercourse, they should not cumulatively produce an excess of fluid; which could hinder conception; see Introduction p. 35.

19 ἵδρωμα τοῦ τόπου: ἵδρωμα is a *hapax* signifying a fluid excretion that is not quite sweat. The moisture referred to here is simply the vaginal lubricant, issuing from the womb (cf. αἱ ὑστέραι ὑγραίνονται, l.24), not the whole body, as is the case for *sperma* (see note on 637a12). In fact, the lubricant produced in the vagina during intercourse is secreted into the vaginal mucosa by Bartholin glands, located near the opening of the vagina. The emission which some women report at orgasm is secreted by Skene glands; see notes on 637a21–8.

19–25 τῷ στόματι σιάλου...διαθέσεως: The simile is very detailed and covers a number of different responses. Saliva produced in the mouth at the expectation of food illustrates an anticipation of enjoyment. Saliva produced when we are chattering and working is a physiological response to the normal working of the body. The production of tears in the eyes illustrates the ability of the part to adjust to the external environment. All three responses are applicable to the healthy womb preparing to conceive.

21 τοῖς ὄμμασι: Eyes used as simile again; cf. 633b20–9 and 634b39–40.

22 πρὸς τὰ λαμπρότερα ὁρῶντες, καὶ ὑπὸ ψύχους καὶ θερμότητος ἰσχυροτέρας: Just as moisture helps the eye get control over a more extreme environment than it is used to, so the moisture produced by the womb enables it to master whatever is presented to it.

ὑπό: Unusually with things, almost personifying the cold and heat.

23 τὰ μόρια: The eyes.

24 ὑγροτέρως: An Ionic form but not unknown in Aristotle; cf. *PA* II.10, 657a2, and III.14, 675a19.

25 ὑγροτέρας διαθέσεως: That is, an overly dry condition of the womb could prevent conception.

26 πάθος: This is something that should happen to promote conception, not pathological.

26–7 θεραπείας ἀεί: Not medical treatment, simply attention, as in 634b30–1, though there the fluid referred to is the woman's *sperma*, not the vaginal lubricant. The word ἀεί may be included to indicate that the woman needs attention after intercourse even if neither of the partners reaches climax, to contrast with the τότε of 634b30, which immediately follows τελέως.

28 πτύσεως: The term πτύσις is used of saliva once it has exited the mouth. So the ἵδρωμα produced by the womb should be emitted into the vagina, but too much of it can prevent the proper mingling of male and female *sperma*. At *HA* VI.18, 572b27–8, Aristotle says a wet womb can "blow away," ἀποφυσᾷ, i.e., fail to hold onto, the *sperma*.

ὑγρασία: This word occurs only once in the Hippocratic Corpus, *Vict.* II.47 (VI.548.3–4) but is very common in Aristotle.

29 καθαρὸν τὸ τοῦ ἀνδρὸς καὶ τῆς γυναικός: In D²'s reading at this juncture only the male contribution has to be drawn into the womb and the fluid it is mixed with is the local ἵδρωμα from the womb—but this contradicts everything else the author says in the treatise about female *sperma*. Either the locution is careless phrasing on Aristotle's part, or he (or a later copyist) failed to realize that the author of *Non Gen.* believed there were two female fluids involved in intercourse. That *sperma* could be used in the singular to refer to the mixture of male and female *sperma* is indicated at 636a10; see note ad loc. *Steril.* 241 (VIII.454.6–456.6) remarks that τὸ ἀπὸ τῆς γυναικὸς μὴ ξυλλαμβάνεσθαι πρὸς τὴν τέκνωσιν, "the <emission> from the woman which goes towards reproduction will not be taken up" if her menses are too moist, and attributes this condition to the illness of both body and womb, τοῦ τε σώματος καὶ τῶν μητρέων νοσεόντων. Cf. 636b37.

IV *In addition to considering the attractive power of the cotyledon, the elasticity of the womb, and the moistness of the vaginal environment during intercourse, a doctor should also consider the effect of intercourse on a woman's body generally.*

635b31–2 τοσόνδε δεῖ κατανοεῖν, τί συμβαίνει: τοσόνδε covers the indirect questions introduced by τί, πῶς, and εἰ in ll.31–5. The prolepsis signifies the scope of what the doctor needs to ascertain. The pronoun either limits the amount the doctor should find out ("this much and no more") or validates seemingly prying questions ("even to this extent"). It would be a strange expression if the intended audience for the treatise were the woman or the infertile couple themselves. κατανοεῖν is used most frequently to indicate an intellectual understanding of some proposition, but it can also be used to indicate a perception of a factual state of affairs (e.g., Thuc. 2.3) or an understanding of facts gleaned from another's account (e.g., Herod. II.28).

33 ἐξανίσταται: This verb is used 3 times in the Hippocratic Corpus. Other than here it appears in the Aristotelian Corpus only in the fragments (3 times).

35 ἐφυγραίνεται: Outside of its appearance in *Non Gen.* (here and at 635a35–40) this verb appears only 5 times, 4 times in the Hippocratic Corpus (*Epid.* I.10 (II.632.5), *Coac.* 297, 396, and 630 (V.650.6, 674.15, and 730.8–9)) and once in Oribasius. In its medical context it normally signifies a loose bowel movement, but that is not what is meant here.

37 προετικὸν εἶναι τὸ σῶμα σπέρματος: The whole body is productive of *sperma*, not just the στόμα of the womb as with the vaginal lubricant; hence emission of *sperma* at the culmination of an erotic dream causes a certain lassitude. This emission has wider effects than the simple moistening of the vagina.

38 τήν τε ποιοῦσαν ποιεῖ ἀσθενῆ: This is a puzzling expression, for which Barnes notes the text as "uncertain." Both Scot and Guil. have lacunae here. ποιεῖ seems to require a predicate adjective and ἀσθενῆ fits both with what precedes and follows. 636b32 says that when the emitted *sperma* comes out of material the body needs, it makes women weaker, ἀσθενεστέρας ποιεῖ. τε is used independently as a conjunction at 635a29 and 636a4. The repeated use of ποιέω, which makes the clause a little odd, reflects the author's enjoyment, but sparing use, of jingles: λυομένῳ λύονται, 635a20; πάσχουσα τὸ πάσχον, 636a25–6.

καὶ σωματωδῶν δ' οὐσῶν ἀσθενεστέρα: καὶ...δὲ takes the previous statement one step further. In *HA* III.20, 521b27, σωματώδης is used to describe the curd as opposed to the whey of milk, at *GA* II.4, 739b26, the bulky part of the milk that is set by rennet while the more fluid part separates off, and at III.11, 761b2, water is said to be less σωματῶδες than earth.

39 ἀνόσως: The only other occurrence of this word before the first century is in *Epid.* I.1 (II.604.2).

ὃν δεῖ: Prolepsis of relative clause.

40 ἄφοδος: This word does not occur in Aristotle but does occur 6 times in the Hippocratic Corpus.

νοσώδης: This means something beyond the loss of strength, since weakness deriving from the healthy production of *sperma* occurs ἀνόσως.

ἦν: Counterfactual force despite the omission of ἄν; see Smyth 2320.

636a2–4 τὸ δέ ποτε καὶ ἰσχύειν μᾶλλον...καὶ τὸ σῶμα ἰσχύει: When drawn in unmixed with the male *sperma* the woman's *sperma* can be incorporated into her own body and does not come back out again. This would be the author's answer to why women do not produce wind-eggs; see the *Dialectic*.

2 [εἶτ'ἐφυγραίνεσθαι]: This has been inserted by a copyist mindful of the author's injunction at 635a38 and 635b35 that the dryness that women experience after erotic dreams should be followed by her becoming moist when the womb releases her *sperma*. But here it is not the womb that has seized the fluid; it has been drawn from the womb (which is therefore dry) and used up on the woman's body. It therefore does not reappear in the woman's vagina.

3 ἀφανίζει: The body is "stealing" the woman's own *sperma*, and this re-appropriation causes the woman's body to gain strength. This is a partial answer to Aristotle's objection that women do not produce "wind-eggs" after they have drawn their own *sperma* unmingled with the male's into their womb, but it does not explain why on other occasions the womb simply releases the woman's *sperma*.

4 πνεύματί τε γὰρ ἕλκει ἡ ὑστέρα: See notes to 634b34 and 637a15–35.

4–5 τὸ προσελθὸν ἔξωθεν αὐτῇ: Note that what has been under discussion in this chapter is the *sperma* that comes from a woman's body and that is described here as coming from outside the womb.

5 ὥσπερ πρότερον εἴρηται: Cf. 634b34–5.

5–6 οὐ γὰρ εἰς αὐτὴν προΐεται, ἀλλ'οὗ καὶ ὁ ἀνήρ: This sentence makes clear that it is the female emission which has been under discussion all along. Dt. compares *GA* II.4, 739a35, and Rose says *HA* X sides with Aristotle against the Hippocratic view of *Genit.* 4; see Rud. p. 19. However, in the *GA* passage, Aristotle attributes the emission of a fluid during sexual arousal in a woman to the στόμα of the womb being open, indicating that he believes that the womb is its source, which is not the case in *Non Gen.*

Following ἀλλ' οὗ καὶ Ald. and Bas. transpose the passage 636b33–637b15, but this is clearly mistaken and was corrected by Bk. See Balme 1991, p. 543 for a lengthy discussion of the ms. history of the transposition and correction.

7 καὶ τὸ σῶμα προσσπαστικὸν τὸ τῆς τοιαύτης: Prolepsis of the adjective, which is a *hapax*. If a woman draws the *sperma* not only into her womb by *pneuma*, but also into her very body, it shows that her body, not just her womb, has attractive power. This attractive power is associated with strength. *Mul.* I.6 (VIII.30.20–2) says women who menstruate less than normal become manlike, ἀνδρικαί, and do not conceive. At *GA* II.7, 747a1–3, Aristotle says "masculine," ἀρρενωποί, women do not menstruate and at *GA* I.18, 725b30–726a6, that fat people (both men and women) are less fertile than others because their seminal residue (i.e., menses in the case of women) gets used up on their own bodies (καταναλίσκεται γὰρ εἰς τὸ σῶμα). So here: women with "strong" bodies are using their own *sperma* deposited in front of their womb for their own bodies, not for the production of children. However, this is only described in relation to a woman's own emissions; there is no indication she can utilize the man's emissions in this way, and *Non Gen.* does not say that women with these sorts of bodies are less fertile than others.

V *Wind-pregnancies caused by an excessively dry womb. Note that the author of* Non Gen. *does not utilize the unfertilized eggs of birds to explain this condition because he is describing a condition involving mixed male and female* sperma.

9–10 and 12 ἐξανεμοῦσθαι: Aristotle uses this verb when reporting the belief that some mares become so desirous of intercourse that they run off to the north or south until they either exhaust themselves or reach the sea, where they thereupon discharge something (τι) called ἱππομανές, the name which is also applied to the growth on a foal's forehead at birth or the fluid mares produce when they are ready to mate (*HA* VI.18, 572a13–28). At *HA* V.5, 541a28, he reports that partridges can become pregnant if they stand downwind of the male. Peck's note to this passage notes other occurrences in ancient literature of the belief that females can be impregnated by the wind. However, none of these are relevant to the condition discussed in *Non Gen.* which develops after intercourse with a man. The condition of wind-eggs (ὑπηνέμια) is also not relevant because they are eggs that have not been fertilized by the male.

Nat. Puer. 30 (VII.532.14–534.10) discusses the case of women who believe they have been pregnant for longer than nine months. The author attributes this to the uterus taking *pneuma* from the κοιλία and swelling up while at the same time the menses begin to collect in the uterus. When these eventually break out, the uterus is cleansed and the στόμα wide open, so the woman easily becomes pregnant but believes her pregnancy began when she first noticed her stomach rise and her menses stop.

The term ἐξανεμωθῇ is used in *Mul.* I.34 (VIII.80.5) and *Nat. Mul.* 69 (VII.402.17) to refer to a woman who is actually pregnant but also suffering from wind in the uterus.

11 πάθος: A pathological use of the term.

11–12 ὅταν συγγένωνται τῷ ἀνδρί, οὔτε προϊέμεναι δῆλαι τὸ σπέρμα: Are we to take the aorist subjunctive here (συγγένωνται) as denoting time prior to or contemporaneous with the main verb δῆλαι (understand εἰσί)? Smyth 2409a indicates it could be either. If προϊέμεναι refers to the female *sperma*, it would seem to be contemporaneous; if it refers to the expulsion of the mixture of male and female *sperma* from the womb after it has been initially taken up, συγγένωνται would signify prior action. If προϊέμεναι referred only to the emission of female *sperma*, this in itself would be sufficient to explain why she did not become pregnant, and since the rest of the paragraph deals with the expulsion of co-mingled *sperma* after it has been taken up by the womb this expulsion has to be the meaning of προϊέμεναι here. The use of the definite article with *sperma* also tends to this conclusion. Because the woman has not clearly emitted the co-mingled *sperma* after taking it up she should become pregnant, but she does not.

12 οὔτε κυΐσκονται: The fact that the woman is not really pregnant is not something that is immediately apparent (see ll.18–23). A "wind-pregnancy" involves some other symptom of pregnancy in addition to the apparent retention of the *sperma*. διὸ καὶ καλεῖται ἐξανεμοῦσθαι. The causal connection of this clause is not clear. Is the author referring to the popular belief that women have been impregnated by the wind (n.b. the term ἐξανεμοῦσθαι is introduced by καλεῖται in l.12), or is he referring to a medical use of the term which reflects a belief that the womb is swollen with air (n.b. αἴρεται in l.22)?

13 πάθους: Here pathological.

13–14 οὐκ: As Dt. saw, the condition depends on the *sperma* not being released immediately.

14–24: Note variations between present and the gnomic aorist throughout this passage.

14–15 τὸ δὲ κατασκελετεύεται…ἐξιόν: If this happens repeatedly, it may be a reason why a woman fails to become pregnant, but it will not always progress to full-blown "wind-pregnancy"; see ll.16–18.

15–16 μικρόν, μικρότητα: Aristotle may be responding to this aspect of *Non Gen.*'s description of "wind-pregnancy" in his description of the uterine mole as εὐμεγέθη in Chapter 7; see note on 638a17.

17 ὑπέρξηρος: This term is used only twice in Aristotle (*Resp.* 14, 477b28 and *Metr.* I.14, 352a7) but 11 times in the Hippocratic Corpus.

19 δοκεῖ κύειν: The symptoms of pregnancy eventually include a swelling of the abdomen (22), but before then women suffering "wind-pregnancy" might feel that their cervix had closed and have suffered suspension of menses, perhaps also such things as morning sickness and pica.

19–20 ὃν ἂν ἔχῃ αὐτὴ πρὸς αὐτήν, ἕως ἂν ἀποβάλῃ: Prolepsis of relative clause. It is not the expulsion of the retained dried out *sperma* which signals that it was not a real pregnancy, because this is not observable. Rather, it is the abatement of all the symptoms of pregnancy without any signs of an abortion or a miscarriage, so that whatever it was that was causing the symptoms of pregnancy remains a mystery. The ancients were well aware of true pregnancies that did not last to term, and the Hippocratics differentiated between them on the length of gestation; see Dean-Jones 1994, pp. 173–6. Here the author of *Non Gen.* is discussing the failure to conceive, not the failure to bring a pregnancy to term, which could have numerous causes, as he briefly notes at 637a35–637b6.

20–1 ὅμοια…πάθη: These are conditions which would be normal, not pathological, in a real pregnancy.

24–5 τὸ δαιμόνιον, θεραπευτόν: *Sac. Dis.* 1 (VI.354.1 and 3–4) implies that by the end of the fifth century BCE a supernatural origin of disease was usually reserved, even among the lay public, for those which were not treatable by medicine; see note on 636b10–13.

26, 32, 37, b10 σημεῖον τοῦ: Used with infinitive. These conditions are not made obvious by the σημεῖα of menses.

26–8 τοῦ τοιαύτας εἶναι: Balme's attempt to explain the argument with the retention of μή seems to me to be misguided in that it requires understanding ὅταν λάβωσι παρὰ τοῦ ἀνδρός as something other than taking the male *sperma* into the womb and συλλάβωσιν as something other than becoming pregnant, which, in the context of this argument, seems to me very difficult to do. The women discussed here are those described in ll.17–18 whose wombs are so dry that they unobtrusively expel the shriveled *sperma* right away without seeming to become pregnant. If their wombs become a little less dry, they will be liable to wind-pregnancies.

27 παρὰ τοῦ ἀνδρός: This phrase does not signify that only the man provides *sperma*. It differentiates a woman who appears not to expel *sperma* from her womb after intercourse and does not become pregnant—which can lead to wind-pregnancy—from a woman who appears not to release her own *sperma* after an erotic dream—which leads to her whole body becoming stronger.

CHAPTER 4

I *After detailing what the attractive powers of the womb should be, the author deals with pathologies of the womb.*

636a28 σπάσμα: Outside of the Pseudo-Aristotelian *Prob.* (V.1 and 39, 880b18 and 885a6) this form is not used by Aristotle, who prefers σπασμός, which he uses 5 times. The Hippocratics also prefer σπασμός, but they use σπάσμα 11 times, including in gynecological contexts at *Aër.* 4 (II.24.10) and *Epid.* VII.73 (V.432.18). Spasm is the closing of the cervix at the wrong time, which would impede conception because the womb could not attract the seed into itself.

29 γίνονται δὲ σπάσματα: Plural verb with neuter plural subject. In both the cases mentioned by the author (inflammation and childbirth) the womb is in a serious condition before spasm supervenes, provoked by the distention of the womb.

29–30 ταῖς ὑστέραις, τῆς ὑστέρας: Note sudden switch from plural to singular.

30 ἐν τῷ τόκῳ: This is not really of interest to our author in this treatise, or at least to Aristotle in his summary of it. There are many other problems that can occur during pregnancy and parturition that are not mentioned. The problems of fertility that are of interest in the treatise as we have it are those that can hamper conception.

31–2 μὴ ἀνοιγομένου τοῦ στόματος: The only time the womb is fully closed is during pregnancy, so spasm during childbirth is the failure of the στόμα to open, whereas outside of pregnancy it is the inappropriate closing of the στόμα.

32–5 τότε ὑπὸ τῆς διατάσεως γίνεται σπάσμα: The τότε is emphasized by the asyndeton and refers only to the spasm arising in childbirth, "At this time the cause is distention."

34–5 ἔχουσα γὰρ σπάσμα φλεγμαίνοι ἂν τότε: This is almost a chiasmus of the sentence at l.32 which explained the reason for spasm in childbirth. Nobody has questioned Dᵃ's ποτε, but this only makes sense if the author was discussing spasm as the cause of inflammation, and the causal relationship is clearly the other way round. Outside of childbirth, there are no cases of spasm which are not caused by inflammation, but there can be cases of inflammation which are not accompanied by spasm; cf. 634a20–6.

35–7 φῦμα…ἐμποδίζει…συλλήψεις: At 633b29 the analogy of an eye had been used to show that while a growth may not prevent a part from performing its ἔργον completely, it would hamper it in some way.

36 φῦμα…ἢ πολλὰ ἑλκωθὲν τὸ στόμα: Aristotle uses the term φῦμα for a growth on an organ at, e.g., *GA* IV.4, 772b29, *PA* III.4, 667b3, but he also uses it to refer to an abscess, e.g., *Resp.* 20, 479b28. In the Hippocratic gynecology φῦμα is used to refer to an abscess within the genital area or the womb itself, caused either by retained menstrual blood or pus; see, e.g., *Nat. Puer.* 15 (VII.496.6), *Mul.* I.2 (VIII.20.13 and 16), *Steril.* 222 (VIII.428.23). For sores on the στόμα they prefer the word φλυκταίνη, e.g. *Mul.* II.173 (VIII.354.3–5). They do, however, frequently discuss an ulcerated στόμα, e.g., *Mul.* I.40 and 49 (VIII.96.8 and 108.3), *Nat. Mul.* 33 (VII.366.14). It seems unlikely that a badly ulcerated cervix would need the further *pathos* of a φῦμα before it caused problems for conception. *Mul.* I.90 (VIII.214.18) uses the phrase ἑλκωθῇ ἢ φλυκταινῶν (though *Nat. Mul.* 108 (VII.422.16) reads ἑλκωθῇ καὶ φλυκταινῶν). The omission of ἢ by haplography after ῇ is easy to account for, and a scribe made sense of the phrase following ῇ by dropping -τόμα and making the clause a participle in agreement with στόματος.

37–8 σημεῖον…συμμύουσα: A growth or a badly ulcerated cervix would be amenable to direct observation either by the woman herself, the doctor, or an intermediary, but such an examination need not be undertaken if the cervix behaves as it should during menstruation and intercourse. Disturbances in this activity might alert a doctor to the possibility of the condition before the growth or ulcers themselves become obvious to the touch. During menstruation and intercourse the concern is only that the womb opens properly, and although just after menstruation was recognized as the best time for conception it was not the only time. The complete closing implied by συμμύω should only occur after conception; cf. 635a30. Here it must mean simply the lessening of the dilation of the στόμα, if it is not a mistaken insertion.

39 χρῆσις: Intercourse is not a common usage of this word. Aristotle qualifies it as τὴν τῶν ἀφροδισίων χρῆσιν at *HA* IX(VII).1, 581b13.

636b1–6 τὸ στόμα συμφύεται...νόσον: In *GA* IV.4, 773a15–20, Aristotle seems to view the condition as entirely congenital. He makes no mention of the possibility that it could be caused by disease.

2 καὶ ἰατὸν καὶ ἀνίατον: Aristotle believed that the condition could reverse itself naturally or the lips of the *stoma* be separated by physicians. However, sometimes the condition was incurable and then, and sometimes after medical intervention, the woman died.

4 οὐδὲν ὧν δεῖ: The clause falls between the two infinitives governing the object; cf. the position of ὑστέρα at 636a38.

5 παρὰ τοῦ ἀνδρός: The author is not denying that the female also emits something when conception takes place. He is here explaining how to eliminate the possibility that the barrier to conception is a womb of which the cervix has closed over. The deposition of seed by the man is simply easier to monitor than a woman's. As in the early diagnosis of a growth on the cervix, intercourse and menstruation afford opportunities to observe the condition.

ἀφιεῖσα: The author's use of ἀφίημι in the rest of the first five chapters suggests that it is the discharge of the menses he is talking about here. It cannot refer to female *sperma* since this does not originate in the womb, so its appearance does nothing to show the womb is open.

6 οὐκ ἂν ἐνσχεθείη: Dᵃ's reading is not tenable. Rud. allows that Dt.'s emendation is ingenious, "sinnreich," but declares the aorist passive out of place here. However, I think the aorist is used because the affliction could have seized the woman some time before the failure to receive and discharge becomes evident, especially if the condition is congenital.

II *Causes of infertility other than conditions of the womb. In* Non Gen. *the author does not consider the possibility that a woman's* sperma *might be infertile, though he seems to countenance the possibility for men.*

ὅσαις: This could mean women or wombs. For purposes of reproduction the author effectively identified the two in Chapter 1; see Rud. p. 35.

τούτων μηδὲν ἐμπόδιον: i.e., everything that has been discussed regarding the womb from Chapter 1 onwards.

7 ὃν τρόπον: Prolepsis.

9 σύμμετροι τῷ ἅμα προΐεσθαι: See 633b13 note ad loc. It is clear here that the way in which the man and woman must be compatible is in the time of emission, which, *pace* Balme, is very different from Aristotle's view that they should be matched in terms of the quality of male heat to the quantity of female material; cf. *GA* I.18, 723a26–30; I.20, 729a17–20; IV.2, 767a15–17; IV.4, 772a2–19; see Introduction pp. 20–4, Rud. p. 21.

10 τούτοις: In sense referring back to ὅσαις at the beginning of the sentence, grammatically including men as part of couples who would remain childless.

10–23: Like the other books in the Aristotelian Corpus, *HA* X was not originally divided into chapters (Beullens and Gotthelf 2007). The 1550 Basle edition was the first to divide the text (into four chapters), and different editors have had different chapter divisions since. This section has been taken as the opening paragraph of Chapter 5 since Bekker, but clearly belongs with the remarks the author has just made on causes of infertility which do not originate in the woman. Chapter 5 is also more of a unity if we remove this section and take it as part of Chapter 4. Because of their lack of ms. authority Balme printed chapter numbers in square brackets within the text rather than in the margin (Balme 2002, pp. 1–2). I have emphasized my chapter divisions to highlight the organization of the text.

10–13 τῷ μὲν οὖν εἰδέναι...γεννῶν: This is the sum total of *Non Gen.*'s remarks on male infertility; see Introduction pp. 36–9.

12 ἄν: Balme takes φαίνοιτο to be an imperatival optative, which is possible, but asking a man to have intercourse with a number of other women (whose fertility and compatibility with him would itself be uncertain) as an experiment does not seem to be an "easy" method to check male fertility. What would be easy is if the man already had children he can point to by other women. Tricot, Louis, and Barnes (who tags the text as "uncertain") all take the sentence to be a conditional of some sort, following either Sn. and Bk.'s addition of ἄν or Pk. and Rud.'s of εἰ. The former of these options, taking ἄν φαίνοιτο in the apodosis, is preferable. Taking φαίνοιτο in either of its meanings in the protasis with εἰ is difficult. The man cannot be said merely to <u>seem</u> to cause other women to conceive, nor would watching a man have intercourse with a woman guarantee that he was the father of the child she bore.

13 πρὸς ἄλλας πλησιάζων καὶ γεννῶν: This, of course, would show that the man was <u>not</u> responsible for the couple's failure to reproduce, which is why Pk. and Dt. emend αἴτια to ἀναίτια in 11. If we want to keep strict logic in the sentence, we could add μή before γεννῶν, but failure to reproduce with other women would still only show that the man was a possible cause; it would not rule out problems on the women's side or serial incompatibility. The sentence is just loosely saying that the doctor does not need to bother entertaining the possibility that the man is infertile if he has fathered children with other women.

τοῦ...ἔχειν: If we retain the mss. reading γεννῶσιν at l.14, this appears to be another genitive articular infinitive citing the cause of the statement; cf. 635a23.

συνδρόμως: The adverb is used by Aeschylus at *Ag.* 1184 but does not otherwise occur in classical Greek.

In the theory of the Hippocratic *Vict.* (I.27 (VI.500.1–22)) the sex and quality of the offspring are determined by the proportions of *sperma* from the mother and the father (both of whom can produce hot and dry male and cold and wet female seed), and the author implies that the window of opportunity in which the proportions will result in the successful conception of either sex is very narrow for everybody (one day each month). But the proportions of heat/cold and dry/wet can be altered by regimen. There is no claim that any particular pairing of man and woman might produce children of only one sex or be irrevocably non-productive if both partners were fertile. *Genit.* 7 (VII.478.16–480.6) argues that the fact that men and women can each be parents of children of different sexes with different partners shows that both men and women produce male and female *gonê*. Aristotle believed it was possible for both partners to be fertile but fail to reproduce because of incompatibility with one another, and that specific couplings would be able to engender only girls or only boys, e.g., *GA* IV.2, 767a14–28, *HA* IX(VII).6, 585b9–14. As with *Vict.* the incompatibility from Aristotle's point of view arose not from timing during intercourse but from the proportion; in Aristotle's theory, the elements which need to be in proportion are the heat in the male semen and the coldness of the female menses, while in *Vict.* the proportionality is between strength and weakness. At *GA* IV.2, 767a25, Aristotle says that changing sexual partners can lead to successful conception for men and women who have been unable to reproduce with their original partners. He does not explain why an incompatibility of proportion cannot be addressed by changing regimen rather than partners, but presumably these would be cases where, e.g., a man produced particularly hot/cold semen so that unless he was paired with a woman who had an exceptional quantity/dearth of menses the window of opportunity for the successful transfer of form would be so slim as to be virtually impossible to hit. When other authors discuss incompatibility, then, they focus on the proportion and relative heat of the male and female contributions. *Genit.* 4 (VII.474.25–476.1) does say that when a man's *gonê* falls into her womb a woman's pleasure "leaps up" (ἐξαΐσσει), but the author also says that it is possible for the woman to climax (ὀργᾷ, 474.20) before the man and does not indicate that this is a barrier to conception. *Mul.* I.17 (VIII.56.21–58.2) says that if the emission of the man runs together (ὁμορροθῇ) on the same side as (κατ' ἴξιν) that of the woman, the woman will get pregnant. However, the author goes on to say that this can happen either straightaway (αὐτίκα) or at a later time (ἐν ὑστέρῳ χρόνῳ), so simultaneity of emission does not seem to be a requirement. Moreover, although the author acknowledges that the woman should be sexually excited for the emission to occur, he simply states that the habit of intercourse will arouse her desire (προθυμίην γὰρ σφίσι ποιέει ἡ μελέτη).

14 πάντων…ὑπαρξάντων: In both male and female cases.

15 εἴπερ γάρ: The author is not suddenly calling the assumption of the whole treatise into doubt. He is using the certainty of the fact that women produce *sperma* to demonstrate how essential it is that the man and woman "keep pace."

16 συμβάλλεται εἰς τὸ σπέρμα καὶ τὴν γένεσιν: The *sperma* referred to here is the mingled male and female *sperma*. If the female emission is identical with menstrual fluid, the requirement that the emissions be coincident makes no sense.

ἰσοδρομῆσαι: At *GA* I.19, 727b10, Aristotle denies the point that the author is making here; see Introduction pp. 19–20.

17 ἐκποιήσῃ: Aristotle does not use this verb anywhere else. It is used twice in the Hippocratics, *Prorrh.* II.3 (IX.10.20) and *Morb.* I.16 (VI.170.5). ἐκ is here acting as an intensifier.

18 αἱ γυναῖκες βραδύτεραι: *Genit.* 4 (VII.474.20) says a woman can emit before a man and it does not seem to cause problems for conception, but there the woman emits her *gonê* directly into her womb and unless the womb is open more widely than usual there is no external fluid to indicate she has emitted. The scope of this remark here is not clear. Female children were expected to develop more slowly in the womb but more quickly after birth. The first is a sign of inferiority because it is a process of a development to something more defined, the second because it is a quicker deterioration; see Dean-Jones 1994, p. 210.

19–21 συζευγνύμενοι οὐ γεννῶσι: Either we must remove the negative before γεννῶντες in l.20 and insert it here or we must assume, as Balme suggests, that ἰσοδρομοῦσι πρὸς τὴν συνουσίαν in ll.20–1 has a different meaning from ἰσοδρομῆσαι αὐτοὺς ἀλλήλοις (24) and ἰσοδρομῆσαι παρ' ἀμφοῖν (17). He believes that ἰσοδρομοῦσι πρὸς τὴν συνουσίαν means equal pace in preparation for coition while the other two expressions mean equal pace in actual emission, which only comes about if the time spent on preparation for emission is unequal. This puts a heavy load on πρός. τὴν συνουσίαν alone is not that different in sense from παρ' ἀμφοῖν and αὐτοὺς ἀλλήλοις, especially when used with the striking verb ἰσοδρομέω. Moreover, the verb ἐντυγχάνω in this context clearly means coition. Balme's generalizing translation "encounter" for ἐντυγχάνω here obfuscates the fact that in his interpretation ἰσοδρομοῦσι πρὸς τὴν συνουσίαν would have had to occur before coition took place and should therefore be in the aorist or perfect. Balme's reading also fails to account for διό, which normally picks up from the statement which precedes it. In his interpretation it would have to refer forward to the following conditional. Moreover, the paragraph is discussing a couple who cannot conceive. Switching the hypothetical couple under discussion to one which can conceive is unnecessary and confusing.

21 ὀργῶσα καὶ παρεσκευασμένη εἴη: In Aristotle's theory, whether or not a woman was inclined to desire intercourse had more to do with the amount of seminal residue present in her body than any thoughts she might have (*GA* IV.5, 774a2–6), and although non-orgasmic pleasure which resulted in the release of the vaginal lubricant could promote conception, a woman could conceive even if she did not enjoy the act of intercourse in which she was inseminated (*GA* I.19, 727b8–12); see Introduction pp. 19–20.

CHAPTER 5

I *This chapter discusses conditions which a couple might think signal infertility but in fact do not. The first is feeling stronger rather than weaker after ejaculation of* sperma.

25 συμβαίνει: Rud. p. 37 identifies the use of this verb with the infinitive as an Aristotelian usage, but it is in fact quite common.

εὐρωστοτέροις: The positive of the adjective is quite common in all periods, but the comparative is found only here and once in Plutarch before Galen, who uses it frequently, so it may have been a medical word.

25–6 μὴ ἰσχύϊ ἀλλ' ὑγιείᾳ: This differentiates the condition from that described in Chapter 3 at 635b31–636a8, where a woman's body became stronger (ἰσχυροτέρα) by absorbing her own *sperma*. At *GA* I.18, 725b8–18, Aristotle argues that most men are exhausted after intercourse, even though only a very small amount of *sperma* is emitted. He acknowledges in a parenthesis that some young men are relieved and feel more comfortable after sex (κουφίζει, εὐημέρει) but says this is only in cases where there is a superabundance of (πλεονάσῃ) *sperma* or it brings away diseased material (νοσώδεις) with it, in which case it is infertile. He could here be paraphrasing this section of *Non Gen.*, but says nothing about women feeling better after night emissions.

26–7 ἠθροισμένον ἐπὶ τὸ τόπον ὅθεν προΐενται: That is, gathered from all over the body to the penis or καῦλος (see below, 637a22–35).

29 ὅταν ἱκανά...ἄχρηστα ᾖ: *Sperma*, as the author explains at the end of the chapter, is drawn from the whole body. Lassitude after sex occurs when the material the body needs for its own maintenance is depleted.

ἐκεῖνα: The pronoun's normal meaning of "former," i.e., it is referring to the emitted *sperma*, not the *sperma* that remains, as Balme takes it.

ἄχρηστα: If the woman could not have used this material in her own body anyway, it may mean that as *sperma* it would not be fertile. At *GA* I.18, 725b15, Aristotle describes seminal material which is νοσῶδες as infertile.

30 πλησμονῆς: Apart from this passage, the word occurs in the Aristotelian Corpus only at *Prob.* X.47, 896a24, though it is very common in other authors including Plato and the Hippocratic Corpus.

636b33–637b15: This section was transposed to follow καί in 636a6 by Ald., Bas., and Fel. The transposition is clearly mistaken. The earlier passage (in Chapter 3) discusses why a lack of enervation after a night emission might indicate an impediment to conception (a woman's body is "stealing" her *sperma*); this passage explains why this is not always the case. Marks in three Greek mss. indicate the similarity in subject matter between the two passages, and this caused Ald., Bas., and Fel. to transpose this passage to the earlier chapter (see Balme 1991, p. 543).

30–637a1 οὐκ ἰσχύϊ...ἀλλὰ κουφότητι: At 636a6 the author indicated that enervation after night emissions in the absence of any disease showed that a woman was fertile. This was contrasted with occasions on which a woman felt stronger (ἰσχύειν μᾶλλον, 636a1), which showed that her whole body was seizing her own *sperma*, which could be an impediment to conception. Here the lack of enervation after night emissions or intercourse is explicitly dissociated from an increase in strength. Her health (ὑγιεία, l.26) has been improved by her being relieved of material her body did not need and which was, in some sense, weighing her down. The author may have thought of this πλησμονή as fluid in nature and not fully assimilated into the woman's body and therefore easy to discharge, in contrast to the σωματώδης form of *sperma* (635b38), which causes most enervation on discharge.

32 ἀπίη: The same Ionicism appears at 635a24; see notes ad loc.

ἀσθενεστέρας ποιεῖ: See 635b38.

33 παύεται δὲ ταχὺ ἂν ἄλλως τις ὑγιάνῃ τὸ σῶμα: This repeats the point made at 635b39 that the loss of strength should be ἀνόσως.

34 σπερμοποιεῖ: A *hapax*. Pseudo-Galen uses σπερματοποιεῖται (*ad Gaurum* VII.2.10).

34–5 τῶν γὰρ αὐξανομένων τοῦτ' ἐστὶ ταχὺ καὶ τῶν αὐξητῶν: This sentence seems to have been included purely to indulge the author's pleasure in jingles and prolepsis. It does not advance the argument, though saying that a woman's *sperma* can cause increase differentiates it from Aristotle's view of female *sperma*. The position of τοῦτ' ἐστὶ ταχὺ causes a chiasmus with the participles.

35 τότε: When they neither perceive a discharge of *sperma* nor feel particularly weakened after intercourse.

36–7 μὴ αἴσθωνται: This must refer to the subjective experience of orgasm. Because the *sperma* comes from an excess, the woman does not experience the sensation of release. This explains why women can become pregnant when they know they have not enjoyed intercourse; cf. Aristotle's remark at *GA* I.19, 727b8–10, that women insist they can become pregnant without feeling pleasure in intercourse, and frequently do not become pregnant when they have (cf. 635b30). Soranus (*Gyn.* I.37.3) says that in women who become pregnant after a rape the sexual appetite (ὄρεξις) must have existed, but been obscured by the woman's resolve (ψυχικῆς κρίσεως).

προϊέμεναι: Various emendations have been suggested for this sentence. Bk. places a full stop after αἴσθωνται. Following the translations Sn. omits δὲ τυγχάνουσιν. Pk. and Dt. insert ἔτι before δὲ τυγχάνουσιν. Rud. suggests transposing to τυγχάνουσιν, δέ but also mentions the suggestion of Danielsson that we should insert προϊέμεναι. This seems to me obviously correct.

II *The previous section explained why women could become pregnant even if they did not feel themselves emitting* sperma. *This section explains how they can become pregnant even if they appear not to draw the* sperma *into the womb.*

636b39–637a9: This passage is repeated at the end of the book after ὅμοιον at 638b37 in Dᵃ, Scot, Guil., and Orib. (chapter 13 in *Lib. Incert.*, Raeder 1933, pp. 101–2). The repetition would seem to have been occasioned by the discussion of cases in which the womb is dry or not dry at 638b33–7. When the text differs between the two, that of the latter passage is occasionally preferable, but this is clearly its correct position. Orib. shows a few alternate readings to that of the second appearance of the passage in Dᵃ.

637a1 ξηρανθῶσι: The woman would only be completely dry if both she and the man had each emitted just enough *sperma* to form a fetus; otherwise there would be some fluid left over. Dryness <u>can</u> be a criterion of conception, but in 635a37 the author says that after an erotic dream a woman should sometimes have to tend to herself as if she had had intercourse with a man and only sometimes be dry, implying that complete dryness after intercourse was not thought of as the norm. At 635b35 one of the things a doctor is told to ascertain after a woman's night emission is if on waking she is at first ξηροτέρα, comparatively, not completely dry. The comparison is with the moistening that should come later, not the state of the woman's vagina before sleep. 636a1 is discussing the womb rather than the vagina, and a condition in which it is not just the womb but the whole body that is drawing in the woman's emission. There is no point in this treatise, then, that asserts that a woman <u>needs</u> to become dry after intercourse in order to become pregnant. *GA* II.4, 739b2–6, appears to support a woman's dryness after intercourse as the necessary state for conception. *Superf.* 26 (VIII.490.6–7) (repeated at *Steril.* 220 (VIII.424.18–19)) says that a woman will know she has taken up her husband's *gonê* if she does not realize her husband has ejaculated until he tells her because she herself feels dry. *HA* IX(VII).3, 583a14, says women do use dryness after intercourse as a sign of conception without any caveat that this is not in fact necessary.

ἐπιδήλως ἀφανισθῆ: The juxtaposition of the two words highlights the oxymoron. The term ἀφανίζει was used at 636a3 to denote an unusual attractive power of a woman's body on her own emission, the only occasion on which the author contemplates the possibility of complete dryness after emission and one that is not necessarily conducive to conception (see note ad loc.).

1–2 τὸ δοθέν: The term τοῦ διδομένου is used of a woman's own emission at 635b2. It does not denote simply the male emission, as the sentences immediately preceding and following make clear.

2 ἐνίοτε: This is a strange word for the author to use since he believes this would be the case more often than not. It is difficult to tell how often the word could have overtones of frequency without knowing the reality of a situation. In the Hippocratic treatise *On Joints* the word seems to be used to mean "often" in situations where we know the circumstances are more likely to happen than not, e.g., *Artic.* 40, 60, 72 (IV.172.14, 256.17, 298.17), cf. Arist. *Plut.* 1125.

3 οὗ ἂν δύνηται ἀφανίσαι καὶ τοῦ ἱκανοῦ: Most editors accept δύνηται for δύναιντο. The male has no role in causing the *sperma* to disappear.

4 σπάσῃ: The singular could refer to either the woman or the womb. The latter is more commonly referred to as the drawing agent.

5 and 13 ἐνδέχεται γίνεσθαι: This is a very common Aristotelian phrase, more common with the earlier form γίγνεσθαι; it is not found in earlier authors.

6 πάθος: In regard to pregnancy, not pathological.

ζῴων: This and ὑῶν in 11 are the only references to animals in *Non Gen*. Because humans do not often give birth to multiple offspring, animal exemplars are needed to illustrate the author's theory of how a single emission of *sperma* can be divided up to produce several offspring none of which lack any bodily part.

7–8 ὅταν ἀπὸ μιᾶς: The ancients believed twinning from superfetation occurred much more frequently than we do, e.g., *Superf.* 1 (VIII.476.1–12). In fact, the assumption that human twins must have arisen from two separate acts of intercourse was so prevalent that *Nat. Puer.* 31 (VII.540.1–542.2) has to argue for the position that they can be conceived from one act of intercourse. At *HA* IX(VII).4, 585a8, Aristotle says of superfetation ἐπ᾽ ἀνθρώπῳ δ᾽ ὀλίγα μέν, γέγονε δέ ποτε, "it is rare in humans, but it has happened occasionally," and relates some anecdotal evidence about the phenomenon. At *GA* IV.5, 773a34–774b4, he has a long and complicated chapter on the topic, and 773b8–11 indicates that he does believe twinning can occur as a result of superfetation, but this is not his primary explanation for twinning. At *GA* IV.4, 771a17–772b6, he explains that multiple births are caused when the female produces more seminal material than is proportionate for an embryo of the εἶδος of the animal and the male *sperma* has enough δύναμις to produce a proportionate number of ἀρχαί for the material.

8 ἐξ οὐχ ἅπαντος: The order is unusual but reflects the author's point that the fetus comes out of the *sperma* but not all of the *sperma*. The unusual order and the fact that in a few lines (at l.12) the author argues that the *sperma* does come from all of the <u>body</u> led Dᵃ to omit the negative.

9 μέρος τι αὐτοῦ ἔλαβέ τις τόπος: The Hippocratics believed that the human womb had two "horns," or pockets, which accounted for twins, and that animals which bore litters had many pockets in their wombs; see note to 635b15–16. Aristotle believed the womb was double but not that this caused twinning (*GA* I.3, 716b32). *GA* I.18, 723b14, states that in regard to multiple births "it is impossible that [the *sperma*] be divided up in the womb," ἐν δὲ ταῖς ὑστέραις χωρίζεσθαι ἀδύνατον, and he repeats his objections to this explanation of multiple birth at *GA* IV.4, 771b27–33. He says there of the theory that it is nothing, οὐθέν ἐστιν. He believes multiple births are the result of the proportionality of female matter to male heat, allowing the instantiation of more than one *eidos*. Van der Eijk 1999, p. 501, believes that the remarks on multiple birth are the only part of the theory of *HA* X that cannot be squared in some way with the theory in Aristotle's later biological works.

9–10 τὸ δὲ περιελείπετο πολλαπλάσιον: πολλαπλάσιον indicates that if there is to be a multiple birth what is left behind after the conception of one fetus must be at least as much again (for twins) or a greater multiple (for triplets or more).

12 δῆλον ὅτι ἀπὸ παντός: For pangenetic theories, see Anaxag. 59 B 10, Democr. DK 68 A 141, Hipp. *Aer.* 14 (II.60.1–5), *Morb. Sacr.* 2 (VI.364.19–20), *Genit.* 3, 8 (VII.474.5–7, 480.7–10), *Morb.* IV.32 (VII.542.3–5), *Vict.* I.7 (VI.480.11). See Dean-Jones 1994, pp. 162–6. The argument here concerns the homogeneity of *sperma*. The immediately following sentence begins: ἀπὸ παντὸς μὲν γὰρ ἐνδέχεται ἀποχωρισθῆναι, "For of course it is possible for an individual to be separated off from all the *sperma*...". The train of thought indicated by μὲν γάρ is inexplicable if the current sentence denied that the *sperma* came from all the body. The omission of the negative by Dᵃ in l.8 (see note ad loc.) can be explained if the author of *Non Gen.* had not used it here or in the following line. It is clear why οὐκ would be inserted here once the treatise was attributed to Aristotle. It is needed to bring the statement into line with his many arguments against pangenesis in *GA* I.18, 722a1-724a14, ending with the statement "it is clear that the *sperma* is not separated off from all the parts," φανερὸν ὅτι οὐκ ἀπὸ πάντων ἀποκρίνεται τὸ σπέρμα τῶν μορίων. But inserting οὐκ here makes *Non Gen.*'s argument unintelligible. He is not arguing for pangenesis. He has assumed this throughout the treatise in his remarks about the enervation and lassitude of the body after emission (635b37, 636b30-5). Here he is stating that while the *sperma* comes from all over the body, when it is divided up into more than one fetus, each fetus will have what is needed for its own body, just as when only one fetus is conceived from a portion of an abundance of *sperma*. The *sperma* does not separate out along the lines of where it originated in the parent's body; see Introduction pp. 68-75.

13 ἐφ᾽ ἑκάστου εἴδους ἐμερίζετο: This is a non-technical use of εἶδος which could have originated either in *Non Gen.* or with Aristotle; it refers to the individual animals, pigs, or humans, within a womb that could be apprehended by the fact that they are discrete shapes. In the Aristotelian sense of εἶδος, however many individual offspring there were in one womb there would be only one form present. In Aristotle's theory the male *sperma* makes no material contribution to the offspring but simply carries the father's form. This is not divided when it informs multiple offspring. It is capable of doing so because it has enough heat to instantiate more than one example of the species' form.

13-14 ἀπὸ παντὸς μὲν γὰρ ἐνδέχεται ἀποχωρισθῆναι καὶ τὸ πᾶν εἰς πολλά: τὸ πᾶν is the entirety of the *sperma* produced by both the man and the woman.

14-15 ὥστε ἅμα καὶ κατὰ μέρος ἀδύνατον: If any given portion of the *sperma* is to contain all the parts of the body, the *sperma* from individual body parts cannot be emitted in discrete portions. The *sperma* is drawn from the body as a unity, homogenized throughout, so that each part of the *sperma* is exactly the same as every other part. The author is arguing against the view of pangenesis as stated at *Morb.* IV.32 (VII.542.3-5), "*sperma* comes from all the parts of the man and the woman," ἀπὸ πάντων τῶν μελέων τοῦ ἀνδρὸς καὶ τῆς γυναικὸς ἐλθὸν τὸ σπέρμα. *Non Gen.* is contrasting ἀπὸ παντὸς τοῦ σώματος with κατὰ μέρος. The author is arguing that since it is not necessary for all the *sperma* to be used to form a fetus, any correctly sized portion of the *sperma* must be capable of engendering an entire body. If there is a multiple conception, the total *sperma* must be a multiple of this correct portion size, but each portion can engender a whole fetus; we do not get one fetus with all the arm *sperma* and another with all the nose *sperma*; nor do we get half-body fetuses if the leftover is not a multiple of the correct portion. *Sperma* is therefore separated from the body as a unity, not part by part. This solution obviates the need for the long note ad loc. in Balme's Loeb edition (pp. 513–15) and his puzzlement over how the last sentence is supposed to follow logically from the one preceding it. It may be relevant that when arguing against Anaxagoras' theory of infinite divisibility at *Phys.* I.4, 187b22–34 Aristotle uses the example of particles in which flesh, blood, and brain are not separate from one another but yet are real and infinite things as something ἄλογον.

III *The author has now disposed of the objections that women sometimes become pregnant even when they feel they have not ejaculated and also when they do not seem to draw in the* sperma. *He ends his treatise with an explanation of how the woman deposits her* sperma *in front of the womb.*

637a15 ἡ γυνὴ προΐεται: As elsewhere in the treatise, it is the woman, not the womb, that is said to emit *sperma*.

16 ὅταν πλησιάσῃ: Is the subject the woman (Balme, Louis) or the man (Barnes, Tricot)? In either case it cannot be assumed that the individual will ejaculate every time they have intercourse, so here πλησιάσῃ must have the implication of climaxing.

σπᾷ: It is clear from the following description of things that draw that the womb is to be understood as the subject of this verb.

17 πνεύματι: Cf. 634b34–5.

17–18 μυκτῆρσιν: The term ῥῖνες was used as an analogy for the cervix in its action of drawing in the *sperma* at 634b35. The use of μυκτῆρσιν here for the same analogy differentiates the cervix and this action from the καῦλος and its action, for which ῥῖνες is used as an analogy in the passage immediately following. At *GA* II.4, 739b11–16, Aristotle likens the womb's attractive power to that of cupping instruments and denies that it can be attributed "as some assert to the parts involved in copulation," ὡς δέ τινες λέγουσι, τοῖς ὀργανικοῖς πρὸς τὴν συνουσίαν μορίοις. In this context it is significant that immediately after his dismissal of what others say about the drawing action of the "parts involved in copulation," Aristotle uses the observation that Nature would be doing something superfluous in having the womb emit *sperma* only to draw it back in to deny the existence of female *sperma*, which he had already argued against at length in *GA* I.19 and 20.

18–19 προσάγεται, ἢ εἴσφυσιν ἔχει ἄνωθεν ἢ κοῖλα ὄντα: Rud. comments that there are many mistakes in this passage, and there have been many scholarly emendations and conjectures. Dt. takes προσάγεται as passive and reads the rest of the clause as ἢ φύσιν ἔχει ἄνω <φέρεσθαι> κοῦφα ὄντα, as if there has been a sudden shift from discussing the nature of the organs that draw things in to the type of stuff that moves upwards. However, if we simply transpose the second ἢ to precede rather than follow κοῖλα ὄντα, the problems are solved. ἄνωθεν is here being used in the sense of ἄνω, and the contrast is between the two ways a hollow container can fill itself. The womb, like the mouth and nose, can be filled by funneling stuff from above, or it can draw it in from below by *pneuma*. In the Hippocratics προσάγεται is used 4 times, once in the passive in discussing the reduction of a dislocation, but the other 3 times in the middle: *Reg.* I.9 (VI.482.16) of an embryo drawing nourishment to itself, *Fist.* 8 (VI.456.6) of bladder attracting phlegm, *Prorrh.* I.145 (V.564.2) of hemorrhages leading to spasm in some people.

εἴσφυσιν: A *hapax*. In this case the root φυσ- has connotations of a crater or calyx shape as in φῦσα (see LSJ) rather than simply denoting a natural outgrowth. In the case of the womb these would be the fallopian tubes (seen or imagined) through which menstrual fluid flows into the womb down from the body.

ἕλκονται: Scal. for ἕλκων ἢ; accepted by most editors even though it involves a swift change from a singular to plural form and the subject is neuter plural.

This is the type of action envisaged by *VM* 22 (II.626.19–22) when it describes shapes that can draw fluids to themselves. Although the *VM* passage cites the necessity of an instrument, a reed, in its analogy, it clearly, like *Non Gen.*, sees the cervix as a part of the womb, not a separable instrument.

19–20 ὡς ἐκ τούτου τοῦ τόπου: Balme believes this phrase, without the insertion of ὡς, refers generally to whatever organ is drawing stuff to itself by means of *pneuma*. He translates "from its present place" and glosses "it uses wind from within itself, as the mouth does" (1991, p. 519, n.a). This may be possible, but it is extremely opaque, even for this author (why not simply say "from itself"?). It seems more likely that the author has already slipped from talking in general terms to talking specifically about the womb and ἐκ τούτου τοῦ τόπου refers to the place in which male and female emit their *sperma*. In the next sentence οὗτος clearly does so.

20 διό: The author returns to the topic announced at the beginning of the paragraph.

21 τοῦτο: i.e., the emission of *sperma*.

21–2 ἔρχεται: The subject here is unstated, but as the καῦλος is compared to the penis it seems reasonable to assume that the author means the subject to be *sperma*, the emission of which is the subject of the immediately preceding infinitive συμβαίνειν.

22–3 ἔχουσι καυλόν, ὥσπερ καὶ οἱ ἄνδρες τὸ αἰδοῖον, ἀλλ᾽ ἐν τῷ σώματι: Although the term καυλός usually refers to a rigid tubular structure such as a plant stem, spear-shaft, or quill of a feather, it can also refer to a more flexible passageway within the body. It is frequently used of the penis itself (not necessarily only when it is rigid), e.g., the Hippocratics use the term of the penis at *Int.* 14 (VII.202.8) and *Alim.* 17 (IX.104.6). At *HA* III.1, 510a26 and 28, the term is used of the canal which carries *sperma* inside the penis. This is probably why the term is used of the corresponding passageway inside the woman. Unless the woman's καυλός mirrored the penis in function, there would be no need to refer to the male organ here because in configuration the καυλός resembles more the nasal passages. The term καυλός is used of the cervix at *HA* III.1, 510b11, but that cannot be its meaning here in a treatise that has talked so frequently in a matter of fact way about the στόμα. Aristotle also used καυλός to refer to the grasshopper's ovipositor in *HA* V.28, 555b21.

23–4 ἀποπνέουσι διὰ τούτου: Asyndeton. The pronoun refers to καυλός, and though it could be assimilated to the neuter because of the intervening αἰδοῖον, the local sense of the preposition requires the genitive here. Most translators take it in the local sense anyway, though Balme translates "because of this."

μικρῷ τε πόρῳ ἀνωτέρωῇ ἠουροῦσιν αἱ γυναῖκες: τε quite commonly links whole clauses or sentences in the Hippocratics, as Smyth notes for Herodotus and Thucydides (2968a). Smyth's note also says τε can be used to link single parallel nouns in poetry. LSJ lists this as a possible use in prose citing Plato twice. In the Hippocratic gynecology I have found at least 8 examples: *Morb.* IV 43 (VII.564.24); *Nat. Mul.* 48 (VII.392.10); *Mul.* I.2, 6, 37, 39 (VIII.18.12, 30.21, 92.10, 96.1); *Mul.* II.119, 133 (VIII.260.15, 294.11). The closest parallels to the *Non Gen.* occurrence are *Nat. Mul.* 48, τὰς φλέβας τὰς ἐν τῇ ῥινί, τάς τε ὑπὸ τοῖς ὀφθαλμοῖς ἀλγεῖν φησιν, "she says that the vessels in her nose and under her eyes hurt," and *Mul.* I.39, πυρετὸς ἕξει αὐτὴν λεπτὸς, θέρμη τε ἀνὰ πᾶν τὸ σῶμα, "a light fever will take hold of her and heat all over her body." Admittedly, with a change of accentuation the τε in the second passage could be connecting a clause ("and she will be hot all over her body") but in the rest of the passage the symptoms are all in the nominative. Elsewhere τε comes at the end of a list in which other elements have been connected by καί. In these circumstances C and θ (the most important mss. for the gynecology of the Hippocratic Corpus) often prefer to omit the τε, but it is telling that they then leave an asyndeton rather than replace it with καί. In these circumstances I prefer to follow Louis and Balme and keep the ms. reading rather than deleting it with Dt. It is the *lectio difficilior* and, in my opinion, makes better sense of the passage.

The μικρὸς πόρος branches off from the καυλός to the outside before the latter reaches the vagina. The position of its opening, "above the place where women urinate," maps on to the clitoris. Votives of female pudenda with a representation of the clitoris have been found at the rural sanctuary of Tessennano near Vulci in Italy (Costantini 1995, plate 42). The clitoris is stimulated like the penis but for the purposes of *Non Gen*.'s theory the *sperma* has to be emitted before the *stoma* of the womb by the καυλός, so the swelling of the μικρὸς πόρος is explained by its emitting *pneuma*. (Aristotle believes the penis emits *pneuma* as well as *sperma* (*GA* II.2, 735a30–736a19). *Genit*. 1 (VII.470.1– 472.4) also describes the *gonê* as foaming when it is agitated.) In many women, but not necessarily all, the nerve roots of the clitoris are connected to Skene's glands, which lie around the base of the urethra and are thought to be the female equivalent of the prostate gland. Many sexologists believe that in women who have these glands there is a connection to the "G-spot," and when the clitoris is stimulated to climax it causes a whitish ejaculate to be emitted from the urethra (Jannini et al. 2002a and b; Wimpissinger et al. 2007; Shafik et al. 2009; Korda et al. 2010; Rubio-Casillas et al. 2011; Salama et al. 2015). It would seem that the author of *Non Gen*. was more interested in the details about where and when women felt pleasure in their sexual experience than his contemporaries, but since he believes the ejaculate is deposited before the cervix rather than around the μικρὸς πόρος it is likely he merely assumed women ejaculated at orgasm by analogy with the male model rather than that women in ancient Greece had more active Skene's glands than modern women. He sees stimulation of the clitoris as the result rather than the cause of sexual excitement.

At *GA* I.20, 728a31–4, Aristotle may also indicate an understanding of the site of female sexual excitement when he states that, during intercourse, women experience "pleasure by touch in the same place as males, and yet they do not emit the fluid from there," τὴν ἡδονὴν τῇ ἁφῇ κατὰ τὸν αὐτὸν τόπον τοῖς ἄρρεσιν· καίτοι οὐ προΐενται τὴν ἰκμάδα ταύτην ἐντεῦθεν. He is aware that women can produce a vaginal lubricant when they enjoy intercourse, so he must think the place in which they feel pleasure is outside the vagina. "The same place as males," then, would seem to refer to the front of the pubes.

Balme believes the womb has to expel *pneuma* (and only *pneuma*) through the καυλός (which he takes to refer to the cervix) before it can "breathe" in and draw in the *sperma*. He see the μικρὸς πόρος as connecting the cervix to the urethra to provide a passage for air during coition. He has an extended note (Balme 1991, pp. 516–17) explaining Aristotle's theory of respiration and arguing that although Aristotle thinks the cycle of normal respiration through the nose begins with the intake of breath, he believes the "respiration" of the womb begins with the expulsion of breath. This seems to be a very detailed working out of a theory when at *GA* II.4, 739b10–16, Aristotle says simply that the womb draws in male semen like a cupping glass, through heat. Furthermore, if *Non Gen.* were an early work of Aristotle, as Balme maintains, it seems unlikely that he would be able to refer in such a condensed way to a refinement of a theory that would not necessarily be known to readers of the treatise.

The Hippocratics knew that the vagina and urethra were separate and give no indication of believing they were connected in any way. Aristotle's understanding of women's genitalia was a little murkier, but it seems more likely that he did not realize that the vagina and urethra were separate passages rather than that he believed there was a connection between the two; see Introduction pp. 12–13.

26 ἔκπτωσις: Because the καυλός is likened to the penis most editors have taken this ἔκπτωσις to be the fluid emission of *sperma*. Scot. translates *exitus spermatis*. The term also seems etymologically fitting for the dropping of fluid out of the καυλός; it seems less suitable as a noun to describe the movement of *pneuma*, to which Balme believes it refers. The term is used frequently in the Hippocratics of more substantial materials than *pneuma*. It is used of a dislocation at *Fract.* 1 (III.412.1) and of the expulsion of the afterbirth at *Aph.* V.49 (IV.550.3). Aristotle uses it for boiling liquid overflowing its container in *Resp.* 20, 480a1, but of heat in *Metr.* II.9, 370a5, and it is used of the rays of the sun in *Prob.* XV.6, 911b5.

27 καθ' ἥν: Feminine, understanding the description of the μικρὸς πόρος as a ὁδός.

ἐκεῖνον τὸν τόπον: The opening of the μικρὸς πόρος, the clitoris.

28 τοῦτο: This refers to the whole situation that has just been described, the fact that there is both a wider and a narrower opening. (Rud., p. 3, takes τοῦτο in l.28 to refer to the καυλός.)

κατὰ τοῦτο: In other respects they are different because the nasal passage is wider to the outside than towards the pharynx.

32 εὐρύχωρον εὔρουν: The opening of the καυλός before the womb has to be wider than that of the μικρὸς πόρος because it must carry *sperma*, but it is still narrower than the vagina itself, which must be able to admit the male's penis.

32–3 ὥσπερ...φάρυγγα: The diameter of the passage is reversed in the case of the nose because the fluid (mucus) flows out through the passage to the outside while the pharynx should ideally admit only air.

This description of the passage by which women deposit their *sperma* in front of their womb concludes what we have of *Non Gen*. Many medical treatises do end abruptly, but for arguments as to why this may not have been the original ending of the treatise, see Introduction, p. 109.

DIALECTIC ON *ON FAILURE TO REPRODUCE*

Aristotle considers the arguments for female sperma *and appends some observations drawn from the animal kingdom which challenge some of the assertions made by the author of* Non Gen.

Topos

This section is placed at the end of Chapter 5 in modern editions. It explains the shape of the argument in Chapters 6 and 7. Aristotle is not concerned to make all the steps of his argument explicit because he is not writing for an external audience. He is engaging in philosophic dialectic with a premise taken from a written text to see to what extent the endoxa *therein can be reconciled with the* phainomena; *see Introduction pp. 43–53 for a fuller description of Aristotelian dialectic.*

637a35–637b6: The argument of this section is very condensed and obscure. Tricot remarks, "Toute la fin du chapitre est obscure. Le texte est peu sûr, et sa reconstitution conjecturale" (1957, p. 714), and Louis, "Tous ce paragraphe est manifestement très abîmé. Le texte est peu sûr et comporte sans doute un certain nombre de lacunes. En tout cas la suite des idées est très obscure et la plupart des constructions sont insolites" (1969, pp. 190–1). Balme describes the argument as "rapid and difficult" (1991, p. 520) and appends a page-long note to explicate the passage (which to my mind raises more confusion than it allays), arguing that the passage is discussing the causes of various illnesses and death in different women, although there has been nothing of a general nosological nature in the rest of the treatise. Barnes comments, "The text of this whole paragraph is uncertain" (1984, p. 990). Rud. goes so far as to say "Ich wage nicht, diesen sehr korrupten Text zu behandeln." Of earlier translations Barnes' comes closest to the purport of Aristotle's argument. Once the role of this paragraph as a *topos* is recognized, the argument becomes clearer.

35–6 ὅ τι συμβάλλεται: There has been no indication earlier in the treatise that there is any question over what a woman's contribution to conception is. Aristotle begins his dialectic with an indefinite pronoun so as not to prejudge the matter. The context and the subordinate causal clause make it clear that it is the contribution of the woman that is the subject here.

36 εἰς τοῦτο: Balme translates this as an adverbial phrase, "to the extent." Louis and Barnes take τοῦτο to refer simply to the place where *sperma* is

emitted, but after the verb συμβάλλω it seems perverse not to take the prepositional phrase as signifying what is contributed to, as is the case at 636b15
and 637b19. If this is the beginning of a *topos*, Aristotle is not thinking simply
of the preceding paragraph but of the premise of *Non Gen.*'s argument that a
man and a woman contribute the same sort of thing to reproduction.

ποιεῖ: When referring to an opponent in a dialectic exchange Aristotle
often simply uses a third person singular verb for which the reader has to
supply the subject (Smith 1999, p. xxvii).

τὸ αἴτιον: We need a direct object for ποιεῖ which can also explain the
following genitive, τῶν αὐτῶν παθημάτων. Scot. once again paraphrases here
(*et hoc valet ad sperma*) and Guil. omits a translation for ποιεῖ and translates the
genitive by an ablative or dative (*eisdem passionibus*) in a lacunose sentence. Dt.
proposed πίστιν τῇ ὑπάρξει, which is adopted by Tricot ("Tout contribue à
faire croire à l'existence..."). Louis marks a lacuna. Balme and Barnes both
translate τῶν αὐτῶν παθημάτων as the direct object of ποιεῖ. I can find no
example of this elsewhere. τὸ αἴτιον gives the requisite sense in the context
of the rest of the passage.

τῶν αὐτῶν παθημάτων: Aristotle is about to say immediately that "the
woman too (καὶ) is emitting a generative fluid," so it is logical to assume that
the entity that suffers the same παθήματα as she does (i.e., enervation following upon emission of fluid during intercourse) is a man. Aristotle notes the
enervation that a man feels after ejaculation at *GA* I.18, 725b16-18.

36–7 ὅτι καὶ ἡ γυνὴ γόνιμον προΐεται: Balme takes ὅτι as correlating to εἰς
τοῦτο and translates, "The woman's contribution brings about the same affections to the extent that she too emits a fertile sperma," where the people who
share the παθήματα are other women. This is circular and redundant given
that *Non Gen.* has been discussing generally what women as a group experience
when they emit *sperma*. If the ensuing argument were about general female
nosology, there would also be no need to emphasize the fertility of the female
emission with the new term γόνιμον. Balme ends his long note on this passage
by saying, "637b6 ff continues the argument by giving evidence that the same
cause (fertile emission) produces the same affections in all female animals." But
in fact Aristotle is going to argue that emission of *sperma* does not produce the
same conditions in all female animals. In the *topos* he is setting up the more
endoxon (see Introduction n. 98) point that if two conditions are different in some
way there is also some difference in the causation of the condition. He will use
the argument to show that the woman's *sperma* is not γόνιμον like a man's.

γόνιμον: Aristotle avoids the term *sperma* here because he does not deny
that women produce a seminal fluid; he is only questioning whether it is "fertile" in the way male *sperma* is. See Introduction nn. 21 and 29.

37 τὰ δ᾽ αὐτὰ αἴτια ταῦτα συμβαίνει: Aristotle is here speaking in the
voice of the author. *Non Gen.* does not differentiate between the generative

power of the man's and the woman's *sperma*. Balme takes ταῦτα to be modifying τὰ δ' αὐτὰ αἴτια and translates "And they (i.e. female diseases generally) are accompanied by these same causes (i.e., the emission of seed)." This is problematic because there has been no prior reference to general female diseases or, in Balme's text, to causes. The reading of Scot. (*eadem*) and the conjecture of Dt. and Louis of ταὐτὰ for ταῦτα, accepted by Tricot, Louis, and Barnes ("And if the causes are the same, the results are the same"), renders a statement with which Aristotle himself would agree, and which he is in fact going to use as his *topos*, but too soon because the next sentence indicates there is something wrong with the statement that preceded it. All three modern translators run into problems trying to make the thought of the next sentence cohere with this statement. Guil.'s *hee* supports Dᵃ's reading ταῦτα.

38 καὶ γάρ...αἴτιον εἶναι: Aristotle is anticipating the fact that there are those who use the condition of uterine mole as evidence that women contribute fertile *sperma* like a man to reproduction, but Aristotle here points out that mole is always a pathological condition which can lead to death—the opposite of a normal pregnancy. Tricot's translation takes the text to be criticizing those who stop at disease or death in their search for a cause ("Et, en effet, ceux qui croient devoir s'arrêter, dans la recherche de la cause, à la maladie ou à la mort, suivant le cas..."); Louis' translation that it is criticizing those who take disease to be the cause of death, or vice versa ("Et en effet, ceux qui estiment à propos de la maladie ou de la mort que l'une est la cause de l'autre..."); and Barnes' translation that the criticism is aimed at those who believe that disease or death could have one cause ("For those who think that one thing can be the cause either of disease or of death..."). It is not clear how any of these interpretations cohere with what has preceded or what follows. Balme translates, "For those too who believe that an illness or a death is due to another thing's cause..." He does not appear to address this clause in his explanatory note.

38–637b1 οὐ θεωροῦσι τὸ τελευταῖον ἐπὶ τὰς ἀρχάς, ὃ δεῖ ὁρᾶν: My argument requires an οὐ here, but the tenor of the argument, especially the final relative clause, implies a negative independent of my interpretation. Both Tricot and Louis take the phrase as negative, though Louis does not add a negative to his text: "ne considèrent que ce qui vent en dernier et ne remontent pas jusqu'aux principes" (Tricot); "n'ont en vue que ce qui vient en dernier, au lieu d'examiner les principes" (Louis). Barnes conjectures the addition of οὐ here.

τὸ τελευταῖον: That female *sperma* causes uterine mole.

τὰς ἀρχάς: This could mean the first principles regarding the parallelism of cause and effect which Aristotle uses to generate his *topos* or, more likely, the starting point of *Non Gen.*'s argument, that the female contribution to reproduction is equivalent to the male, and should therefore be a source of life.

ὃ δεῖ ὁρᾶν: θεωροῦσι implies a more thoroughgoing consideration of a statement, ὁρᾶν the remembering of the premises on which the statement was based.

1–2 τοῖς μὲν γὰρ...πάντα: The contrast with the following τοῖς δὲ οὐδὲν implies a πάντα here. Barnes adds πάντα to πρῶτα, but I suspect πρῶτα supplanted πάντα under the influence of ἀρχάς.

τοῖς μὲν...τοῖς δὲ...τῶν δέ: This is a generalizing statement, applicable for a comparison of the similarities and differences between a man and a woman's conditions after a seminal emission and between those of avian wind-eggs and human uterine mole. The *Dialectic* is using the fact that wind-eggs have little in common with moles to argue that male and female *sperma* are also different.

4 διὰ πάντων...παθημάτων: The term πάθημα does not occur in *Non Gen.*; see Introduction n. 208. All females of sexually dimorphic species can reproduce when their generative fluid combines correctly with the males, because in this case all the causes are the same.

5–6 διὰ πολλῶν...μηδέν: Between normal reproduction, a condition which all female animals share because the basic causes are the same, and wind-eggs in birds, which has no analogy in women, there are a number of conditions which are more or less analogous for different female animals, e.g., the similarities and differences between vivipara and ovipara or between a woman's night emissions and the fluid produced by female animals when they are ready for mating.

CHAPTER 6

I *Aristotle begins applying the* topos *by describing the behavior of some female animals that could be put forward as evidence that they were undergoing the same conditions as males in producing* sperma.

637b6 τὰ ζῷα: Humans are not here included in this designation.

6–7 ὅταν ὀχευθῆναι δέηται: Aristotle believes female emission in animals is tied to a compulsion to use up material in forming a baby rather than an amatory desire to emit material as a male does. Women do not have to have the ἐννοίας ἐπιτηδείας *Non Gen.* referred to in 636b22. A physical necessity, rather than careful preparation, causes the psychological affect. At *GA* IV.5, 774a2–6, Aristotle says bearing several children can blunt a woman's appetite for intercourse because it uses up her seminal material, which is what produces the desire. But by "seminal residue" here Aristotle is referring to menstrual fluid, not the fluid produced in a woman by sexual excitement or during night emissions, which is what *Non Gen.* equates with female *sperma*.

If women's night emissions and the emissions by female animals when they need to be mated play the same causal role in reproduction, according to the argument about sameness of causes that Aristotle has just enunciated in the *topos*, women who produce this fluid will experience all the same παθήματα as birds who emit their *sperma* into themselves and eventually produce eggs even if they do not mate with a male. He will show that there is no human comparandum to wind-eggs, therefore women's night emissions, and the moisture they produce when aroused during intercourse, are not equivalent to a female bird's seminal emission.

7 αἱ ἀλεκτορίδες: *HA* VI.2, 560b30–561a3, uses pigeons rather than hens to illustrate birds' desire for mating.

8 ὑφιζάνουσιν: A *hapax* for Aristotle, used by Euripides (Rud. p. 29).

8–9 τοῦτο δὲ ποιεῖται ἄλλα ζῷα: *HA* VI.18, 572a8–b30 describes the behavior of mares, cows, bitches, and sows when they desire intercourse. At *HA* II.1, 500b10–11, Aristotle says female sheep protrude and widen their genital organ when they want to mate. *HA* V.5, 541a11–25, says female oviparous fishes follow the male when they want to mate, and that in the breeding season female as well as male quadrupeds produce a liquid round their genitals and smell the genitals of the opposite sex.

9–11 εἰ δὴ ταὐτά...τὰ αἴτια συμβαίνοντα: Aristotle repeats the point made in the *topos*. The logic of the argument demands that the αἴτια are the same as well as the πάθη.

11 ἥ γε ὄρνις: The particle emphasizes that birds are the best illustration of the claim that female animals emit their contribution to conception when sexually excited because they lay eggs even if they have not been mated with a male.

12 σημεῖον δὲ τούτου: A common locution in the Aristotelian Corpus. It occurs 19 times in this order or as τούτου δὲ σημεῖον; otherwise it does not appear before Polybius in the third century BCE.

13 πίπτει ὑπ' ἄλλην: At *HA* VI.2, 560b30, when discussing pigeons, Aristotle says αἱ θήλειαι ἀλλήλας ἀναβαίνουσιν.

14 ὑπηνέμια: These are unfertilized eggs, which never hatch into live chicks but do eventually "die" and become rotten. Their name reflects the folk belief that the wind could impregnate certain female animals (see note to 636a9–10). They were very important to Aristotle's theory in illustrating that the female could instil a type of soul (nutritive) into her seminal residue but not the full form; see, e.g., *GA* II.5, 741a19–32, III.1, 750b3–751a24, *HA* V.1, 539a31–b1, VI.2, 559b21–560a20. This is not the condition of "wind-pregnancy" discussed in Chapter 3 of *Non Gen*.

14–15 ἐπιθυμοῦσα καὶ τοῦ ἀφεῖναι τότε, ὡς ἀφεῖσα ὅταν καὶ τῷ ἄρρενι συνῇ: The passage 636b33–637b15 that was mistakenly transposed to follow ἀλλ᾽ οὗ καὶ at 636a6 by Ald. and Bas. (see note ad loc.) ended at ἄρρενι. Bk.

returned the text to its correct order but mistakenly left the word ἀνήρ from 636a6 following ἄρρενι (see Balme's extended note explaining the editorial history of this transposition, 1991, p. 543). Tricot, Louis, and Barnes all read the line with ἀνήρ as referring to homosexuality, e.g., Barnes: "showing that she wants then to emit and actually emitting—as happens when a man has intercourse with another male." This reading is encouraged because without ἀνήρ, as the mss. stand, ὡς ἐπιθυμοῦσα suggests that the hen's desire to emit is a mere appearance which only comes to fruition when she is actually with the male. Accepting Balme's explanation for the misplaced ἀνήρ and substituting the ὡς from before ἐπιθυμοῦσα for the καί before ἀφεῖσα gives the required sense. The comparison is between two different times a hen emits (τότε, ὅταν), not between two animals who engage in homosexual activity.

16–18 ποιεῖ δὲ τοῦτο...αὐτόματοι ἔγκυοι: At *HA* V.1, 539a30–b14, Aristotle discusses animals which reproduce "spontaneously," but grasshoppers are not among them, and at *HA* V.28, 555b17–556a8 he discusses the reproduction of grasshoppers beginning with the assertion:

αἱ δ' ἀκρίδες ὀχεύονται μὲν τὸν αὐτὸν τρόπον τοῖς ἄλλοις ἐντόμοις, ἐπιβαίνοντος τοῦ ἐλάττονος ἐπὶ τὸ μεῖζον (τὸ γὰρ ἄρρεν ἔλαττόν ἐστι).

Grasshoppers copulate in the same way as other insects, with the smaller (for the male is smaller) mounting the larger.

He does not mention the possibility of spontaneous or parthenogenetic reproduction in this discussion either. The current passage is not evidence that he once believed grasshoppers could reproduce without a contribution from the male. Aristotle introduces it as a premise with which the author of *Non Gen.* might be expected to agree as it adds weight to his claim that women emit *sperma* like that of a man. Rud. notes that πειράομαι with the genitive *rei* is not found elsewhere in Aristotle and thinks this reference is probably taken from elsewhere. This could be a quotation by Aristotle himself or a later interpolation. Given the use made of the grasshopper example later in the passage, I prefer the first possibility.

19 συμβάλλεται εἰς τὸ σπέρμα: Here τὸ σπέρμα means the initial mixture of male and female *sperma* as at 636b15. Aristotle is still arguing on the premises of the author of *Non Gen.*

19–20 εἴ γε καὶ ἐφ' ἑνὸς γένους: This is not "an interpolated gloss" or "a feeble parenthesis" as Balme states (1991, pp. 524–5). It is what the Answerer thinks he has demonstrated, but in fact it shows that he is not heeding the principle of cause and effect enunciated in the *topos*. Even if grasshoppers were parthenogenetic, the fact that their emission of *sperma* into themselves resulted in an actual pregnancy would show that it was a different αἴτιον than the hen's *sperma*, because it produced a different condition, viable offspring rather than wind-eggs. At this point, though, Aristotle is still presenting the *endoxon* that females produce the same sort of *sperma* as males, as a proponent of the theory would.

21 ᾠόν: Dt.'s conjecture for ζῷον is correct; otherwise there is a flat contradiction in terms.

21–2 τοῦτο...ἦλθεν: In the mss. reading τοῦτο cannot refer to either the grasshopper pregnancy or the wind-eggs because neither of them came from both parents. Dt.'s conjecture οὐ for καί gives the requisite meaning. Female grasshoppers can produce live young parthenogenetically. This shows that female sperma is γόνιμον, though in other animals it has to be mingled with the male to produce live offspring.

22–3 οὐδὲ τὰ ἀπὸ τοῦ ἄρρενος ἅπαντα γόνιμα: If a hen has already shown herself to be fertile by laying wind-eggs, failure for the fertilization of the eggs after mating must either lie entirely on the male's side or the incompatibility of the male and female *sperma*.

συναρμοσθῇ: This is not *Non Gen.*'s vocabulary of "keeping pace," ἰσοδρομῆσαι. This vocabulary is more in line with the Aristotelian idea of συμμετρία, e.g., *GA* IV.2, 767a14–35, than that of *Non Gen.*'s simultaneous emissions. Aristotle may have chosen a more generic term to cover both *Non Gen.*'s and his own concept of the harmonization of *sperma*.

24 ἔτι γυναῖκες ἐξονειρώττουσι: The ἐπεί of the mss. would leave this as a subordinate clause without a main clause. Balme reads it as "For," as if the sentence is giving an explanation for what has preceded, but there is no real connection between the two statements. The emphatic placement of γυναῖκες as second word in the sentence makes it clear that Aristotle has finished outlining the argument drawn from birds and is returning to evidence for female *sperma* that can be drawn from humans. Here he simply paraphrases the arguments found in *Non Gen.* One of his favorite formulae to introduce a new argument is ἔτι with or without further particles. He uses the same formula to introduce successive arguments in theories with which he disagrees; e.g., at *GA* I.17, 721b17, when introducing the second argument of pangeneticists he states, "Further, mutilated offspring come from mutilated parents," ἔτι τὸ ἐκ κολοβῶν κολοβὰ γίνεσθαι.

25–6 ταὐτὰ παθήματα: This is the argument made in *Non Gen.*, though not with the term παθήματα. Aristotle nowhere says intercourse drains a woman's strength; only childbearing eventually uses up her seminal residue, *GA* IV.5, 774a2–6.

26–7 δῆλον τοίνυν: That is, to the author of *Non Gen.* and others who share his assumptions about female *sperma*.

26, 27, and 28 ὀνειρωγμόν, ἐξονειρωγμῷ, ἐξονειρωγμούς: In all its references to nocturnal emissions, *Non Gen.* did not use this term. Nor is it a Hippocratic term. ἐξονειρώττ- is the more common root. It is not clear why Aristotle uses this form here.

27–8 τότε: That is, when they become sexually excited during intercourse with a man. In a dream emission there is nothing to contribute to.

28–30 ὅτι μετὰ...συγγένωνται ἀνδρί: The similarity between a woman's moistness after an erotic dream and that after intercourse is taken to parallel the similarity between wind-eggs and fertilized eggs and therefore to demonstrate her contribution to conception. Aristotle is going to show that the parallelism is spurious.

31 πρόεσις σπέρματος: Aristotle summarizes the conclusion others come to from the foregoing evidence. He is laying out the evidence for the ἔνδοξον espoused by his Answerer, while at the same time he is preparing to undercut this conclusion.

II *Why, then, do quadrupeds not reproduce parthenogenetically, or at least produce wind-eggs?*

32 προΐενται δ' οὐκ εἰς αὐτὰς τὰς ὑστέρας: D^a has αἱ ὑστέραι in the nominative case as the subject of προΐενται, which requires emending the simple pronoun αὐτάς found in D^a to the reflexive αὑτάς. It also requires either emending ἕλκει in the following line to ἕλκονται and again αὐτάς to αὑτάς, unless we assume a subject change from the womb to the woman. However, throughout *Non Gen.* the author never states that the womb emits *sperma*; he always uses the locution "the woman emits" and makes clear that the female *sperma* comes to the womb from outside, e.g., 634b30–635a2, 635a34–5, 635b2 and 38, 636a5, 636b27, 637a2–5 and 15–17. He believes the *sperma* was delivered to the womb via the woman's interior καυλός. Aristotle discusses this possibility nowhere else in his corpus, perhaps because he believed his animal dissections had empirically disproved the existence of such a structure so there was no need for its dialectical refutation. When arguing against the identification of the vaginal lubricant as female *sperma* at *GA* II.4, 739b16–20, he argued that if the <u>womb</u> emitted *sperma* outside itself it would then have to draw it back in, which would be superfluous, and Nature does nothing superfluous. However, in this dialectic Aristotle is arguing from the premises of *Non Gen.* itself and he reflects the author's understanding in his *topos* at 637a37, ἡ <u>γυνὴ</u> γόνιμον προΐεται.

33 ἕλκει εἰς αὐτάς: Guil. and most editors have taken the womb to be the continued subject and emended ἕλκει to ἕλκονται and αὐτάς to αὑτάς. Scot took the woman to be the subject of both *eicit* and *attrahit*, though he also includes a rather strange *ipsum*. If women are the subject of προΐενται, it is easier to countenance the abrupt change to the singular in ἕλκει, particularly following the singular ὁ ἀνήρ, rather than an abrupt change of both subject

225

and number with no other indication, and αὐτάς can stand unaspirated. This would then foreshadow the comparison between ἡ μὲν ὄρνις εἰς τὴν ὑστέραν προῖεται (637b35–6) and εἰς ὃν καὶ τὸ θῆλυ προῖεται (637b38–638a1).

ὡς: The following sentence begins ἢ ὅτι, which is the standard way to begin an answer in the *Prob.* after a question has been posed (even if there are no alternative answers), so we need an interrogative here. Scal. and Sn. conjecture ὡς for Dᵃ's ὤν, Pk. and Dt. πῶς οὖν. Aristotle uses ὡς as an interrogative at *EN* IV.8, 1128a1. This is Aristotle's first participation in the dialectic as Questioner.

35–7: In Aristotle's mature biological theory most female animals retain their seminal fluids in their wombs; after it has left the body it is not usually suitable for reproduction. (Some fish are exceptions; see *GA* I.21, 730a18–24.) The reason birds produce wind-eggs is that their wombs are higher in their body and closer to the ἀρχή of the heart and therefore hotter; see *GA* III.1, 750b12–17. Here, however, Aristotle is arguing in terms with which the author of *Non Gen.* could be assumed to agree, albeit with a view to using quadrupeds to discredit *Non Gen.*'s whole argument. The phrasing shows that Aristotle is contrasting the site of the emission—into the womb in birds, outside the womb in quadrupeds—not whether or not the emission remains in the womb or is emitted from it.

37 διὸ...τὴν γῆν ἐκχεῖ: Aristotle is framing the response that he believes the Answerer could give to his objection. Hens do not have a space in front of their wombs into which they emit as women do. If they did, at least occasionally their wombs would fail to take up their *sperma*, as they sometimes fail to take up the male's, and their *sperma* would immediately flow away unused. This does not happen. This different αἴτιον explains, from the Answerer's point of view, why quadrupeds do not experience a πάθημα analogous to wind-eggs even though they produce γόνιμον σπέρμα.

37–638a1 τοῖς δὲ τετράποσιν...καὶ τὸ ἄρρεν: Aristotle allows that quadrupeds do have a space before the womb and that this is where a man and a woman emit in sexual intercourse, but in the following chapter he proceeds to undermine the conclusion that the emission on the woman's side is her seminal secretion.

1 ὅπερ: The relative has no antecedent, but this is easily understood to be the unexpressed object of προῖεται, ἀφίησιν, and ἐκχεῖ in what precedes. From what follows it becomes clear that Aristotle is referring only to the female emission here.

τοῖς μὲν ἄλλοις: Quadrupeds generally.

1–2 τῶν ἄλλων ὑγρῶν: As Answerer Aristotle adds a further αἴτιον to explain why quadrupeds and women do not produce something akin to wind-eggs. The fluid which is produced during sexual excitement prior to climaxing mixes with the female's ejaculated *sperma* and prevents it from being drawn into the womb, just as can happen with the mingled *sperma* of a man and a woman, 635b29.

4 συμπέττει: This is a favorite word of Aristotle to describe the gestation process. He believes menstrual fluid and male *gonê* each have their ability to generate because of the level of "concoction" they have each reached, i.e., the amount of innate heat to which they have each been subjected. Males are innately hotter than females, so their seminal residues can instantiate sentient soul while the female can concoct her residue only to the point of instantiating nutritive soul. Birds lay eggs as an evacuation of their seminal residue, but it contains no more different type of soul than does women's menstrual fluid. There is no inkling of this process in the first five chapters of *Non Gen.*

4–5 διότι...εἶναι: In the case of birds, both Aristotle and his Answerer would agree on this, even if it is not true of grasshoppers, so the πάθημα of wind-eggs shows why it is that quadrupeds do not reproduce parthenogenetically. But this has not answered the question why they do not produce something like wind-eggs.

CHAPTER 7

I *Aristotle turns to confuting the premises he has adduced as Answerer to support* Non Gen.*'s claim that the fluid women emit when sexually excited is* sperma. *He begins by asking why other animals do not produce wind-eggs and offers uterine mole (see note to l.11) as a possible candidate.*

638a5 ἔστι δ' ἐνστῆναι: This is a common Aristotelian term when raising an objection, e.g., *APr.* II.26, 69b6 and *APo.* I.10, 76b26; *Top.* II.3, 110a27 and VIII.2 and 10, 157b8 and 160b36; *Rhet.* III.18, 1419a17; here it articulates the objection to the previous explanation that female quadrupeds do not produce something analogous to wind-eggs because they do not emit *sperma* directly into their wombs.

5–6 δῆλον...ἄνωθεν: See 634b30. If women can draw their emissions into their womb, as *Non Gen.* has argued their dryness on awakening from an erotic dream shows they do, why do quadrupeds not do this?

7 διὰ τί: This is a phrase that is used to introduce 98 percent of the problems in the *Prob.*, Mayhew 2011, p. xiii, n. 1.

γεννᾷ αὐτὰ καθ' αὑτά: Here Aristotle means generation up to a point, the equivalent of wind-eggs.

8 μιχθέν: Aristotle does not believe that the male and female seminal fluids are mixed together outside the womb before being drawn in; he is using *Non Gen.*'s own theories to undermine this very claim. If the womb draws in mixed male and female *sperma*, why would it not also draw in a female's unmixed *sperma*, and why then do other animals not become pregnant after the fashion of wind-eggs in birds?

9 ἀμιγές: Pk.'s emendation for αἱ αἶγες is surely correct. Balme's defense of αἱ αἶγες is based on the argument that the subject of this sentence has to be something other than the human female because it has been granted that women can draw their own *sperma* unmixed into their womb after a night emission. But the further question here is why they do not develop something akin to wind-eggs after this has happened. The Answerer's response to this is going to be that women do produce something analogous to a wind-egg— the uterine mole. No more is said about quadrupeds in this connection after this point as Aristotle becomes fully engaged in the problem of the mole. However this comes about in the human female, why it does not occur in quadrupeds is going to be a problem for any theory. Aristotle probably allows the response because at this stage, if it can go undetected for years, he cannot disprove that animals also suffer from mole. He acknowledges this possibility in *GA* IV.7, 776a8–14:

> ἀπορίαν δ' ἔχει διὰ τί ποτ' ἐν τοῖς ἄλλοις οὐχὶ γίγνεται ζῴοις, εἰ μή τι πάμπαν λέληθεν. αἴτιον δὲ δεῖ νομίζειν ὅτι μόνον ὑστερικόν ἐστιν ἡ γυνὴ τῶν ἄλλων ζῴων καὶ περὶ τὰς καθάρσεις πλεονάζει καὶ οὐ δύναται πέττειν αὐτάς· ὅταν οὖν ἐκ δυσπέπτου ἰκμάδος συστῇ τὸ κύημα, τότε γίγνεται ἡ καλουμένη μύλη ἐν ταῖς γυναιξὶν εὐλόγως ἢ μάλιστα ἢ μόναις.

> But in this there is a puzzle as to why it (mole) does not occur in other animals, unless in some way it has gone completely undetected. We must assume the reason to be that women alone among animals are liable to conditions of the uterus and with regard to menstrual material produce it in excess so that they are unable to concoct it. And so, if the so-called mole develops whenever the fetation is set from some under-concocted fluid, it logically occurs either primarily or exclusively in women.

αὐτῶν: Although the subject of ἕλκει in l.7 is ἡ ὑστέρα, in l. 8 and here it is τὰ θήλεα. The author of *Non Gen.* did not think female *sperma* originated in the womb, and Aristotle recognized this.

10–18 αἷς…συναποθνήσκει: Many edd. suspect there is a lacuna at the beginning of this sentence, but this is not necessary (other than perhaps inserting δέ) if we read this sentence as the Answerer's reply to the question just posed by the Questioner: women __do__ produce something akin to wind-eggs when they draw in their unmixed *sperma*—a uterine mole. The author of *Non Gen.* had said at 636a2–4 that when women drew in their own *sperma* and did not release it they were using it up on their own bodies. He did not discuss the condition of mole. Aristotle is still advancing the argument along lines that would seem to support the ἔνδοξον of *Non Gen.* See Introduction pp. 66–7 for the relationship of this case history of the uterine mole to the virtually verbatim account in the *GA*.

An hydatiform mole is recognized today as a clump of growing tissue formed from a fertilized ovum which lacks any chromosomes of its own, an empty egg, so the mole contains only DNA from the father. Left untreated the condition is almost always resolved by a spontaneous abortion of a mass of tissue that does not resemble a fetus. Occasionally, though, the condition can become chronic and invasive and serious complications, including cancer, can supervene. Causes of mole are unclear, but they are more prevalent among women under 20 who suffer from bad nutrition. These conditions would have been more prevalent in ancient Greece than the modern West, so it is possible that the hydatiform mole underlies the ancient view of uterine mole, but it does not account for the idea that the condition could become chronic but benign and end after several years with an abortion.

10 κυούσαις: In the *GA* Aristotle describes uterine mole as a type of pregnancy: γίνεται μὲν ὀλιγάκις ταῖς γυναιξί, γίνεται δέ τισι τοῦτο τὸ πάθος κυούσαις, "This condition occurs seldom in women, but it does occur in those who are pregnant." He believed it was formed from the mixture of male and female seminal residues but that the woman's womb could not produce enough heat to maintain the development of a fetus. At *GA* IV.7, 776a1, the mass in the womb is called a κύημα, his term for the earliest stages of the embryo (*GA* I.20, 728b34). *GA* III.1, 750b10, refers to unfertilized eggs of fish and birds as σύστασις κυημάτων, but this is clearly an exception. Peck 1965, pp. lxix–lxx, says the term "covers all stages of the living creature's development from the time when the 'matter' is first 'informed' to the time when the creature is born or hatched." At *GA* IV.7, 776a4 Nature is said to be unable to perfect her work and bring generation to completion, οὐ δύνασθαι τελειῶσαι οὐδ' ἐπιθεῖναι τῇ γενέσει πέρας, a phrase which Aristotle is unlikely to have used if generation had not even started.

ἔτη πολλά: Aristotle is differentiating the symptoms of uterine mole from *Non Gen.*'s description of "wind-pregnancy" in humans, which passes quickly. Rather, once mole has started it becomes a chronic condition lasting many years.

10 τίκτουσι γάρ... 638b37 στόμα ὅμοιον: This passage, with the omission of 638a26–b7, is quoted by Orib. (chapter 13 in *Lib. Incert.*, Raeder 1933, pp. 101–2); see note on 636b39–637a9. With the exception of the datives for the genitives in l.12, there are no readings from the *GA* version of the case history.

11 μύλην: The term refers to a hard formation of some sort in a woman's womb. It can also refer to a millstone or a kneecap, which may give some idea of the shape it was conceived to be by ancient Greeks, unless the term was associated with underdone meat; see note to 638b18–20. The Hippocratics recognize the condition at *Mul.* I.71 (VIII.148.24–150.23, repeated at *Steril.* 233 (VIII.446.7–448.7)) and *Mul.* II.178 (VIII.360.18–362.2); see Dean-Jones 2018. In the first case the author attributes the condition to excessive menses receiving a small amount of diseased *gonê* (πολλὰ τὰ ἐπιμήνια ἐόντα γονὴν ὀλίγην καὶ νοσώδεα ξυλλάβωσιν). He says the condition can last two, sometimes three years, and that if there is only one σάρξ the condition is invariably fatal, but if there are many there can be a bloody and fleshy discharge which can save the woman as long as it is not excessive. The second passage says the condition can be caused by thick *gonê* (πάχεος γονῆς ἐνεχομένης) but says nothing about its duration or consequences if not cured. In neither case is it clear whether the *gonê* is male, female, or both. The first explanation bears some resemblance to Aristotle's account in *GA*, but neither conforms to the suggestion put forward here that it is in some way equivalent to a wind-egg. At *Epid.* V.25 (V.224.6–13) there is a case history of a woman who from her youth had pain whenever she had sexual intercourse and never became pregnant. At age 60 she experienced strong pains like those of labor and from the *stoma* of the womb passed a rough stone as big as a spindle-whorl. From then on she was healthy.

11–12 συγγενομένης τῷ ἀνδρὶ καὶ δοξάσης συλλαβεῖν: The fact that the woman had recently had intercourse is presented as a coincidence which led to her believing she was actually pregnant. Aristotle believes the preceding intercourse is more than a coincidence himself, but here he is presenting uterine moles as the Answerer's possible suggestion of a human equivalent to a wind-egg.

12–13 ὅ τ' ὄγκος...κατὰ λόγον: *Non Gen.* 636a21–3 says that the symptoms of "wind-pregnancy," ἐξανεμοῦσθαι, mimic those of true pregnancy, but says that the condition is not a pregnancy, 636a12. This condition does develop from the mixture of both male and female *sperma* after intercourse.

15–16 ἕως δυσεντερίας: Uterine mole is not a condition which can resolve itself, unlike *Non Gen.*'s "wind-pregnancy," 636a17, 20, 23.

17 εὐμεγέθη: In contrast to the resolution of wind-pregnancy in *Non Gen.*, where the retained *sperma* becomes so small, μικρόν, through being dried out, κατασκελετεύεται 636a14–15, that it slips out without the woman noticing, 636a14–16. This adjective is not present in the almost verbatim account of uterine mole in *GA* IV.7, 775b34, because there the contrast with "wind-pregnancy" was not necessary; see Introduction p. 67.

17–18 συγκαταγηράσκει: See Rud. p. 17.

II *Aristotle has established from the* phainomena *that the condition of uterine mole exists. The fact that no analogue to the* παθήματα *of either wind-eggs or uterine mole can be identified in quadrupeds argues against the fluid they produce in their vagina when "in heat" being identified with the* αἴτια *that cause these conditions in birds and women. Aristotle will now proceed to consider whether wind-eggs and uterine mole are in fact the same* πάθημα. *He will begin by considering the* endoxon *that they are analogous and the mole is caused by a particularly hot and dry womb.*

638a18–20 πότερον δέ: Aristotle is here returning to his role as Questioner. He regularly uses this locution to introduce a question subsequent upon a previous question, e.g., *De an.* II.2, 413b13, *GA* II.1, 735a4, *Metaph.* VII.2, 1028b13. He never uses the phrase πότερον δή.

θερμότητα...θερμὴ καὶ ξηρά: At *GA* IV.7, 776a1–3, Aristotle deals summarily with the suggestion that uterine mole is caused by heat:

καὶ οὐ διὰ θερμότητα, ὥσπερ τινές φασιν, ἀλλὰ μᾶλλον δι' ἀσθένειαν θερμότητος.

And it does not come about through heat, as some people say, but rather through a weakness in heat.

At *GA* IV.7, 775b34–6, before dismissing the possibility of heat as a cause of a uterine mole, Aristotle describes its hardness, and at 776a8 attributes this to a lack of concoction (ἀπεψία), that is a lack of heat. In his comments on *Non Gen.* Aristotle does not introduce the hardness of the mole due to μωλύσεως, under-cooking, until 638b10–15, perhaps because he did not want to prejudge the matter or because he had not come to any definitive conclusion at this point. However, when he compares a uterine mole, μύλη, to underdone meat, μώλυνσις, at *GA* IV.7, 776a9, it may indicate that there was believed to be an etymological connection between the two states which would favor a popular assumption that a uterine mole was caused through a lack rather than an excess of heat.

21 ἀνελέσθαι καὶ φυλάξαι πρὸς αὐτήν: *Non Gen.* said excessive dryness—636a13 λίαν ξηρά, 17 ὑπέρξηρος, which while not heat itself is readily attributable to heat—caused "wind-pregnancy," but did not believe the womb was able to hold onto the *sperma* in these conditions. Aristotle is attempting to explain why mole could become chronic; see Introduction pp. 61–3.

22 ἐὰν μὴ μεμιγμένον ἐστὶ τὸ ἀπ' ἀμφοῖν: Sylb., Sn., and Dt. emended ἐστί and ἐνδέξαιτο of D^a (and Orib.) to the subjunctive ᾖ and ἐνδέχηται (Sylb.) or ἐνδέξηται (Sn. and Dt.). Rud. comments that it is not easy to see how ᾖ could become ἐστί and mentions two places where all the mss. of Aristotle show ἔαν/ἄν with the indicative, *Rhet.* II.25, 1402b30 (aorist passive) and *Poet.* 25, 1460b22 (as here, with the perfect passive), though he attributes the moods to the slightly later date at which he believes the "Autor-Kompilator" was working (1911, pp. 39–40).

23 θατέρου: The argument shifts from focusing exclusively on the woman's *sperma*; see Introduction pp. 59–60.

26 ἐμμένει: After ἐμμένει the equivalent of 19 Bk. lines are missing from Orib. This may have been caused by the copyist's eye skipping from the πολὺν δὲ χρόνον of l.a26 to the χρόνον ποιοῦσι πολύν of b7, but it is more likely that in the context of assembling passages on human reproduction, Orib. saw no need to copy out a discussion of the causes of a bird laying eggs.

27 καὶ διότι: διότι anticipates διόπερ in l.35. Clearly, the laying of wind-eggs in birds is being contrasted to, not paralleling, the mole becoming a chronic condition in women.

ἡ μὲν ὄρνις: μὲν anticipates the δέ in l.31, contrasting the conditions which cause the bird to lay eggs with those that bring about labor in viviparous animals. Neither of these conditions is applicable to the uterine mole.

28 οἰγνυμένης: The repletion of the bird's womb causes the womb passively, and the bird actively (see note on l.30), to expel the eggs.

30 ἀλλὰ καὶ τὸ σῶμα προετικὸν γενόμενον ὅτε ἐπληροῦτο: Something has to be supplied as the subject of ποιεῖ in l.31. It cannot be the womb itself because that is the object. The other options would be the bird or the bird's body. If we assume the subject is ὄρνις, we have to emend προετικὸν γενόμενον in l.30 to the feminine form. It seems simpler to follow Scal., Sn., and Dt. and emend κατά to καὶ τό and take σῶμα as the subject throughout. In this case καί would indicate that the body had become expulsive in addition to something else, that something else being the womb. If the womb did not open, the bird could not push out her eggs. If the bird does not push, all of the eggs would not necessarily be expelled from an open womb.

31 οὐκέτι...ἀντισπαστικήν: Taking the adverb with the adjective rather than the verb. Nothing has been said to explain how the bird's body would cause her womb to be retentive, only the role it plays in causing the womb to release the eggs.

ὅσα δὲ ζωοφορεῖ: The only other time Aristotle uses this term (in noun form) is to refer to the Zodiac at *Mu.* 2, 392a11. He referred to viviparous animals as τὰ ζῳοτοκοῦντα. Neither the verb nor the noun is seen again until the second century BCE.

32 δύναμιν: The word appears to be used in a typical Aristotelian sense. It indicates that Aristotle is thinking more and more in terms of his own theory, abandoning framing the reply to the objection in the language of the original Answerer.

32–3 ἄλλοτε ἀλλοίας δεῖσθαι τροφῆς: Aristotle believed this is what caused birth in all animals, including chicks hatching from their shell; cf. *GA* IV.6, 774b11–14, 35–6, IV.8, 777a22–7. The laying of eggs is not birthing.

33 ἐπιφλεγμαίνουσά τι: A *hapax* for Aristotle, found 3 times in the Hippocratics. The unprefixed form is extremely common in the Hippocratic Corpus and is found 6 times in Aristotle. The prefixed form is not seen again until the first century CE, when it becomes relatively common. At 638b8–9 Aristotle indicates it is movement alone which causes labor, and at *GA* IV.8, 777a22–7, he says that the insufficiency of nourishment causes the birth of young animals by causing the collapse of blood vessels in the umbilical cord. Nowhere in the Aristotelian or Hippocratic corpora is birth explained as the result of inflammation, and it is hard to see what Aristotle had in mind here. It may be an explanatory interpolation from a copyist who misunderstood his remark about inflammation in l.35. It cannot be a reference back to the discussion of spasm in *Non Gen.* Chapter 4 because there inflammation and the excess material during childbirth caused the womb <u>not</u> to open.

33–4 τακτὸν τὸν τόκον: For ταὐτὸν τόκον. It is possible that the reading in the mss. means to parallel the phenomenon of birth in vivipara with the laying of eggs in birds, a parallelism with which Aristotle disagrees in the rest of his biology but which he seems to have assumed for the purposes of framing the argument here. But even in the context of the sometimes telegraphic form of his argument this would be a very condensed expression.

34 ὁμαλῶν: That is, unlike a fetus, which will eventually be given birth because it needs a different type of nourishment, there is no change in development which instigates the ejection of a uterine mole from a womb. Nor, however large the mole grows, will the womb open and the body push it out as in birds.

35 δεῖ γὰρ ὃ βαρύνει τὴν ὑστέραν οὐδὲν ποιεῖν αὐτὴν φλεγμαίνειν: φλεγμαίνειν is regularly intransitive in Aristotle and the Hippocratics. In *Non Gen.* cf. 634a23 and 636a35. If simply carrying a weight in the womb caused inflammation, fetuses would never be brought to term. This does not say that it is inflammation which causes birth. It is a reference to the fact that what brings about a resolution of mole is a supervening illness, such as dysentery, which could cause inflammation. But if a copyist took it to mean inflammation was what caused birth it would explain the puzzling ἐπιφλεγμαίνουσά τι in l.33.

37 ἐὰν μὴ δι᾽ εὐτύχημα ἀσθενήματος...δυσεντερίας: Ironic humor. *Mul.* II.116 (VIII.252.10) says that a certain form of leukorrhea which brings great suffering is difficult to cure in older women ἢν μή τι εὐτύχημα τῶν αὐτομάτων λύσῃ γενόμενον.

III *Aristotle now considers whether the cause of mole is not rather a womb which is not quite hot enough to concoct a fetus from the fluid in the womb, his solution to the problem in* GA.

638b2–3 ἢ μᾶλλον...οἷον μύει: This sentence appears as a third alternative to heat and cold as possible causes of mole in Dᵃ. Guil. has *aut magis propter humiditatem, quoniam et est repletio, uelut...* followed by a lacuna and does not have a second *aut* before beginning the consideration of cold as a cause of mole. The entire sentence is omitted in Scot. It is unlikely that Aristotle would introduce a third alternative in less than ten words between the discussions of heat and cold without expanding upon the circumstances that would cause such an accumulation of fluid to develop into a mole. If we take the words as the beginning of the discussion of causation by coldness, the sentence as a whole provides the cause and also gives an object for ἀφεῖναι and πέψαι.

ὑγρότητα: This generic term for fluid is used in *Non Gen.* to refer solely to menses at 634a15 and 23, solely to female *sperma* at 635a40, and solely to the vaginal lubricant at 635b31. Because of its lack of specificity the term could also be used for mingled male and female *sperma*, however these are to be identified, which must be its meaning here; see Introduction p. 19. Aristotle is here, then, moving towards the explanation for mole found in *GA*, but here the lack of heat is associated with the womb itself. In *GA* it is the lack of heat in the κύημα itself, brought about by the amount of menstrual fluid in proportion to the heat carried by the male semen.

πλήρωμα: This is cited as one of the symptoms of mole in *Mul.* I.71 (VIII.150.8). It is also listed as a symptom of inflammation of the womb which can give the false impression of pregnancy at *Mul.* II.169 (VIII.348.13) and *Nat. Mul.* 11 (VII.326.21). In the discussion of spasm in Chapter 4 it is the amount of fluid in pregnancy, πληρώματος πολλοῦ, that can cause the στόμα not to open for childbirth, 636a31–2.

3–4 ἢ ὅταν...πέψαι: This is what Aristotle claims causes uterine mole in *GA* IV.7, 776a1–8. If the heat of the male semen completely fails to master the woman's seminal residue, there will be no conception and the menses will simply flow away from the female taking the male semen with them. If the male semen is hot enough, it will "concoct" or "cook" the menstrual fluid by passing over the form into it and an animal will develop. The ratio of heat in the male semen to the amount of menstrual material determines where on the continuum from complete monstrosity to a perfect reproduction of the father the animal falls, *GA* IV.3 and 4. A uterine mole is formed when the semen is just hot enough to set the menses but there is too much menstrual fluid (GA IV.7, 776a12) for it to pass on any sort of ἀρχή that could direct development.

5–6 τὰ ἐν ἑψήσει...παχυτῆτα: Aristotle discusses the process of boiling at *Metr.* IV.3, 380b12–381a22. There he says that boiling concocts by drawing the moisture out of a thing where roasting (ὀπτάω, which can also mean broiling or frying, cooking by dry heat generally) causes the thing being roasted to draw moisture to itself, so that boiled meats are drier than roasted. Not everything is able to be boiled, only those things which can get thicker, smaller, or heavier, παχύτερα, ἐλάττω, βαρύτερα. He goes on to discuss, μώλυνσις, under-boiling or simmering (the term parboiling means to cook a thing in actual boiling water for a shorter than normal period of time, the opposite of what Aristotle is talking about), which is due either to the lack of heat in the surrounding liquid or the amount of moisture in the thing being boiled. For the argument to make sense we have to assume that ἐν ἑψήσει in the phrase ἐν ἑψήσει πολὺν χρόνον means simmering, not actual boiling for a long time since Aristotle has just said that the womb does not have enough heat to πέψαι, and if something was actually boiled for a long time it would be overcooked, not undercooked. Aristotle also says that μώλυνσις results in lack of concoction rather than overcooking at *GA* IV.7, 776a8, ἀπεψία γάρ τις καὶ ἡ μώλυνσίς ἐστιν.

We are then faced with the question of whether τὰ δ' ἑψόμενα means things that are actually boiled or things that are simmered. If the former, ταχυτῆτα seems more appropriate. Aristotle is saying that in cooking food by boiling there is a point at which it is ready (πέρας), and if the water is actually boiling, this point will be reached in a specific, relatively short, amount of time. This requires τὰ δ' ἑψόμενα to be in sharp contrast to τὰ ἐν ἑψήσει πολὺν χρόνον, which remain the same, i.e., never reach a point of readiness. If τὰ δ' ἑψόμενα is referring to the same things as τὰ ἐν ἑψήσει πολὺν χρόνον, then we should read παχυτῆτα, as in the *Metr.* passage. The process of simmering explains why uterine mole is χρόνιον, why it develops to a certain consistency and stays that way, why there is no development towards readiness however long it stays in the womb. πέρας and παχυτῆτα are both hendiadys which would explain the corruption.

6 αἱ δὲ τοιαῦται ὑστέραι: That is, wombs which keep the *sperma* "simmering" for a long time.

7 ἀκρόταται: The "extreme" type of womb is that which can cause the condition to last a long time, which would seem to require that the extremity be one of neither heat nor cold but, paradoxically, of a state between the two. At 638b18 and *GA* IV.7, 775b25, Aristotle comments that uterine mole occurs ὀλιγάκις.

It is at the end of this line that the text resumes in Orib.

8–9 οὐ κινούμενον…ἔμβρυον: Here there is no mention of inflammation having a role to play in prompting labor; see above, ll.31–4. *Nat. Puer.* 30 (VII. 530.20–532.14) *Oct.* 1 (VII.436.8–14) also attributes birth to the greater movement of the fetus looking for food, which causes a rupture of the membranes. On ancient conceptions of childbirth, see Hanson 1991, pp. 87–96, Dean-Jones 1994, pp. 211–15, Demand 1994, pp. 71–86. At *GA* IV.6, 775a4–9, Aristotle says male fetuses move about more than female and on this account are more frequently born deformed. At *HA* IX(VII).4, 584a26–34, he attributes the shorter birthing time of male babies to their greater movement. Sometimes, he says, even so slight a movement as the fetus turning its head can make a woman think she is beginning labor.

διὰ τὸ ζῆν: This explains the source of the movement, not a separate reason once labor begins for the expulsion of the embryo.

10 σκληρότης: As in the *Metr.* passage, this is associated with simmering rather than boiling.

μωλύσεως: The word appears in *GA*'s discussion of uterine mole as μωλυνόμενα and as μώλυνσις at IV.7, 776a2 and 8. Outside the Aristotlelian canon, the word appears more often without the nu; see Bonitz 471 and 479. The assonance with μύλη may have caused the association of the condition with undercooking.

11–12 ὥστε πελέκει οὐ δύνανται διακόπτειν: Aristotle discusses the hardness of the uterine mole and the difficulty (n.b. not impossibility) of cutting it with an axe at *GA* IV.7, 775b34–6, immediately following his remarks on the uterine mole lasting into old age and death for some women, but it is not a very close echo of the Greek here: τὰ δὲ θύραζε ἐξιόντα τῶν τοιούτων γίνεται σκληρὰ οὕτως ὥστε μόλις διακόπτεσθαι καὶ σιδήρῳ. It is interesting that the attempt was made, as it was presumably only for empirical reasons. There is no pragmatic reason to assail a uterine mole with an axe.

12–14 τὰ μὲν οὖν ἐφθά…σκληρά: Boiling makes things thicker, παχύτερα; it does not necessarily make them harder, but nor does it necessarily make them softer. Some things become softer in boiling, e.g., vegetables, but Aristotle would not say that boiling makes all things softer. There is no answering δέ to give μέν the necessary partitive sense; this has to be implied from the locution καὶ πάντα. However, Aristotle is even less likely to say that all things that have been concocted become softer. Concoction creates bone from blood. Either Aristotle is being extremely sloppy with his terms here, or there is something wrong with the text, or this is a copyist's mistaken gloss.

IV *The rarity of uterine mole and the condition that is often mistaken for it.*

638b15 ὅ τι πολλοὶ ἰατροὶ ἀγνοοῦντες: Rud. p. 17 sees here a formal echo of *Mul.* I.2 τῶν ἰητρῶν πολλοὶ ἤδη οὐκ εἰδότες (VIII.20.14), but competition among doctors in the Hippocratic Corpus is not rare and Aristotle elsewhere comments that not every doctor is always right (*Rhet.* I.15, 1375b20–3; see Dean-Jones 2003, pp. 99–108). Although the author of *Non Gen.* does not discuss uterine moles, the πάθος which he names "wind-pregnancy" and attributes to the shriveling and unnoted emission of male and female *sperma* at 636a9–28 has the symptoms Aristotle is about to describe. He is going to argue that this condition in fact has very little to do with the womb, and nothing to do with *sperma*, so the author of *Non Gen.* is to be included among the ἀγνοοῦντες on this point at least.

16–17 τάς τε κοιλίας ἐπαιρομένας: In *Non Gen.*'s description of "wind-pregnancy" it was the womb which was said to rise, αἴρεται ἡ ὑστέρα (636a22). Aristotle is correcting that observation. The Hippocratics frequently refer to the womb, especially in contexts of pregnancy, as γαστήρ, so when in discussing the condition caused by πλήρωμα, *Mul.* II.169 says ἡ γαστήρ... ἀείρεται (VIII.348.12) and *Nat. Mul.* 11 ἡ γαστὴρ...φυσᾶται καὶ μεγάλη γίνεται (VII.326.18–20), it is not clear whether they would agree with *Non Gen.* or Aristotle.

17 ὕδρωπος: A bodily humor found throughout ancient medical texts. The only other time Aristotle uses it is in describing women's labor at *HA* IX(VII).9, 587a6. It is also used at *Prob.* VII.8, 887a23. Aristotle uses the term ὑδρωπιῶσιν at *GA* V.8, 789b14, in discussing the use of the lancet to draw the fluid from a dropsical patient.

ἐπιμηνίων: Although the word is used frequently by Hippocratic authors, the only other time Aristotle uses it is at *Metaph.* XII.6, 1071b30.

σχέσιν: This word appears 5 times in the Aristotelian fragments, but nowhere else in his extant works. It is used 12 times for the retention of various fluids in the Hippocratics, e.g., blood *Ulc.* 26 (VI.430.18), urine *Artic.* 48 (IV.216.3), diarrhea *Aph.* VII.79 and 80 (IV.604.10). It may be that Aristotle is quoting from a medical source here.

19 σύρρους: A *hapax* when used as a noun; Plato uses it as an adjective; see Rud. p. 28. The term is used in later medical texts.

20 περιττωμάτων: This word does not appear in the Hippocratic Corpus outside the Pseudo-Hippocratic *Epistulae*. It is not common before Aristotle, but becomes extremely common for any bodily residue after him; see Introduction pp. 103–4. Orib. adds καὶ λέπτων and Guil. *subtiles* under the influence of παχυτέρων, but the comparison is with ὑδαρῶν.

21 τὸν περὶ τὴν κοιλίαν τόπον: Aristotle is making it abundantly clear he is not talking about the womb here.

τοιαῦται: Aristotle is talking about the nature of women who develop the condition called "wind-pregnancy" by *Non Gen.*, which had attributed the condition to excessive dryness, 636a13 and 17. Reading the feminine plural here makes the plural ὦσιν (omitted in some of Dᵃ's apographa) easier.

22 ταῦτα γάρ: This sentence accounts for why the condition is at first taken to be pregnancy rather than a pathological condition.

24 οὐδεμίαν ἄλλην ἐπισπῶνται νόσον: Further explanation of why the condition is identified as pregnancy rather than a pathological condition. Note the use of a plural verb with neuter plural subject.

25 πήρωμά τι: This is an Aristotelian term (not used before him) meaning a mutilated or deformed animal, here clearly one that is lifeless in the womb, though the condition for which it is used as an analogy is not in the womb.

26 καταμηνίων: Aristotle's normal term for the menses.

τὸ δεῦρο...θηλάζωνται: Aristotle uses the simile of suckling because in that condition menses are directed away from the womb to the breasts, close to the area of the body in which he believes this πάθος has its seat.

καταναλίσκεσθαι: In the Hippocratic Corpus this term is found exclusively in the first two books of *Vict.*, where it is used 17 times to mean consume, usually for purposes of nourishment.

28 ὀλίγα: The womb must be open for this to happen, which is significant in differentiating the condition from both pregnancy and mole see 638b36.

28–9 τὸν μεταξὺ τόπον τῆς ὑστέρας καὶ τῆς κοιλίας: Yet another emphatic indication that Aristotle is not talking about the womb.

31 ἂν μύλη ᾖ θιγγανομένης τῆς ὑστέρας: The verb θιγγάνω must refer to the palpation of the womb. More than a visual examination is needed to differentiate mole from both true pregnancy and wind-pregnancy. Scot and Guil. both describe the womb being touched in the passive voice, Guil. using the ablative absolute. Scal., Buss., and Dt.'s conjectures have the woman doing the touching. This may be correct, but it would presumably be under a doctor's guidance because Aristotle is discussing the mistaken identification of the condition by doctors, not by women themselves, and is here emphatically contrasting active palpation of the womb with the simple visual inspection (ἴδωσι, l.16) of the doctors who identify the condition as mole too quickly; see note to 635a8.

33–4 θερμή τε καὶ ξηρά: It does not make sense for the womb to be described as both hot and cold to the touch. ψυχρά was probably imported from l.36 as Rud. suggests. This may have been influenced by the section explaining mole in the *GA* where Aristotle had said the womb was both hot enough to have retained the *sperma*, but cold enough to prevent complete concoction. For purposes of the examination, however, what would be registered is that the womb was hotter than a non-pathological womb.

35 τὸ στόμα τοιαύτη οἷα ὅταν κύωσιν: That is, it will be closed, not as in the previously described condition.

36–7 ἀεὶ τἰὸ στόμα ὅμοιον: That is, open.

Aristotle began the Dialectic *to query* Non Gen.'s *assumption that the fluid produced by women when they reach orgasm is equivalent to male semen. He does not come to any explicit conclusions, but he begins to develop some tentative theories:*

1) *When considering why birds produce wind-eggs Aristotle wonders whether it is because they inject their* sperma *directly into their wombs. In* GA *he will attribute the production of wind-eggs to the fact that the bird's uterus is high in her abdomen, close to the diaphragm. There is no indication of that explanation here.*

2) *The fluid produced by quadrupeds when they are in heat is not equivalent to* sperma *because they produce neither wind-eggs nor uterine moles. In the* GA *he will attribute this to the fact that they do not produce as much menstrual fluid as women and are not susceptible to diseases of the uterus, but he does not raise that issue here.*

3) *Uterine moles are not analogous to wind-eggs because women do not develop a mole unless they have had intercourse. He does not say this explicitly, as he does in the* GA, *because here he puts forward the theory from the point of view of the Answerer, who is arguing that moles do not develop from mingled male and female* sperma, *but his only example of a woman who suffered a mole was a woman who had had intercourse, and he describes the condition as being mistaken for a normal pregnancy, which would not happen if the woman had not had intercourse.*

4) *Uterine moles are more likely caused by lack than excess of heat. He is more definite about this fact in the* GA. *The condition called wind-pregnancy in* Non Gen. *is a pathological condition and is not discussed in the* GA.

In the GA *Aristotle says he has dealt with the uterine mole in the* Prob. *No such problem has survived. The* Dialectic *would appear to be preliminary to a full discussion of the uterine mole. It was written at a time when Aristotle was uneasy about the claim that women ejaculated at orgasm but before he was ready to assert categorically that women do not contribute* sperma *to conception in the way men do.*

BIBLIOGRAPHY

Anagnostopoulos, G. (2009) "Aristotle's Works and the Development of his Thought," in Anagnostopoulos, G. (ed.), 14–27

(ed.) (2009) *A Companion to Aristotle*, Oxford: Blackwell

Andorlini, I. (2009) (ed.) *Greek Medical Papyri II*, Florence: Istituto Papirologico

Aubert, H. R. and Wimmer, C. F. H. (1866) *Aristoteles Thierkunde*, Leipzig: Wilhelm Engelmann

Balme, D. M. (1985) "Aristotle *Historia Animalium* Book Ten," in Wiesner, J. (ed.), *Aristoteles, Werk und Wirkung, vol. I*, Berlin: De Gruyter, 191–206

(1987) "The Place of Biology in Aristotle's Philosophy," in Gotthelf, A. and Lennox, J. (eds.), 9–20

(1991) *Aristotle: History of Animals Book VII–X*, Cambridge, Mass.: Harvard University Press

and Gotthelf, A. (2002) *Aristotle, Historia Animalium vol. I: Books I–X: Text*, Cambridge: Cambridge University Press

Barnes, J. (1980) "Aristotle and the Methods of Ethics," *Revue Internationale de Philosophie* 34: 490–511

(1984) "History of Animals Book X," in Barnes, J. (ed.), *The Complete Works of Aristotle*, Princeton: Princeton University Press, 984–93

(1997) "Roman Aristotle," in Barnes, J. and Griffin, M. (eds.), *Philosophia Togata II: Plato and Aristotle at Rome*, Oxford: Clarendon Press, 1–69

Berger, F. (2005) *Die Textgeschichte der* Historia Animalium *des Aristoteles*, Wiesbaden: Ludwig Reichert

Berrey, M. (2014) "The Hippocratics on Male Desire," *Arethusa* 47: 287–301

Beullens, P. (1999) "A 13th-Century Florilegium from Aristotle's *Books on Animals*," in Steel et al., 69–95

Beullens, P. and Bossier, F. (2000) *Guilelmus de Moerbeka:* De historia animalium, 2 vols. Leiden: Brill, new edn forthcoming

Beullens, P. and Gotthelf, A. (2007) "Theodore Gaza's Translation of Aristotle's *De Animalibus*: Content, Influence, and Date," *GRBS* 47: 469–513

Bolton, R. (1987) "Definition and Scientific Method in Aristotle's *Posterior Analytics* and *Generation of Animals*," in Gotthelf and Lennox, 120–66

(1990) "The Epistemological Basis of Aristotelian Dialectic," in Devereux, D. and Pellegrin, P. (eds.), *Biologie, Logique et Métaphysique chez Aristote*, Paris: Éditions du Centre National de la Recherche Scientifique

Bos, A. P. and Ferwerda, R. (2007) "Aristotle's *de Spiritu* as a Critique of the Doctrine of *Pneuma* in Plato and his Predecessors," *Mnemosyne* 60.4: 565–88

(2008) *Aristotle on the Life-Bearing Spirit (de Spiritu)*, Leiden: E. J. Brill

Buck, C. D. (1955) *The Greek Dialects: Grammar, Selected Inscriptions, Glossary*, Chicago: University of Chicago Press

Byl, S. and de Ranter, A. F. (1990) "L'étiologie de la sterilité feminine dans le Corpus Hippocratique," in Potter, P., Maloney, G., et Desautels, J. (eds.), *La maladie et les maladies dans la collection hippocratique*, Québec: Éditions de Sphinx, 303–22

Campese, S., Manuli, P., and Sissa, G. (1983) *Madre Materia*, Turin: Boringhieri

Cohoe, C. (2017) "Why the View of the Intellect in *De anima* I.4 isn't Aristotle's Own," paper presented at the Society for Classical Studies Annual Convention, Toronto, January 8

Connell, S. (2016) *Aristotle on Female Animals: A Study of the* Generation of Animals, Cambridge: Cambridge University Press

Constantini, S. (1995) *Il deposito votivo del santuario campestre di Tessennano*, Rome: G. Bretschneider

Cooper, G. L. III, after Krüger, K. W. (1998) *Attic Prose Syntax*, vol. II, Ann Arbor: University of Michigan Press

Cooper, J. M. (2009) "Nicomachean Ethics VII.1–2: Introduction, Method, Puzzles," in Natali, C. (ed.), *Aristotle's Nicomachean Ethics Book VII*, Oxford: Clarendon Press

Craik, E. (2006) *Two Hippocratic Treatises:* On Sight *and* On Anatomy, Leiden: Brill

Dean-Jones, L. (1992) "The Politics of Pleasure: Female Sexual Appetite in the Hippocratic Corpus," *Helios* 19: 72–91

(1994) *Women's Bodies in Classical Greek Science*, Oxford: Clarendon Press

(2003) "Written Texts and the Rise of the Charlatan in Ancient Greek Medicine," in Harvey Yunis (ed.), *Writing into Culture: Written Text and Cultural Practice in Ancient Greece*, Cambridge: Cambridge University Press, 97–121

(2017) Review of Connell (2016), *Ancient Philosophy* 37: 475–8

(2018) "The Persistence of the Hippocratic Definition of Uterine Mole," in Lorenzo Perilli (ed), *Ippocrate e gli Altri*, Rome: École Française de Rome, unpublished paper delivered at Colloquium Hippocraticum XVI, Rome, October 2018

Demand, N. (1994) *Birth, Death and Motherhood in Classical Greece*, Baltimore: Johns Hopkins University Press

Denniston, J. D. (1954) *The Greek Particles*, Oxford: Clarendon Press

Dittmeyer, L. (1907) *Aristotelis de Animalibus Historia*, Leipzig: Teubner

Dorandi, T. (1991) "Den Autoren über die Schulter geschaut," *Zeitschrift für Papyrologie und Epigraphik* 87: 11–33

Düring, I. (1950) "Notes on the History of the Transmission of Aristotle's Writings," *Götesborgs Högskolas Årsskrift* 56: 37–70

(1957) *Aristotle in the Ancient Biographical Tradition*, Göteborg: Studies of the University of Göteborg

Faraone, C. A. (1999) *Ancient Greek Love Magic*, Cambridge, Mass.: Harvard University Press

Filius, L. (2007) "The Arabic Translation of the *Historia Animalium* of Aristotle," in Vrolijk, A. and Hogendijk, J. P. (eds.), *O Ye Gentlemen: Arabic Studies on Science and Literary Culture in Honor of Remke Kruk*, Leiden: Brill, 25–33

(2018) *The Arabic Version of Aristotle's* Historia Animalium: *Book I–IX of Kitab al Hayawan*, Leiden: Brill

Flemming, R. (2013) "The Invention of Infertility in the Classical Greek World: Medicine, Divinity and Gender," *Bulletin of the History of Medicine* 87: 565–90

Föllinger, S. (1996) *Differenz und Gleichheit: das Geschlechterverhältnis in der Sicht griechischer Philosophen des 4. bis 1. Jahrhunderts v. Chr.*, Stuttgart: F. Steiner

Frede, D. (2012) "The *Endoxon* Mystique: What *Endoxa* Are and What They Are Not," *Oxford Studies in Ancient Philosophy* 43: 185–215

Gershenson, D. E. and Greenberg, D. A. (1962) "Aristotle Confronts the Eleatics," *Phronesis* 7: 137–51

Gignon, O. (1987) *Aristotelis Opera III: Librorum deperditorum fragmenta*, Berlin: De Gruyter, 502–3

Gohlke, P. (1949) *Die Lehrschriften VIII.1: Tierkunde*, Paderborn, Ferdinand Schöningh

Gotthelf, A. and Lennox, J. (eds.), (1987) *Philosophical Issues in Aristotle's Biology*, Cambridge: Cambridge University Press

Gottschalk, H. B. (1990) "The Earliest Aristotelian Commentators," in Sorabji, R. (ed.), *Aristotle Transformed: The Ancient Commentators and Their Influence*, London: Duckworth, 55–82

Grensemann, H. (1982) *Die gynäkologischen Texte des Autors C nach den hippokratischen Schriften* de Mulieribus *I, II und* de Sterilibus, Wiesbaden: Steiner

Hanson, A. (1990) "The Medical Writer's Woman," in Halperin, D., Winkler, J. J., and Zeitlin, F. (eds.), *Before Sexuality*, Princeton: Princeton University Press, 309–38

(1991) "Continuity and Change: Three Case Studies in Hippocratic Gynecological Therapy and Theory," in Pomeroy, S. B. (ed.), *Women's History and Ancient History*, Chapel Hill NC: University of North Carolina Press, 73–110

Hatzimichali, M. (2013) "The Texts of Plato and Aristotle in the 1st c. BC," in Schofield, M. (ed.), *Aristotle, Plato and Pythagoreanism in the first century BC*, Cambridge: Cambridge University Press, 1–27

Housman, A. E. (1922) "The Application of Thought to Textual Criticism," *Proceedings of the Classical Association* 18: 67–84

Irwin, T. (1988) *Aristotle's First Principles*, Oxford: Clarendon Press

Jacob, C. (2004) "Questions sur les questions: Archéologie d'une pratique intellectuelle et d'une forme discursive," in Volgers, A. and Zamagni, C.

(eds.), *Erotapokriseis: Early Christian Question-and-Answer Literature in Context. Contributions to Biblical Exegesis and Theology* 37, Leuven: Peeters, 25–54

Jannini, E., Simonelli, C., and Lenzi, A. (2002a) "Sexological Approach to Ejaculatory Dysfunction," *International Journal of Andrology* 25: 317–23

(2002b) "Disorders of Ejaculation," *Journal of Endocrinological Investigation* 25: 1006–19

Keyt, D. (2017) *Nature and Justice: Studies in the Ethical and Political Philosophy of Plato and Aristotle*, Leuven: Peeters

King, H. (1983) "Bound to Bleed: Artemis and Greek Women," in Cameron, A. and Kuhrt, A. (eds.), *Images of Women in Antiquity*, London: Croom Helm, 109–27

(1989) "The Daughter of Leonides: Reading the Hippocratic Corpus," in Cameron, A. (ed.), *History as Text: The Writing of Ancient History*, London: Duckworth, 13–32

(1998) *Hippocrates' Woman*, London: Routledge

Korda, J. B., Goldstein, S. W., and Somner, F. (2010) "The History of Female Ejaculation," *Journal of Sexual Medicine* 7: 1965–75

Leith, D. (2009) "Question-Types in Medical Catechisms on Papyrus," in Taub, L. and Doody, A. (eds.), *Authorial Voices in Greco-Roman Technical Writing. Antike Naturwissenschaft und ihre Rezeption, AKAN-Einzelschriften* 7, Trier: Wissenschaftlicher Verlag, 107–23

Lennox, J. (1996) "Aristotle's Biological Development: The Balme Hypothesis," in Wians, W. (ed.), 229–48

Leroi, A. M. (2014) *The Lagoon: How Aristotle Invented Science*, New York: Viking

Lloyd, E. A. (2005) *The Case of the Female Orgasm: Bias in the Science of Evolution*, Cambridge, Mass.: Harvard University Press

Louis, P. (1964) *Aristote: Histoire des animaux*, Paris: Les Belles Lettres

Mansfeld, J. (1990) "Doxography and Dialectic: the *Sitz im Leben* of the 'Placita'," *ANRW* II: 36.4, 3193–208

(1992) "*Physikai Doxai* and *Problêmata Physika* from Aristotle to Aëtius (and beyond)," in Fortenbaugh, W. W. and Gutas, D. (eds.), *Theophrastus: His Psychological, Doxographical, and Scientific Writings*, New Brunswick NJ: Transaction Publishers, 63–111

Manuli, P. (1983) "Donne mascoline, femmine sterili, vergini perpetue: la ginecologia greca tra Ippocrate e Sorano," in Campese et al., 149–204

Mayhew, R. (2004) *The Female in Aristotle's Biology: Reason or Rationalization*, Chicago: University of Chicago Press

(2011) *Aristotle: Problems Books 1–19*, Cambridge, Mass.: Harvard University Press

McMahon, J. M. (1998) *"Paralysin Cave": Impotence, Perception, and Text in the Satyrica of Petronius*, Leiden: Brill

Moraux, P. (1951) *Les listes anciennes des ouvrages d'Aristote*, Louvain: Éditions universitaires de Louvain

Nussbaum, M. C. (1982) "Saving Aristotle's Appearances," in Schofield, M. and Nussbaum, M. C. (eds.), *Language and Logos. Studies in Ancient Greek Philosophy Presented to G. E. L. Owen.* Cambridge: Cambridge University Press, 267–93

Nutton, V. (2013) *Ancient Medicine,* 2nd edn, London: Routledge

Owen, G. E. L. (1961) "τιθέναι τὰ φαινόμενα," in *Aristote et les problèmes de méthode.* Paris: Nauwelaerts, 83–103

Peck, A. L. (1942) *Aristotle: Generation of Animals,* Cambridge, Mass.: Harvard University Press

Peng, R. D. and Hengartner, N. W. (2002) "Quantitative Analysis of Literary Style," *The American Statistician* 56: 175–85

Perelli, L. (2012) "Writing, Preserving and Disseminating Scientific Knowledge," *Manuscript Culture* 5: 20–32

Prentice, W. K. (1930) "How Thucydides Wrote His *Histories,*" *Classical Philology* 25: 117–27

Rubinelli, S. (2009) *Ars Topica: The Classical Technique of Constructing Arguments from Aristotle to Cicero,* Heidelberg: Springer

Rubio-Casillas, A. and Jannini, E. A. (2011) "New Insights from One Case of Female Ejaculation," *Journal of Sexual Medicine* 8: 3500–4

Rudberg, G. (1911) *Zum sogenannten zehnten Buch der aristotelischen Tiergeschichte,* Uppsala: Skrifter utgifna af Kungl, Humanistiska Vetenskaps-Samfundet, 13.6

Runia, D. (1999) "The *Placita* Ascribed to Doctors in Aëtius' Doxography on Physics," in van der Eijk, P. (ed.), *Ancient Histories of Medicine: Essays in Medical Doxography and Historiography in Classical Antiquity,* Leiden: Brill, 196–206

Salama, S., Boitrelle, F., Gauquelin, A., Malagrida, L., Thiounn, N., and Devaux, P. (2015) "Nature and Origin of 'Squirting' in Female Sexuality," *Journal of Sexual Medicine* 12: 661–6

Sato, R. L. (2002) "Adolescent Gynaecology," in Yamamoto, L. (ed.), *Case Based Pediatrics for Medical Students and Residents,* University of Hawaii, www.hawaii.edu/medicine/pediatrics/pedtext/pedtext.html, accessed 10/16/2017

Shafik, A., Shafik, I. A., El Sibai, O., and Shafik, A. A. (2009) "An Electrophysiologic Study of Female Ejaculation," *Journal of Sex and Marital Therapy* 35: 337–46

Sharples, R. (2010) *Peripatetic Philosophy 200 BC to AD 200: An Introduction and Collection of Sources,* Cambridge: Cambridge University Press

Smith, R. (1999) "Dialectic and Method in Aristotle," in Sim, M. (ed.), *From Puzzles to Principles? Essays on Aristotle's Dialectic,* Oxford: Lexington Books, 39–55

Smyth, H. W. (1920) *Greek Grammar,* Cambridge, Mass.: Harvard University Press

Spengel, L. (1842) *De Aristotelis Libro Decimo Historiae Animalium et Incerto Auctore Libri Peri Kosmou Commentario*, Heidelberg: G. Richard

Steel, C., Guldentops, G., and Beullens, P. (1999) *Aristotle's Animals in the Middle Ages and Renaissance*, Leuven: Leuven University Press

Stevens, P. T. (1936) "Aristotle and the Koine," *CQ* 30: 204–17

Thesleff, H. (1966) "Scientific and Technical Style in Early Greek Prose," *Arctos* n.s. 4: 89–113

Totelin, L. (2009) *Hippocratic Recipes: Oral and Written Transmission of Pharmacological Knowledge in Fifth and Fourth Century Greece*, Leiden: Brill

(forthcoming) "Do No Harm: Phanostrate's Midwifery Practice," in Nutton, V. and Totelin, L. (eds.), *Behind and Beyond: Studies Presented to Elizabeth Craik*

Tricot, J. (1957) *Aristote: Histoire Des Animaux*, Paris: Librairie Philosophique

van der Eijk, P. J. (1999) "*On Sterility* ('*HA* X'), A Medical Work by Aristotle?" *CQ* 49: 490–502

(2001) *Diocles of Carystus: A Collection of the Fragments with Translation and Commentary, vols. I & II*, Leiden: Brill

(2016) "On 'Hippocratic' and 'Non-Hippocratic' Medical Writings," in Dean-Jones, L. and Rosen, R. (eds.), *Ancient Concepts of the Hippocratic*, Leiden: Brill, 17–47

van Oppenraay, A. M. I. (1999) "Michael Scot's Arabic-Latin Translation of Aristotle's *Books on Animals*. Some Remarks Concerning the Relation between the Translation and its Arabic and Greek Sources," in Steel et al., 31–43

(2003) "The Reception of Aristotle's *History of Animals* in the Marginalia of Some Latin Manuscripts of Michael Scot's Arabic-Latin Translation," *Early Science and Medicine* 8, 387–403

von Staden, H. (1992) "Jaeger's 'Skandalon der historischen Vernunft': Diocles, Aristotle, and Theophrastus," in Calder, W. M. (ed.), *Werner Jaeger Reconsidered*. Proceedings of the Second Oldfather Conference, University of Illinois: Atlanta, 227–65

Wians, W. (1992) "Saving Aristotle from Nussbaum's *Phainomena*," in Preus, A. and Anton, J. P. (eds.), *Aristotle's Ontology*, Albany: University of New York Press, 133–49

(ed.) (1996) *Aristotle's Philosophical Development*, London: Rowman and Littlefield

Wimpissinger, F., Shifter, K., Grin, W., and Stackl, W. (2007) "The Female Prostate Revisited: Perineal Ultrasound and Biochemical Studies of Female Ejaculate," *The Journal of Sexual Medicine* 4: 1388–93

Winkler, J. J. (1989) *The Constraints of Desire: The Anthropology of Sex and Gender in Ancient Greece*, New York: Routledge

INDEX LOCORUM

Although in my text the various passages from *HA* X are usually cited as coming from *Non Gen.*, *Topos* or *Dial.*, the Bekker page numbers are listed after *HA* X in the Aristotle section.   References to *HA* X itself refer either to the whole book, or to references by other secondary authors.

INDEX LOCORUM

253

WORD INDEX

LILIANE BODSON AND ALLAN GOTTHELF

This index is excerpted from the full word index in Balme's 2002 Cambridge Classical Texts and Commentaries edition of the HA, which was in turn based on the full index to the present text of HA in Liliane Bodson, *Index verborum in Aristotelis* Historiam animalium. *Listes de fréquence. Relevé inverse des lemmes. Relevés des zoonymes, phytonymes, toponymes, théonymes, anthroponym.es* (Hildesheim: Georg Olms, 2004). In the present index, all words are included except articles, conjunctions, particles, prepositions, and the verbs εἶναι and γί(γ)νεσθαι. (The prepositions ἕνεκα and χάριν are retained for their philosophical interest.)

The index is verbal rather than conceptual. Information on the general principles of the full index and their application to the present index may be found in Bodson's introduction to the full index. A conceptual index, in English, to the whole of *HA*, prepared by A. Gotthelf, may be found in vol. III of the Loeb edition: Aristotle, *History of Animals Books VII–X*, ed. D. M. Balme (Cambridge MA and London: Harvard University Press, 1991). Due to emendations a few words from the list in Balme are omitted and a few added.

ἀγαθός 635a29, 36
ἀγγεῖον 635b14
ἀγνοεῖν 638b15
ἄγονος 637b23
ᾄδειν 637b16
ἀδυναμία 637b26
ἀδυνατεῖν 633b22
ἀδύνατος 633b24, 635a1, 636b39,
    637a15
ἀεί 634a9, 38, 635b27, 34, 37, 636b28,
    638a34, b36
ἀήρ 637a30, 33
ἀθροίζειν, -εσθαι 636b26
αἰδοῖον 637a23
αἴρειν, -εσθαι 636a22
αἰσθάνεσθαι 636b36
αἰτία 635a1
αἴτιος 633b13, 16, 17, 634b3, 13,
    636a13, b7,11, 15, 637a36, 37,
    38, b2, 10
ἀκολουθεῖν 634b4
ἄκοπος 633b20, 24
ἀκριβῶς 633b28
ἀκρίς 637b16
ἄκρος 638b6
ἄκων 635b4

ἄλγημα 635a12
ἄλγος 635a27
ἀλέα 633a16
ἀλεκτορίς 637b7
ἀληθής 638a5
ἀλλήλων 633b13, 636b9, 13,
    19, 23
ἄλλοθι 634b8
ἀλλοῖος 635a14, 28, 638a32
ἄλλος 633b18, 634a2 (*bis*), 17, 22, b2,
    635a19, b16, 636b11, 12, 637b9,
    13, 16, 38, 638a1 (*bis*), 4, 13,
    b24, 35
ἄλλοτε 638a32, b19, 20
ἄλλως 636b33
ἄλυπος 633b19
ἀλύπως 633b26
ἅμα 634a6, 635a19, 636b9, 30, 38,
    637a14
ἀμιγής 638a9
ἀμφινωμᾶν 633a26
ἀμφότερος 636b8
ἄμφω 633b13, 636b17, 37, 637b22, 24,
    31, 638a4, 22, 24
ἀνάγκη 634a18, 29, 636b23
ἀναιρεῖν, -εῖσθαι 635a1, 638a21

WORD INDEX

WORD INDEX

WORD INDEX

265

WORD INDEX

φαίνειν, -εσθαι 635a35, 636a26, 33, 37, b4, 12, 637a10, b10, 20, 23, 27
φανερός 633b18, 634a5, 637b6, 30
φανερῶς 635a10, 12, 636a22
φάρυγξ 637a29, 33
φάσκειν 638a5, 638b16
φαῦλος 635b14 (bis)
φλεγμαίνειν 634a23, 636a35, 638a35
φλεγμασία 634a21, 635a4, 636a29, 33
φλεγματικός 634a26
φοινικοῦς 634b19
φοιτᾶν 634b16, 635a11
φορά 635b20
φύειν, -εσθαι 634a24, 635b26, 637a21
φυλάττειν, -εσθαι 638a21
φῦμα 636a35
φυμάτιον 633b29
φῦσα 635b4
φύσις 635a3, 4, b8, 11, 39, 636a25, 638b21

χαλεπός 634a5, 636b3, 638b30
χρή 634a11
χρῆσις 636a39
χροιά, χροία, χρόα 635a11
χρονίζειν, -εσθαι 638b17
χρόνιος 638b4
χρόνος 634a13, 35, 636a19, 22, 638a14, 26, b5, 7
χώρα 635b9

ψῦχος 635b22
ψυχρός 638b3, 19, 33, 36
ψυχρότης 638b23

ὠδίς 638b8, 9
ᾠόν 637b21
ὡς 634a30, 34, b11, 24, 29, 32, 635a32, 34 (bis), 636b37, 637b15, 24, 25, 27, 33, 638a35
ὥσπερ 633b18, 27, 634a22, b31, 635b5, 19, 28, 636a5, 637a17, 19, 20, 22, 32, b30, 638a22, 25, b1, 4, 25, 27

GENERAL INDEX

Page numbers in bold are in the translation; with 'n' are notes.